Medicolegal Aspects of Alcohol Determination in Biological Specimens

Edited by
James C. Garriott

PSG Publishing Company, Inc.
Littleton, Massachusetts

Library of Congress Cataloging-in-Publication Data

Medicolegal aspects of alcohol determination in biological specimens.

Includes index.
1. Alcohol in the body—Measurement. 2. Alcoholic beverages—Analysis. 3. Chemistry, Forensic.
I. Garriott, James C. [DNLM: 1. Alcohol, Ethyl—analysis. 2. Forensic Medicine—methods. QV 84 M4895]
RA1061.5.M43 1987 614′.1 86-30496
ISBN 0-88416-717-8

Published by:
PSG PUBLISHING COMPANY, INC.
545 Great Road
Littleton, Massachusetts 01460

Printed in the United States of America.

International Standard Book Number: 0–88416–717–8

Library of Congress Catalog Card Number: 86–30496

Last digit is print number: 9 8 7 6 5 4 3 2 1

CONTRIBUTORS

Randall C. Baselt, Ph.D.
Director
Chemical Toxicology Institute
Foster City, California

Barbara Basteyns, B.S.
Supervisor Toxicology Section
State Laboratory of Hygiene
Madison, Wisconsin

Richard Baxter, B.S.
Department of Public Safety
Austin, Texas

George E. Browne, B.S.
Manager of Breath Test Services
Scientific Director Breath Test Program
Austin, Texas

Yale H. Caplan, Ph.D.
Office of the Chief Medical Examiner
Baltimore, Maryland

Janet E.L. Corry, Ph.D.
Ministry of Agriculture, Fisheries, and Food
London, England

Ivan E. Danhof, Ph.D., M.D.
Professor, Retired
Department of Physiology
University of Texas Southwestern Medical School
Grand Prairie, Texas

Kurt M. Dubowski, Ph.D.
Director, Toxicology Laboratories
Distinguished Professor of Medicine
University of Oklahoma College of Medicine
Oklahoma City, Oklahoma

Patricia H. Field, Ph.D.
Chief, Toxicology Section
State Laboratory of Hygiene
Madison, Wisconsin

James C. Garriott, Ph.D.
Chief Toxicologist
Bexar County Medical Examiner's Office and Regional Crime Laboratory
San Antonio, Texas

David R. Harper, Ph.D.
The Metropolitan Police Forensic Science Laboratory
London, England

Barbara R. Manno, Ph.D.
Professor
Director, Clinical Toxicology Laboratory
Department of Pharmacology and Therapeutics
Louisiana State University Medical Center
Shreveport, Louisiana

Joseph E. Manno, Ph.D.
Professor
Department of Pharmacology and Therapeutics
Chief, Section of Toxicology
Director, Clinical Toxicology Laboratory

Louisiana State University
Medical Center
Shreveport, Louisiana

Bill H. McAnalley, Ph.D.
Carrington Laboratories
Research Facility
Dallas, Texas

Morton F. Mason, Ph.D.*
Department of Pathology
University of Texas Health
Science Center at Dallas
Dallas, Texas

Nancy Berk Pilchen
Former Legislative Analyst,
Office of Federal Affairs
National Safety Council
Washington, D.C.

Richard F. Shaw, B.S.
Chief Toxicologist
San Diego County Coroner's
Office
San Diego, California

Alvin Weathermon, B.A., B.S.
Department of Public Safety
Austin, Texas

*Deceased

CONTENTS

PREFACE

Forensic alcohol analysis is without question the most frequently performed of all analyses in forensic laboratories, and likewise is the most commonly used laboratory result in courts of law. Alcohol-related litigation most frequently pertains to arrests of drinking drivers, but also includes industrial accidents as well as aircraft and public transport accidents.

There were 46,200 motor vehicle–related deaths and 1,700,000 disabling injuries in the United States in 1984. Estimated losses from these were $47.6 billion. Most studies of motor vehicle fatal or nonfatal accidents show drinking driver involvement in more than half, and in some studies the figure is as high as 75%. Studies of homicides, suicides, or victims of other forms of violent death also show that greater than half involve alcohol.

In death investigation, it is often that an alcohol analysis is the first and sometimes sole chemical analysis performed. All 50 states of the United States, as well as most countries of Western Europe and other parts of the world, have statutes regulating driving a motor vehicle under the influence of alcohol and often other laws governing use of alcohol, such as public intoxication and intoxication in the workplace.

Thus testing for use of alcohol in deceased individuals or in living individuals under a variety of circumstances is nearly universal. Whether such testing is performed on body fluids such as blood or urine, or breath in living individuals or on body fluids or even organs in deceased individuals, it is often extremely important and even critical that the alcohol analyses be performed accurately and correctly and that they be properly interpreted.

As a forensic toxicologist, the editor has often been called upon to interpret alcohol concentrations found in autopsy specimens or in mishandled blood specimens, and sometimes had to conclude that the results were meaningless or had been misinterpreted due to factors discussed at length in the ensuing chapters. In discussing alcohol litigation with attorneys, pathologists, physicians, or other laboratory specialists, we are often asked for a reference to a book that explains the science of alcohol: its disposition in the body, decomposition influences, legal considerations, and many other facets. Unfortunately, the answer is usually that "no such book exists."

The goal of the authors of this work is to provide at least a piece to begin to fill this gap in the world alcohol literature. It is recognized that not all topics could be covered and that more comprehensive and continuing updated coverage of topics is desirable and necessary, and it is hoped that future editions of this work will address those needs.

J.C.G.

ACKNOWLEDGMENT

Many individuals deserve some measure of credit for the fruition of this "alcohol" book. Firstly to be thanked are the authors, who gave so unselfishly of their time and expertise and then patiently and sometimes painfully waited through the delays we encountered before publication. Special indebtedness is owed to Randall C. Baselt, who provided a confident, supporting hand through the whole process of its development.

Marie G. McQueen of the Bexar County Medical Examiner's Office is responsible for typing and retyping our manuscripts and for performing many of the multiple chores necessary for any publication. Her patient dedication and efforts were indispensable and are sincerely appreciated.

Lastly, if this work were to be dedicated to anyone, I would unhesitatingly offer it to the memory of the late Rolla N. Harger, who devoted many years of research to the pharmacology and toxicology of alcohol, and to his colleague, Robert B. Forney, who has devoted much of his life to teaching forensic toxicology as well as pursuing alcohol research. Their enthusiasm stimulated my interest (and that of many other of their students, including some authors of this book) in the science of ethyl alcohol, beginning with a Breath Alcohol Training Session they taught for the Indiana State Troopers in 1961. Their pioneering works and research efforts are often cited in these pages.

James C. Garriott, PhD

1

Chemistry of Alcoholic Beverages

Bill H. McAnalley

Alcoholic beverages include wines, beers, and spirits. Wines are made from fermenting fruits, berries, honey, and even milk. Beers are produced from fermenting grains, and spirits are distilled from wines and beers.

Ethyl alcohol is the alcohol of "alcoholic" beverages. It is also known as drinking alcohol, grain alcohol, and ethanol. Fermentation of sugars by yeast is the oldest synthetic chemical process used by man and therefore ethyl alcohol is the oldest synthetic organic chemical produced by man (Morrison and Boyd, 1983).

During fermentation, sugar is converted to drinking alcohol, and carbon dioxide is released as gas bubbles, for example, as in carbonated drinks. This chemical change was a great mystery to ancient man because the mixture appeared to be boiling without heat. Knowledge resulting from the study of wine fermentation was a major contributor to the early development and progress of the modern sciences of microbiology and biochemistry.

Understanding the "mysteries" that baffled the artisan winemaker began in the 1860s when Louis Pasteur discovered that alcoholic fermentation could occur only in the presence of small living "ferments" or, as they are known today, yeasts.

In 1897, Edward Buchner reported that yeasts could be broken up and that the cell-free yeast juice could ferment sugar. Later, the yeast juice was found to contain enzymes which are responsible for the conversion of sugars to alcohol and carbon dioxide.

The learning process of mankind is exemplified by beverage making. The natural course of events in acquiring knowledge begins with "magic" which, with more understanding, becomes an art, and with further understanding, a science.

DESCRIPTION AND HISTORY OF COMMON ALCOHOLIC BEVERAGES

The liquor industry is almost as old as man himself. A description of alcoholic beverages and some knowledge of their history are useful in understanding their chemical make-up. The first beverages were made from fruits (wine) or grains (beer). Later, distillation was developed and utilized in beverage production in order to achieve a more potent drink.

Wine is the term used for an alcoholic beverage that is made from fruits, herbs, berries, milk, or even from flowers, but generally refers to products made from fermented grapes. Wines are classified according to color — red, rosé (pink), and white. Contrary to popular belief, white or red grapes can be used to make red or white wines. Both red and white grapes have color pigments (white grapes produce dark seedless raisins). The length of time the grape skins are left in the fermenting *must* (grape juice) determines the color of the wine. In general, red wines are produced by fermenting the must with the skins; for a rosé wine the skins are left in for part of the fermentation; the skins are removed before fermentation for white wine.

The taste is classified as sweet or dry with varying degrees of each. Sweet wines are higher in sugar content than dry wines. Also, high acidity may contribute to the dryness of a wine.

Wines are also classified as table, sparkling, or fortified wines. In table wines the alcohol content ranges from about 7% to 15% and they may be white, rosé, or red. Sparkling wines are usually white but may be red or rosé with an alcohol content similar to table wines. Fortified wines may be red or white with a higher average alcohol content ranging from 16% to 25%. The higher alcohol content is provided by adding brandy or some distilled spirit. Fortified wines with added flavoring are called aromatic wines.

Paleontologists have found evidence of grape stems and skins that apparently were from grapes crushed by prehistoric man. Egyptians credit Osiris and the Greeks credit Dionysius with the gift of wine, but the Hebrews claim that Noah first introduced it. Numerous references in the Bible indicate that not only wine but stronger beverages were made. Different Hebrew words were used to describe the wines — *yayin* for common wine, *homer* for fresh, unmixed wine, *tiros* for strong wine, *meseg* for mixed wine, and *sekhor* for strong drink.

Indeed, the church had the single greatest influence on the development of wines. The priests needed wine for the sacramental functions and their major efforts were directed toward improving the vines and the quality of the wine. Padre Junipero, a Dominican missionary, planted the first vines in California, bringing them from Spain. Today, wine is defined as the fermented juice of grapes and other fruits.

Beer is a malted and hopped (the addition of hops, an herb), somewhat bitter beverage. Malt can be made from cereal grains such as rice and wheat, but barley is the main cereal employed. Barley is dried until the moisture content is 12% to 14% and then stored for at least 4 weeks to overcome its natural dormancy and to render it suitable for uniform germination. Gibberellic acid may be added to speed up the germination rate, and potassium bromate may be added to restrict rootlet formation, which means less sugar energy is used in root production.

During germination, enzymes convert the starches to sugars which are required for fermentation. The maltster knows when to stop the germination process and grind the plant embryo into malt which can then be used to produce beer.

The art of brewing is as old as recorded history — over seven thousand years. Archeologists have found hieroglyphics which represent brewing. Also, from analysis of beer jugs, they have found that barley has been used to produce beer for centuries. The Egyptians made *beer* from corn, the Chinese made *samshu* and the Japanese made *sake* from rice, while the Russians made *quass* or *kvass* from rye.

William Penn was probably the first to operate a large commercial brewery in America. Beer played an important part in American history. The Pilgrims on the *Mayflower* would have continued their journey to Virginia but instead landed at Plymouth Rock because, as recorded in their journal, "We could not now take time for further search and considerations, our victuals being spent, especially our beer." (Grossman and Lembeck, 1983)

Distilled spirits are alcoholic beverages in which the concentration of ethyl alcohol has been increased above that of the original fermented mixture. The principle of alcoholic distillation is based upon the different boiling points of alcohol (173.3°F or 78.5°C) and water (212°F or 100°C). When the alcohol-containing mixture is heated above 173.3°F, the alcohol begins to vaporize and can be separated from the water.

Distilled spirits have fewer congeners than beer or wine because many substances will not vaporize in the distillation process and are left behind. However, some of the volatile congeners with low boiling points will be concentrated much like the ethyl alcohol.

The first mention of distillation is attributed to Albukassen, an Arabian alchemist of the tenth century. It probably originated with the Arabs or Saracens, as they gave us the words alcohol and alembic, the latter meaning "still." Distilled spirits are called ardent spirits which comes from the Latin *adere*, meaning "to burn." A popular Spanish brandy is called *aguardiente* (burning water). The following are common examples of distilled spirits.

Absinthe was developed by Dr Ordinaire, a French physician and pharmacist, while he was exiled and living in Switzerland. It was one of the most potent alcoholic beverages, with an alcoholic content of 68% by volume. Oil of wormwood was the chief flavoring ingredient and other minor ingredients included licorice, hyssop, fennel, aniseed, and star anise. Henry Louis Pernod purchased the formula from Dr Ordinaire and it was first produced commercially in 1797. It was yellowish-green in color and turned to a cloudy opalescent white when mixed with water. Wormwood came to be considered dangerous because it was thought to cause hallucinations, mental deterioration, and sterility.

In 1908, Switzerland, and in 1915, France, prohibited the sale of absinthe. Other countries soon followed suit. Today, similar beverages, lower in alcohol content and without wormwood, are sold under trade names such as Pernod and Ricard.

Aquavit is a clear to pale-yellow, dry liquor ranging in alcohol content from 42% to 45% by volume. It is distilled from fermented potato or grain mash and then redistilled in the presence of various flavoring agents to extract their flavors. Flavoring agents include lemon and orange peel, caraway or cumin seed, cardamom, and aniseed. In Sweden the beverage is called *snops* and the equivalent Danish product is called *schnapps*.

Brandy is an alcoholic liquor distilled from wine or various fermented fruit juices. Reportedly, the best brandies are the cognac and armaqnac named for the two French regions where they are produced. Most spirits today are distilled in continuous stills. True cognac comes from the traditional pot-still type of distillation. In this process, the first and last runs of brandy are discarded and only the middle or heart is retained.

The history of brandy making can be traced to a Dutch shipmaster who hit upon the idea of concentrating wine to reduce freight charges. His plan was to concentrate wine by eliminating the water in France and transporting the spirit to Holland where it could be diluted with water. The Dutch liked the taste of the concentrate, however, and decided it would be a waste of water to try to return it to its original state. The new product was called *brandewyn*, a Dutch word for "burned wine."

Gin is a distilled liquor usually made from grain and flavored principally with the juniper berry which is responsible for its name. Juniper in French is *genièvre*. The name was altered by the Dutch to *genever* and shortened by the English to gin.

Gin producers use botanicals such as orris, angelica, licorice root, caraway, coriander, cardamom, anise, fennel, and orange and lemon oils to provide a unique flavor to their product.

Franciscus Sylvius, a professor of medicine at the University of Leyden in Holland, invented gin. His objective was a medicinal product. He felt that by redistilling pure alcohol with the juniper berry he could obtain the natural diuretic properties of the plant in an inexpensive form. In the seventeenth century, English soldiers, returning home, brought back gin and in no time it became the national drink of England, a position it still holds today.

Vodka is a clear beverage without much taste or flavor of its own and an alcohol content of 33% to 45% by volume. Potatoes are frequently used in Russia and Poland to produce vodka while cereal grains are more frequently used in the United States.

Vodka combines well with other beverages without imparting much flavor of its own. This makes vodka drinks such as the screwdriver, made with orange juice, and the bloody mary, made with tomato juice, very popular. Some vodkas are flavored with buffalo grass, lemon peel, berries, peppercorns, or caraway.

Vodka originated in Russia during the fourteenth century. *Vodka* means "little water" in Russian.

Liqueurs are flavored and sweetened distilled beverages with an alcohol content ranging from 24% to 60% by volume. Liqueurs are usually produced by combining a basic spirit such as brandy with herbs and fruits and sweetening them with a syrup at a concentration of 2.5% or more by volume.

Fruit liqueurs are produced by the infusion method whereby fruit is steeped in the spirit, which absorbs the color, flavor, and aroma.

Plant liqueurs are made by percolating or distilling a beverage in the presence of plants, seeds, roots, or herbs. In the percolator the plant material is placed in the top section and the bottom section holds the beverage. The process is much the same as that of percolating coffee.

Popular liqueur flavors are apricot, pineapple, crème de cacao, mint, and coffee (Kahlua). Ocha is a Japanese liqueur flavored with green tea. The British make Drambuie with a Scotch whiskey base. Cherry Herring (made from cherries) comes from Denmark, Triple Sec and Grand Marnier (both made from orange peel) are produced in the Cognac region of France, and Galliano is made in Italy; the United States produces Creme Yvette and Forbidden Fruit, among others.

Okolehao, also referred to as Oke, is a product of Hawaii. Okolehao was first made about 1790 by an Australian, William Stevenson, who cooked the sacred ti root and allowed the mash, rich in fructose, to ferment in the bottom of a canoe. Next, he distilled the fermented mash using the ship's cooking pot and a water-cooled gun barrel for a coil. Today, a modern distillery is used. Okolehao is not aged but is filtered through charcoal.

Pulque is the fermented juice of the mezcal plant, which is a species of *Agave*. It is distilled to make a brandy called maguey. In Mexico a species of *Agave* (*A atrovirens*) is known as *maguey*. The best mezcal is grown near Tequila, Mexico, and it is used to make the pulque which is distilled to make tequila, named for the city near which the natural plant is grown.

Rum is any alcoholic beverage made from distillates of sugar cane, molasses, or other sugar cane products. It has been made in the West Indies for more than 300 years. Aroax is a rum produced in Java and owes many of its characteristics to the wild yeast, *Saccharomyces vordermanni* which is used in its production.

Whiskey: The word "whiskey" comes from the Scottish and Irish word *usquebaugh* (pronounced us kwĭ-bo), meaning "water of life." Scotch whisky is obtained primarily from barley. The grain is soaked in water and when the sprouts are about three quarters of an inch long they are transferred to a kiln. The green malt, as the sprouts are called, is placed on a screen directly above a peat fire which provides the acrid and oily smoke which gives Scotch whisky part of its unique flavor.

Until 1853, Scotch whiskies were either straight malt or straight grain whiskies. Then Andrew Usher and Company began the practice of blending malt and grain, achieving blended Scotch whisky. A Scotch whisky blend can easily contain thirty to forty malt whiskies with five or more grain whiskies. The secret of fine Scotch whisky lies in the art of the blender. The depth of color is governed by the amount of caramel and burned sugar used to produce a uniform color.

Two different yeasting processes are currently used in America: sour mash and sweet mash. In the sour-mash process, at least one quarter of the fermenting mash comes from a previous distillation and is mixed with fresh mash and allowed to ferment from 72 to 96 hours. Sweet mash, also known as a yeast mash, is processed totally from fresh mash and allowed to ferment from 36 to 50 hours. The acid pH of sour mash inhibits bacterial contamination, making it easier to control than sweet mash, which must be processed above 80°F to help avoid contamination.

Canadian whisky, contrary to popular belief, is not a rye whiskey but is made from corn, rye, wheat, and barley, with no one grain making up more than 50% of the whole.

Scotch whisky gets its smoky flavor from peat, a partially carbonized vegetable matter, usually mosses, found in bogs. Irish whiskey has a similar barley malt character without the smoky flavor. Scotch and Irish whiskies are lighter in body than American straight whiskies because they are aged longer — 7 to 12 years. Maturation in previously used cooperage, wooden containers, requires a longer period. American whiskies are charred in new oak cooperage which makes an earlier maturation possible. However, the longer maturation period practiced in Ireland and Scotland allows for formation of more esters which provide greater depth of flavor.

FERMENTATION

In general, alcoholic beverages can be produced from any substance that contains sufficient sugar or starch. Beverages fall into three basic categories: (1) fermented beverages which are made from agricultural products such as grapes or other fruits and grains, (2) distilled or spirituous beverages, and (3) compounded beverages which are made by combining fermented and/or distilled beverages with flavoring substances (Grossman et al, 1983).

The chemical process of fermentation was formulated by Gay-Lussac in 1810; one molecule of sugar (glucose) was shown to result in two molecules of ethanol and two molecules of carbon dioxide. This equation can be written as:

$$(C_6H_{12}O_6) \rightarrow 2(CH_3CH_2OH) + 2(CO_2)$$

Theoretically, 180 g of glucose should produce 92 g of ethanol and 88 g of carbon dioxide which would yield 51.1% of the weight of sugar fermented as ethanol. The actual yield is only 48% because the yeast uses energy to produce a series of compounds other than alcohol, and some sugar is used to synthesize new yeast cells. By-products include acetaldehyde, higher molecular weight alcohols (fusel oil), and other fermentation and flavoring chemicals.

The conversion of sugar to alcohol requires at least a dozen enzymes in a sequence of chemical reactions called the Embden-Meyerhof pathway. The 6-carbon sugars are converted to fructose-1,6-diphosphate which is split into two 3-carbon triose phosphates. These are dihydroxyacetone phosphate and glyceraldehyde-3-phosphate, which are converted to two molecules of pyruvic acid. The pyruvic acid is converted to acetaldehyde and carbon dioxide as gas bubbles. The acetaldehyde is converted to ethanol, drinking alcohol.

Some glycerin is produced in every wine fermentation, ranging from 0.2% to 1.5%. More may be produced in the presence of high amounts of bisulfite. Glycerol is slightly sweet and contributes to the "body" of wine. Some pyruvic acid is converted to alanine, an amino acid, and a small amount of pyruvic acid is changed to lactic acid. A portion of the acetaldehyde is converted to acetic acid (vinegar). Undesirable bacterial contamination can result in too much acetic acid and ruin the wine.

It is the minor constituents that are of major importance to the flavor and aroma of alcoholic beverages. These important esters and other aromatic components determine the quality and distinctive characteristics of the various beverages. Fusel oils, including 5-carbon or amyl alcohols, 4-carbon butanols, and 3-carbon propyl alcohols compose less than 0.1% of wine. Also, some yeast cells die and "leak" or break up (autolyze) and contribute constituents to the solution. In addition to yeast, other microorganisms produce flavor substances.

As an alternative to sugar, beverages can be made from grains rich in starch, which converts to sugar. In order for grain starch to be converted to sugar, the grains are allowed to sprout which results in an enzyme called amylase. This phenomenon was first understood in the 1930s and the enzyme was then called diastase, from the Greek *diastasis* meaning "separation." Today, in the beverage industry, amylase and diastase are used interchangeably. Amylase acts to separate large starch molecules into the simple sugar maltose. Once this step has occurred, the sugar can be converted to alcohol by the familiar process of fermentation. This process is illustrated schematically in Figure 1-1.

Yeasts

The flavor composition of beverages is markedly altered by the yeast fermentation process. Generally, the dominant beverage flavor constituents are formed during yeast fermentation (Schreier, 1979). The yeast species can affect the flavor and chemical composition considerably. For example, the amount of D(−)-lactic acid depends on the yeast species. *S rose* forms relatively small amounts of lactic acid (about 100 mg/L) whereas the formation of lactic acid is much higher (about 1800 mg/L) when *S veronae* is used. The common beverage

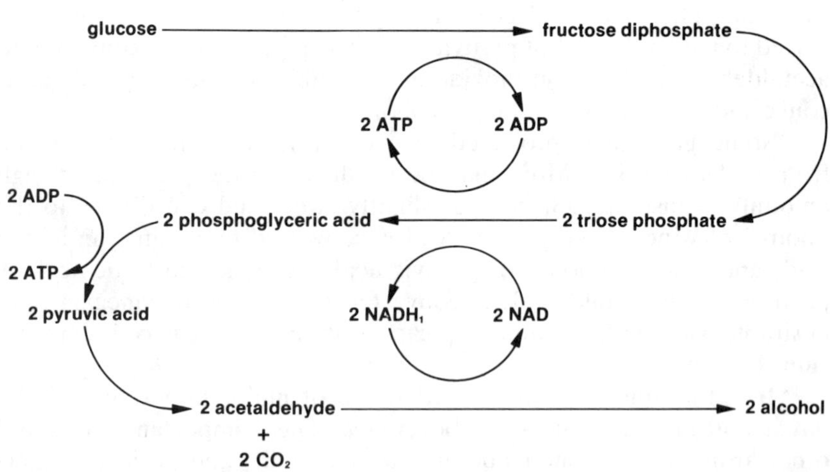

Figure 1-1 Diagram of fermentation

yeasts are *S carlsbergensis* (lager beer), *S cerevisiae* (ale), and the sulfur dioxide–resistant *S ellipsoideus* (California wine).

Bacterial Contamination

The alcohol fermentation process must be carefully guarded against undesirable microorganisms which can impair the quality of or even spoil te beverage. Bacteria such as Enterobacteriaceae, originating in the intestine of warm-blooded animals, have been found in beverages (Van Vuuren et al., 1981). These microorganisms can affect the congener content by producing different chemical substances which, in turn, can be used to detect bacterial contamination. For example, D(−)-lactic acid is formed by yeasts but L(+)-lactic acid is produced by bacteria (Schreier, 1979). High amounts of acetic acid also indicate spoilage, usually by *Acetobacter* (Kupina et al., 1982).

NUTRITIONAL VALUE OF ALCOHOLIC BEVERAGES

There is general agreement among nutritionists that the modern Western diet contains too much alcohol (Chatton and Ullman, 1984). Alcohol provides 7 calories/g compared to 9 calories/g for fats and 4 calories/g for protein and carbohydrates. The caloric values of some common beverages are provided in Table 1-1.

Some people survive almost completely on alcoholic beverages. Excessive intake can contribute to malnutrition in several ways. It may depress appetite, displace food, or affect gastrointestinal absorption or digestion. Through its effect on the liver, it can alter the utilization of nutrients.

As a general rule, distilled beverages contain few, if any, vitamins and minerals, but beers and wines can contain significant amounts.

Carbohydrates

Distilled beverages do not contain carbohydrates unless they are added after distillation because sugars do not vaporize during the distillation process. Beers and wines contain varying amounts of carbohydrates.

Approximately 50% of the energy obtained from the average American diet comes from carbohydrates (Guthrie, 1983). It is now recommended that this amount be decreased to 40% with dietary fat and protein each providing 30% of the remaining calories (Chatton and Ullman, 1984).

Table 1-1
Caloric Content of Some Common Alcoholic Beverages

Beverage	Calories
Beer (8 oz)	110
Ale (8 oz)	150
Gin (1 oz)	
80 proof	65
86 proof	88
Rum (1 oz)	70
Whiskey (1 oz)	80
Wine (3 oz)	
Red	145
White	90
Vermouth, sweet (1 oz)	50
Manhattan (3 oz)	165
Martini (3 oz)	140

From Guthrie, 1983.

The average adult consumes approximately 300 g of carbohydrates each day. This is the amount of carbohydrates contained in approximately 15 quarts of beer or wine that is 2% carbohydrate. A quart of one of the very sweet liqueurs contains approximately 300 g of carbohydrate. The carbohydrate content of several types of beverages is given in Table 1-2.

Proteins

The recommended daily allowance of protein for the average adult is 44 g for women and 56 g for men. Little of this can be obtained from alcoholic beverages because alcohol causes protein to precipitate. In wines and beers this precipitate is usually filtered out during bottling. Protein is not volatile and therefore is not found in distilled beverages.

Table 1-2
Carbohydrate Content of Selected Beverages

Beverage	Total Carbohydrates (%)	Source
Beers	2.1–8.3	Pirola, 1978
Wines	2.0–12.0	Ondus et al, 1983
Sprite	10.3	Ondus et al, 1983
Cola	12.3	Ondus et al, 1983
Apple juice	10.4	Ondus et al, 1983
Liqueurs	2.5–35	Grossman and Lembeck, 1983

Wines contain from 0.1 to 2.0 g/L and beers from 0.63 to 6.2 g/L of protein (Pirola, 1978).

This means that an adult would need to consume several gallons of beer or wine each day to get the recommended daily allowance (RDA) of protein. For example, a man would need to drink from 9 to 90 quarts of beer daily. As you can see, beer is not rich in protein, and wine and other alcoholic beverages usually contain even less. For this reason many alcoholics are protein-deficient which can severely restrict the immune system and other natural functions of the human body.

Fats

The fruits and grains used to make beverages are very low in fat. They are selected for their carbohydrate content and for this reason most alcoholic beverages contain little or no fats. Beer contains the most fat with an average fat content of 0.06% (Watt and Merrill, 1963).

Vitamins and Minerals

Only beers and wines contain vitamins. They are not usually found in distilled beverages. The RDA for various vitamins can be compared to their content in selected beverages by referring to Tables 1-3 and 1-4. The reader will note that beers contain more B vitamins than wines in most cases, but nicotinic acid is the only vitamin that is in sufficient quantity to meet the RDA. Both wines and beers contain extremely variable amounts of minerals. Many lay reports state that various beverages are high in some vitamin or mineral, but one cannot rely on obtaining vitamins or minerals from alcoholic beverages.

Table 1-3
Vitamin Content of Wines and Beers (μg/L)

Vitamins	Wines*	Beers*	Recommended Daily Allowance (mg)†
Thiamine (vitamin B_1)	0–240	20–60	1.0–1.50
Riboflavin (vitamin B_2)	60–220	300–1200	1.2–1.7
Pantothenic acid	70–450	400–900	4.0–7.0
Pyridoxine (vitamin B_6)	220–820	400–900	1.8–2.2
Nicotinic acid	410–960	5000–20,000	1.3–1.9
Cobalamin (vitamin B_{12})	0.009–0.025		0.003
Folic acid	15–21		0.4
Biotin	0.6–4.6	0–15	0.1–0.3

*From Pirola, 1978.
†RDA-9th Rev. 1980
NTL-AC. Science

Table 1-4
Mineral Content of Wines and Beers (mg/L)

Mineral	Wines*	Beers*	RDA (mg)†
Chloride	10–80	—	1700–5100
Calcium	29–99	20–70	800–1200
Copper	0–9	T–0.40	2–3
Iron	0–20	T–0.64	10–18
Potassium	180–1620	130–1040	1875–5625
Sodium	10–200	68–550	1100–3300
Fluoride	1–10	0.1–0.9	1.5–4.0
Phosphate	30–900	50–300	800–1200
Magnesium	10–350	50–300	300–400
Manganese	T–51	—	2.5–5.0
Iodide	T†	—	0.15
Chromium		0.5–22.0 μg/L	0.05–0.2
Selenium		0.2–2.50 μg/L	0.05–2.0

*From Pirola, 1978; Zee et al, 1983; Robberecht et al, 1984.
†RDA = recommended daily allowance; T = trace amounts.

ANTIMICROBIAL PROPERTIES OF ALCOHOLIC BEVERAGES

Both antibiotic (Asmus et al., 1983) and antiviral properties (Konowalchuk and Speirs, 1976) have been attributed to nondistilled alcoholic beverages. Lincomycin is a medium-spectrum antibiotic that is produced during fermentation of beers and wines. A mixture of lincomycin A and lincomycin B is produced with a reported total concentration ranging from 340 to 10,020 mg/L in alcoholic beverages (Asmus, 1983).

The recommended oral dose of lincomycin for adults is 500 mg every six to eight hours (Weinstein, 1975). A comparison of the recommended oral dose with the reported fermentation concentrations supports the anecdotal reports that certain alcoholic beverages may have antibiotic properties.

Lincomycin was first isolated from soil collected near Lincoln, Nebraska, and the drug was first reported in the literature in 1962. The adverse effects are diarrhea, nausea, vomiting, skin rashes, and vaginitis (Weinstein, 1975). Because of the possible unwanted effects, there are few if any valid reasons to use lincomycin (Sonde and Mandell, 1980).

Antiviral activity has been demonstrated in a variety of wines, and in grape juice the activity was demonstrable in fractions of juice varying in molecular weight from 1000 to 30,000 as determined by membrane filtration (Konowalchuk and Speirs, 1976).

This area of study is fascinating and further research could explain some of the varying effects observed in different individuals. For example, as many as 20% of patients who take lincomycin orally have diarrhea as a side effect (Weinstein, 1975), and many beverage drinkers report having diarrhea from drinking certain alcoholic beverages. These studies also support the practice of the Egyptian warriors who were instructed to mix wine with their drinking water to disinfect it and reduce illness.

CANCER AND ALCOHOL

Epidemiologic studies find that alcoholics are at higher risk of getting cancer (Hoeft, Obe, 1983). Some tests implicate acetaldehyde as the mutagen (Obe, 1980). Some of the nonvolatile residues have been shown to induce mutations (Hoeft, Obe, 1983).

The high incidence of esophageal cancer in certain areas has been correlated with the mutagenic activity of acrolein, butyrolactone, furfural, and glycidol, usually found in certain brandies (Loquet et al., 1981).

The Institute of Public Health in the Netherlands found that beer was the major source of nitrosamine, contributing, in the late 1970s, 71% of the average daily intake (Stephany and Schuller, 1980). As a result of concern over this carcinogenic activity, the beverage manufacturers have taken steps to remove the suspected carcinogens or reduce them to acceptable levels.

ETHYL ALCOHOL CONTENT

By definition, any drinkable liquid containing from 0.5% to 95% ethyl alcohol is an alcoholic beverage. Prior to scientific methods, beverage strength was measured by mixing equal amounts of spirit and gunpowder. When ignited, if the mixture did not burn it was too weak. If it burned too rapidly it was too strong; an even blue flame meant the beverage was proved. Today, we know this concentration to be about 50% alcohol, and the term *proof* is used to describe the strength of alcoholic beverages. Proof is just about twice the percentage of the alcohol concentration of a beverage. For example, 50% alcohol by volume equals approximately 100 proof. (Since alcohol causes water to contract, 50 parts alcohol + 53.73 parts H_2O gives *not* 103.73 parts mixture, but 100. Proof is slightly more than double.) The ethyl alcohol content of some selected beverages is provided in Table 1-5.

CONGENERS

Ethyl alcohol is the major physiologically active component of most alcoholic beverages. Together with water, it makes up the greater part

Table 1-5
Ethyl Alcohol Content of Selected Beverages

Beverage	%
Beers (lager)	3.2–4.0
Ales	4.5
Porter	6.0
Stout	6.0–8.0
Malt liquor	3.2–7.0
Sake	14.0–16.0
Table wines	7.1–14.0
Sparkling wines	8.0–14.0
Fortified wines	14.0–24.0
Aromatized wines	15.5–20.0
Brandies	40.0–43.0
Whiskies	40.0–75.0
Vodkas	40.0–50.0
Gin	40.0–48.5
Rum	40.0–95.0
Aquavit	35.0–45.0
Okolehao	40.0
Tequila	45.0–50.5

From Grossman and Lembeck, 1983

of the alcoholic drink. The remaining fraction is collectively made up of compounds called *congeners*. Although quantitatively small, congeners play a crucial and often overlooked role in the social use and abuse of alcoholic beverages.

Congeners may be highly volatile (easily evaporated) compounds consisting of a variety of alcohols (in addition to ethanol), acids, aldehydes, ketones, and esters. Other components of alcoholic beverages, sometimes also termed congeners, include carbohydrates, tannins, phenols, metals, coloring agents, vitamins, minerals, histamine, and other pharmacologically active agents. Current data indicate that the congener content of commercial alcoholic beverages differs significantly for each type of beverage (Greizerstein, 1981).

Congeners are responsible for the variable taste, aroma, and color of different beverages. Some have nutrient and medicinal effects and others may have toxic effects, even though quantities may be small. Some congeners are derived from primary plant materials, some from the fermentation process, and others come from the aging process, for example, by contact with wooden containers.

Consumers of alcoholic beverages have noticed for years that certain beverages appear to have a more pronounced effect than others, immediately upon consumption as well as in the postdrinking period. Prior to 1958, no literature existed concerning the analysis of alcoholic beverages by gas liquid chromatography (Carrol, 1970). In the 1960s, with new analytical techniques and with increased knowledge of the effects of alcoholic beverages, the question of the relationship between the congeners and the effects of the beverage became subject to experimental inquiry. The nature of these congeners and other components of alcoholic beverages is the subject of this chapter.

CLASSIFICATION OF CONGENERS

Hundreds of different chemicals have been detected in alcoholic beverages (Schreier, 1979). With today's advanced analytical equipment, thousands of congeners can be identified in beverages, but full understanding of their significance will take many years of research.

The congeners can be classified in accordance with the analytical methods used for their analysis. They can be divided into acid, basic, and neutral fractions designated as volatile, semivolatile, and nonvolatile. The nonvolatile fractions can be divided into minerals, vitamins, carbohydrates, and proteins.

Modern analytical methods can be used to identify congeners responsible for the taste and quality of a beverage (Marais et al, 1981), and its chemical components can be used to identify the geographic region in which the beverage was produced (Brown and Clapperton, 1978; Marais et al, 1981).

In this section only the major volatile congeners and those having the greatest impact on the quality and character of the beverage will be discussed.

Volatile Congeners

The many volatile congeners which, in addition to ethyl alcohol, make up an alcoholic beverage are responsible for its taste and aroma and many of them can have pharmacologic effects.

While thousands of different volatile congeners may be found in various beverages at one time or another, several have been found to be consistently present. Acetaldehyde, ethyl acetate, ethyl formate, and the small aliphatic alcohols make up the major volatile congener content of beers, wines, and distilled spirits.

Alcohols In addition to ethyl alcohol, more than 45 different alcohols have been identified in alcoholic beverages (Schreier, 1979). When starch is the sugar source, a mixture of primary alcohols is produced, consisting mostly of isopentyl alcohol with smaller amounts of *n*-propyl alcohol, isobutyl alcohol, and normal butyl alcohol. This mixture is commonly called fusel oil from the German *Fusel*, meaning inferior liquor (Morrison and Boyd, 1983).

Methyl alcohol is the simplest, lowest molecular weight alcohol, yet it is the most toxic of all, due to its metabolic products. Methyl alcohol is also known as methanol, wood spirit, carbinol, wood alcohol, methylol, and colonial spirit. Severe poisoning and death have occurred primarily from ingestion of beverages adulterated with methyl alcohol.

Typically, within 18 to 48 hours after ingestion, the victim develops acidosis, nausea, abdominal pain, headache, shortness of breath, and blurred or double vision. Severely poisoned individuals become comatose and may die, and those who recover can be left blind (Proctor and Hughes, 1978). In the body, methanol is oxidized to formaldehyde and formic acid. Both of these metabolites are very toxic (Cleland and Kingsbury, 1977). Ethyl alcohol competes with methyl alcohol for the alcohol metabolizing system. For this reason, ethyl alcohol is given in the treatment of methyl alcohol poisoning. The best treatment so far is a combination of hemodialysis to remove the methanol, and the administration of ethanol to inhibit the metabolism of methanol and reduce the rate of production of the more toxic metabolite. Sodium bicarbonate is used to correct the acidosis.

Ethyl alcohol (ethanol, ethyl hydroxide, grain alcohol, methyl carbonol) is an irritant to the eyes and mucous membranes, and causes CNS depression. The second smallest alcohol next to methanol, it is a clear, colorless, flammable liquid with a burning taste. Ethyl alcohol is rapidly oxidized in the body and converted to carbon dioxide and water. It has also been found in public drinking water samples in concentrations of 5 μg/L. The Environmental Protection Agency (EPA) has established 26 mg/L as the estimated permissible concentration in drinking water (Cleland and Kingsbury, 1977).

N-*propyl alcohol* (ethylcarbinol, propanol) is a potent narcotic similar to ethyl alcohol. It is slightly more toxic than isopropyl alcohol and at very high dosages has produced cancer in rats. Public drinking water samples have been shown to contain 1.0 μg/L; the EPA has established 6.9 mg/L as the estimated permissible concentration in water (Cleland and Kingsbury, 1977).

Isobutyl alcohol (isobutanol, 2-methyl-1-propanol) is a clear, sweet-smelling liquid. It acts as a narcotic at high concentrations, and is more toxic than *n*-butyl alcohol. Isobutyl alcohol, like ethyl alcohol, causes CNS depression. The EPA has established as the estimated permissible concentration in drinking water 2.07 mg/L (Cleland and Kingsbury, 1977).

N-*butyl alcohol*, also known as *n*-butanol, is a colorless volatile liquid; the estimated permissible concentration for drinking water is 2.07 mg/L (Cleland and Kingsbury, 1977).

Isopentyl alcohol (isomyl alcohol, isobutyl carbinol) has a disagreeable, pungent odor. Like the other alcohols, it causes CNS depression.

The EPA has set 5.0 mg/L as the estimated permissible concentration in drinking water (Cleland and Kingsbury, 1977).

Fermentation has been taking place since yeast first appeared on the earth, and, as mentioned above, many of the alcohols are found in drinking water supplies. It is interesting to compare the EPA criteria to the actual concentrations found in alcoholic beverages (Table 1-6). Many beverages exceed the recommended water limits for the congeners.

Aldehydes Only a few aldehydes have been detected in alcoholic beverages. Probably, because of the sulfur dioxide treatment, many of the aldehydes are converted to bisulfite addition products which, because of their high water solubility, escape detection. Twenty-seven aldehydes have been identified in grapes (Schreier, 1979).

Acetaldehyde (acetic aldehyde, ethanal, ethyl aldehyde) is colorless with a fruity aroma and is found in most alcoholic beverages. Like drinking alcohol, acetaldehyde is a CNS depressant. It has been found in public drinking water supplies at concentrations of 0.0001 mg/L; the EPA's estimated permissible concentration in drinking water is 2.45 mg/L (Cleland and Kingsbury, 1977).

Only trace amounts of the other aldehydes have been reported in beverages. Cinnamaldehyde, which is used commercially as a flavoring agent, has been detected in wines (Schreier, 1979).

Esters The aroma of beverages is strongly influenced by esters developed during the yeast fermentation. Predominantly, ethyl, isobutyl, and isopentyl esters have been detected, but the list of identified esters surpasses 100 (Schreier, 1979). Some common esters with their reported concentrations are given in Table 1-7. Ethyl acetate and ethyl formate are potentially pharmacologically active.

Ethyl acetate (acetic ester, ethyl ethanoate) has a potent fruity odor. It causes extreme depression of the CNS and in high doses induces narcosis.

Ethyl formate (formic ether, ethyl methanoate) is used as a solvent for cellulose nitrate, in synthetic flavors, and as a fumigant. It also causes CNS depression.

Alcohols, Aldehydes, and Esters

Up to the present, most alcohol research has been conducted on ethyl alcohol since it is the alcohol found in beverages in the highest concentration. However, people do not drink pure ethyl alcohol. Alcoholic beverages contain other alcohols as well as aldehydes and esters that have effects similar to ethyl alcohol.

Generally speaking, these can produce gastric irritation when swallowed and, in higher doses, cause headache, nausea and vomiting.

Table 1-6
Alcohol Content of Beverages Compared to EPA Water Criteria (mg/L)

Beverages	Ethyl Alcohol	Methyl Alcohol	*N*-propyl Alcohol	Isobutyl Alcohol	*N*-butyl Alcohol	Isopentyl Alcohol
Beers	33,000–40,000	6–27	16–124	15–109	1–6	44–248
Wines	88,000–144,000	96–329	46–67	54–109	2–15	115–166
Distilled spirits	153,000–392,000	3.3–220	1–122	1–296	1–17	1–381
EPA*	26.0	3.6	6.9	2.07	2.07	5.0

*EPA's estimated permissible concentration in drinking water (Cleland and Kingsbury, 1977)
From Greizerstein, 1981.

Table 1-7
Common Esters Found in Alcoholic Beverages (mg/L)

Compound	Concentration Range
Ethyl formate	T–166.0
Ethyl acetate	T–285.0
Isobutyl acetate	T–0.2
Isopentyl acetate	T–8.0
Hexyl acetate	0.1–2.0
2-Phenethyl acetate	T–2.6
Ethyl propionate	T–1.2
Ethyl 2-hydroxypropanoate	10–400
Ethyl hexanoate	0.1–2.0
Ethyl octanoate	0.2–1.5
Ethyl laurate	T–0.4
Diethyl succinate	0.8–20.0

T = trace.
From Schreier, 1979; Greizerstein, 1981.

The *higher molecular weight* alcohols are absorbed more slowly than ethyl alcohol so their effects are felt later than those of ethyl alcohol. Also, the body cannot eliminate these alcohols as quickly as it eliminates ethyl alcohol so their effects last longer. This helps explain the common complaint of some drinkers that when they drink a particular beverage, they wake up drunk the next day.

The individual and total congener content of some common beverages is provided in Table 1-8. Because of their volatility, congeners are evaporated along with ethyl alcohol during distillation, giving distilled beverages the highest concentration of congeners compared with other beverages. However, by taking into account the standard drink sizes for beers (12 oz), wines (4 oz), and distilled beverages (1.5 oz), beers and wines contain the highest congener content on a per drink basis.

This is consistent with studies showing that beer and wine produce the most severe hangovers (Haag et al, 1959), and that the severity of the hangover is greater after drinking whiskey than after consuming equivalent amounts of vodka (Chapman, 1970), which contains less congeners.

The threshold limit values (TLVs) are provided at the bottom of Table 1-8 to help evaluate the relative protency of the congeners. It will be noted that ethyl alcohol is the least hazardous alcohol, based on the TLVs. For example, the average adult inhales approximately 10 m^3 of air in eight hours (Cleland and Kingsbury, 1977), and the TLV for ethanol is 1900 mg/m^3. Thus in eight hours an average adult could consume 1900 $mg/m^3 \times 10\ m^3$/eight hours = 19,000 mg/eight hours. This

Table 1-8
Congener and Ethanol Content per Standard Drink of Beer (mg/12 oz), Wine (mg/4 oz) and Distilled Spirits (mg/1.5 oz)

	Total Congener Content	Acetaldehyde	Ethyl Formate	Ethyl Acetate	Methanol	*N*-propanol	Isobutanol	*N*-butanol	Isopentanol	Ethanol
Beers										
Budweiser	142.5	12.2	13.9	6.8	6.7	42.3	37.1	0.6	22.9	13,600
Michelob	48.6	3.5	9.2	2.6	2.3	8.0	5.4	1.6	16.0	13,600
Miller	64.3	4.6	14.1	3.0	9.2	5.4	5.0	1.7	21.3	13,000
Genesee	55.1	4.7	7.6	3.3	6.2	8.5	9.6	0.2	15.0	12,300
Genesee Cream	76.9	7.5	11.3	3.1	2.4	12.0	13.1	1.2	26.4	11,900
Michelob Lite	120.1	4.5	4.0	1.1	2.1	8.1	13.9	1.9	84.5	11,300
Wines										
Taylor Tawny Port	93.7	14.1	7.5	3.4	36.5	6.1	6.8	0.4	18.9	16,400
Widmer port	115.8	29.6	4.1	10.0	37.4	7.2	10.8	1.7	15.0	16,400
Martini & Rossi dry vermouth	108.4	26.0	17.8	2.8	33.2	7.6	7.2	0.7	13.1	15,900
Cinzano sweet vermouth	58.6	7.7	2.9	1.7	14.2	6.1	9.6	1.1	15.3	14,000
Gallo burgundy	62.9	8.1	4.0	1.2	17.2	5.3	6.1	0.2	20.8	10,900
Almaden rosé	77.3	9.0	18.9	2.0	10.9	7.2	12.4	0.5	16.4	10,000

Distilled Spirits										
Smirnoff vodka (100 proof)	8.5	0.4	0.7	0.2	1.6	2.1	3.3	0.1	0.2	16,700
J & B scotch	20.3	1.2	0.6	0.8	2.4	2.6	5.8	0.1	6.8	14,100
Coronet brandy	36.5	1.1	0.9	0.4	9.4	3.4	4.4	0.7	16.2	13,900
Gordon's Dry Gin	6.8	0.5	0.9	0.3	1.0	3.4	0.1	0.1	0.7	13,800
Smirnoff vodka (60 proof)	15.7	0.4	1.9	0.2	1.6	4.4	7.0	0.1	0.2	13,600
Bacardi light rum	16.8	0.6	0.8	0.3	5.6	3.4	2.5	0.1	3.6	13,500
Chex vodka (60 proof)	9.2	0.3	0.7	0.3	0.8	3.3	0.1	0.1	3.8	13,400
Hiram Walker whiskey	11.5	1.9	2.6	0.4	1.5	1.2	1.5	0.1	2.4	13,400
Dewar's scotch	48.6	1.1	1.5	0.4	2.4	5.2	12.6	0.2	25.2	13,300
Schnapps	12.8	0.2	0.5	0.1	0.7	2.4	5.7	0.1	3.2	10,200
Amaretto liqueur	13.2	0.7	0.9	0.1	1.1	0.1	10.5	0.1	0.1	6,500
TLV mg/m^3		360	300	1400	260	500	300	450	360	1,900

TLV = threshold limit values; see text.

From Greizerstein, 1981.

is a little over 0.5 oz in eight hours, and would result in no detectable effects.

Threshold limit values are the concentration limits set by the National Institute for Occupational Safety and Health as permissible exposure limits (Proctor and Hughes, 1978). The TLV for ethanol (1900 mg/m^3) is four to seven times higher than that for other congeners, which reflects their higher potency.

The total amount of congener per drink, as shown in Table 1-8, varies from 6.8 mg/L to 48.6 mg/L in distilled beverages and from 48.6 mg/L to 142.5 mg/L for beers and wine. Many investigators feel that the effects of these congeners need to be considered when assessing health problems caused by excessive alcoholic beverage consumption (Greizerstein, 1981).

Common Acids

Over 130 different acids have been identified in alcoholic beverages. The predominant acids in grapes are malate, tartrate, and citrate acids, with malate and tartrate acids accounting for over 90% of the total acid content. Many acids are natural by-products of alcohol fermentation.

Acetic acid is a normal by-product of yeast metabolism during the early stages of alcohol fermentation. It is found in good wines and may range in concentration from 300 mg/L to 500 mg/L. Higher concentrations indicate spoilage by microorganisms, usually *Acetobacter*. This can make the wine undrinkable. The legal limit of volatile acidity in California is 1200 mg/L for red wine and 1100 mg/L for white wine (Kupina et al, 1982).

Generally, the dominant flavor constituents of wine are formed during yeast fermentation with the formation of the volatile acids. The acid content of wine is used to differentiate between species or varieties of grapes, fruits, and growing conditions. Naturally occurring acids such as transgeranoic acid that are not produced or changed by fermentation are used for this purpose (Schreier, 1979). Some common acids in alcoholic beverages are listed in Table 1-9.

Ketones

3-Hydroxy-2-butanone (acetoin) and the diketones are produced during the fermentation process. The acetoin concentration is usually in the range of approximately 2 to 32 mg/L but sherry can contain up to 350 mg/L (Schreier, 1979). Mainly, they contribute flavor to the beverages but they can have pharmacologic properties. Acetone, for example, like ethyl alcohol, depresses the CNS.

Table 1-9
Common Acids in Alcoholic Beverages (mg/L)

Compound	Biogenesis	Concentration
Acetic acid	F, B	T–1000
Succinic acid	F	100–2000
Malic acid	G	500–5000
Tartaric acid	G	1000–2000
Citric acid	G	130–400
Pyruvic acid	F	8–50
2-Hydroxpropenoic acid	B	0.1–3000
Gluconic acid	D	T–2500
Galacturonic acid (0-Coumaric)	F, D	10–2000
Lactic acid	Beers	500–800

F = yeast fermentation; B = bacterial origin; G = grapes; D = other origin; T = traces.
From Schreier, 1979; Pirola, 1978.

Phenols VOLATILE

Both volatile and nonvolatile phenols have been detected in alcoholic beverages (Lehtonen, 1983b). Phenols produce a smoky aroma in alcoholic drinks and other foods. Scotch whisky owes some of its smoky character to phenolic compounds (Lehtonen, 1983a).

The nonvolatile phenolic compounds enter distilled beverages during the aging process by alcoholysis of lignin in the oak barrels. Lignin dissolves in the beverage and then decomposes into many phenolic compounds (Otsuka and Imai, 1964).

The volatile phenols found in beverages include phenol, *o*-cresol, *m*-cresol, *p*-cresol, guaiacol, *p*-ethylphenol, *p*-ethylguaiacol, eugenol, and *p*-(*n*-propyl)-guaiacol in concentrations ranging from 0 to 2 mg/L (Lehtonen, 1983a). Lehtonen also found that the cresols occurred only in Scotch, Spanish, and Japanese whiskies as a consequence of the raw materials used, especially peated malt. Also, *p*-(*n*-propyl)-guaiacol was found only in dark rum.

The nonvolatile phenols in distilled alcoholic beverages have been detected in concentrations ranging from 0 to 11 mg/L. Gallic acid and syringaldehyde were the main components (Lehtonen, 1983b). In addition, vanillic acid, syringic acid, vanillin, and ferulic acid were the minor phenolic compounds detected. High concentrations of nonvolatile phenols have been detected in wines in ranges of 0 to 123.9 mg/L with catechin, epicatechin, and caftaric acid making up the major phenolics, while gallic acid, couteric acid, astilbin, and engeletin were the minor phenols.

As little as 1 g of phenol may be lethal (Proctor and Hughes, 1978). Symptoms of phenol poisoning include anorectic weight loss, weakness, and liver and kidney damage. The cresols have approximately the same toxicity as phenol, causing CNS depression, mental confusion, and liver and kidney damage. Also, certain individuals become hypersensitive to cresol (Proctor and Hughes, 1978). It is apparent that phenolics can play a significant role in the effects of congeners from different alcoholic beverages.

Vasoactive Congeners

TYRAMINE Some alcoholic beverages contain tyramine (Lovenberg, 1974) and histamine (Schreier, 1979). Both are vasoactive and can affect blood pressure. The enzyme monoamine oxidase metabolizes primary amines such as adrenaline in the body. Drugs that inhibit monoamine oxidase were the first antidepressants. Severe hypertensive reactions have occurred in patients treated with such drugs who then consumed tyramine in certain wines (eg, Chianti) (Goth, 1978). Tyramine levels range from 2 to 10 mg/L in beer, and from 0 to 25 mg/L in wine (Lovenberg, 1974).

HISTAMINES Selected alcoholic beverages can exert potent histamine activity (Ough, 1971; Trethewie, 1979; Parodi et al, 1980). As little as 0.1 mg of histamine phosphate injectd intravenously causes a sharp decline in blood pressure, tachycardia, elevation of the CSF pressure, flushing of the face, and headache (Goth, 1978). In asthmatics it may precipitate a severe asthmatic attack. Histamine taken by mouth is less effective because much of it is metabolized before it can enter the main blood stream.

The headache and flushing sometimes experienced after ingestion of some alcoholic drinks may be partly due to their histamine content. As a general rule, a histamine headache is not produced when the histamine level in beverages is less than 2 mg/L, even in subjects prone to migraine (Trethewie, 1979). Wine containing 8 mg/L has been shown to cause headaches (Shinohara and Watanabe, 1981; Trethewie, 1979). The histamine content of some alcoholic beverages is shown in Table 1-10.

Maturing wine in wood can reduce the histamine content. For example, an Australian red wine matured in wood contained negligible histamine levels, whereas the same wine not matured in wood contained 5 mg/L histamine (Trethewie, 1979).

Toxic Metals

Both the type and amount of metal must be considered in evaluating its toxicity. A small amount may be essential and excessive amounts

Table 1-10
Histamine Content of Selected Alcoholic Beverages

	Histamine (mg/L)		
	Range	*Average*	*No. of Samples*
Chilean wines	0.0–22.0	—	100
French wines	0.1–30.0	5.4	60
California wines	0.1–15.5	—	300
Fruit wines	—	0.56	
Dessert wines	—	2.60	
Chianti Becchi	—	2.60	3
Bourgueil wine	—	15.10	2
Moselle wine	—	0.04	1
Swedish beer	2.6–4.7	3.8	6
Danish beer	3.2–15.0	7.8	5
Brandy	—	0.0	
Scotch whisky	—	0.0	

From Ough, 1971.

can be toxic. For example, marginal chromium deficiency leads to impaired glucose and lipid metabolism.

In one study, 12 oz (355 mL) of ordinary beer would supply 7% of the minimum recommended safe and adequate intake of chromium (Anderson, 1983). In another study of 74 different beers, approximately 12 oz contained 5% of the chromium and 1% of the selenium recommended as the minimum safe and adequate intake (Robberecht et al, 1984).

Food and drink account for the major portion of man's daily intake of lead and arsenic. The maximum allowable limit has been gradually reduced as scientists learn more about the health effects of these two metals. The EPA has set 0.05 mg/L as the drinking water limit for lead and 0.10 mg/L for arsenic, and the Australian National Health and Medical Research Council has reduced the lead and arsenic maximal residue limits in wine to 0.20 mg/L and 0.10 mg/L, respectively (Handson, 1984).

In a recent survey of 27 table wines, the average concentrations of lead and arsenic were 0.31 mg/L and 0.08 mg/L, respectively, for wines from vineyards that had used a lead arsenate compound for caterpillar control, and 0.03 mg/L (lead) and 0.01 mg/L (arsenic) in control vineyards (Handson, 1984). Wine samples that contained 50 mg/L have been implicated in arsenic poisoning in humans (Houser and Vitek, 1979; Gerhardt et al, 1980).

Since moonshine (illegally distilled whiskey) is still consumed in many areas of the United States and other parts of the world, the potential for toxicity from trace elements in this beverage is very real. In a recent study of 12 samples, lead and arsenic were found in potentially toxic concentrations (Gerhardt et al, 1980).

CONGENERS FROM SPICES AND HERBS

"Secret" herbs and spices are used to give alcoholic beverages the variety of flavors unique to each. Just as water is used to extract flavoring chemicals from coffee and tea, alcohol and water are used to extract chemicals from herbs and spices in concentrations that water alone would not extract.

The congeners extracted from many herbs and spices in alcoholic beverages are reported to have pharmacologic effects. The beverage consumer may not know that a beverage contains these natural products which can affect his health in many different ways. Some of these agents are listed here along with some of the health effects associated with them. The chemical composition of many herbs and spices is not known and the effect of many of the known chemical constituents is unknown. The information on flavoring agents is abstracted from a pharmacognosy text (Tyler et al, 1981).

Angelica (gin): A volatile oil constitutes 5% of angelica. It is used medically as a bronchial tonic, a diaphoretic (an agent that increases perspiration), a diuretic, and in the treatment of rheumatism. Both the dried fruit and the root are used but the chemical composition of angelica is unknown.

Anise or *aniseed* (gin, aquavit) is one of the oldest known medicinal plants, mentioned by Dioscorides of Anazarbos, Pliny, and Theophrastus. It contains 1% to 3% volatile oil consisting of 80% to 90% anethole. It is used as a carminative (an agent that relieves flatulence) and for the relief of colic and griping. Its most common use is as a flavoring agent. Anethole is (E)-*p*-propenylanisole, but the Japanese anise is very poisonous and contains a toxin called hananomin.

Cacao (liqueurs) is made from the seeds of *Theobroma cacao*, a tropical American tree (*theobroma* is Greek for "food of the gods"). The seeds contain 35% to 50% fixed oil, about 15% starch, 15% protein, 1% to 4% theobromine, and 0.07% to 0.36% caffeine. Theobromine is a diuretic and smooth muscle relaxant. It is used in the treatment of cardiac edema and angina pectoris. The usual dose is 200 mg three times a day. Caffeine is also a diuretic, but also has a stimulant effect.

Caraway (gin, aquavit, vodka) is used for its flavor and as a carminative. The volatile oil is about 50% (+)-carvone and 50% (+)-limonene.

Cardamom (gin, aquavit) is also used as a carminative. The volatile oil contains 26% to 40% cineole, 28% to 34% (+)-terpinyl acetate, 14% limonene, 3% to 5% sabinene, and 8% linalyl acetate.

Coriander Oil (gin) is used, like caraway and cardamom, as a flavoring agent and carminative. The oil contains (+)-linalool, limonene, α-pinene, γ-terpinene, *p*-cymene.

Fennel (gin) is also a carminative and the oil contains 50% to 60% anethole, (+)-fenchone and (+)-pinene.

Hops (beer) contain β-myrcene and esters of myrcenol and linalool. In addition, they contain humulon and lupulon, which are resins with bacteriostatic properties. Hops also have sedative properties, which are attributed to humulon and lupulon.

Hyssop (absinthe) is described in the Bible and has been used in folk medicine for fever, rheumatism, and to remove the discoloration from a black eye. Hyssop contains cadinene, pinene, (−)pinocampheol, and pinocamphone.

Juniper (gin) is used to flavor beverages and in the over-the-counter (OTC) drug market as a diuretic. It contains pinene, myrcene, limonene, and terpineol.

Licorice or *glycyrrhiza* (gin, liqueurs) contains glycyrrhizin which is fifty times sweeter than sugar. Other constituents include liquiritin, rhomnoisoliquiritin, and the coumarin derivatives herminarin and umbelliferon. Licorice is a demulcent and expectorant. It is used in dermatology for its anti-inflammatory properties. Glycyrrhizin can increase sodium and fluid retention. Therefore persons with cardiac problems should avoid consumption of significant amounts of licorice.

Nutmeg (eggnog) contains myristicin and elemicin. Myristicin has been used to help control diarrhea. Large doses can cause flushing of the skin, tachycardia, dry mouth, and have an hallucinogenic effect.

Wormwood (absinthe) has a long history of use for indigestion, flatulence, and as a diaphoretic. It was used to flavor absinthe, a beverage thought to cause acute and chronic toxicity. It contains thujone which causes trembling, stupor, convulsions, dementia, and even death. Today, most countries prohibit its use (Grossman and Lembeck, 1983).

SEMIVOLATILE CONGENERS

In reviewing the literature, it seems that the semivolatile congeners have been largely overlooked. Samples of beers, wines, and distilled spirits were examined, using the method described in the appendix. Only the major peaks were identified and they are listed in Tables 1-11 through 1-16.

The significance of these congeners remains to be determined. The content and concentration of the semivolatile constituents are as variable as the volatile and nonvolatile congeners of alcoholic beverages.

Table 1-11
Semivolatile Congeners in Selected Wines (mg/L)

	Rosé			
Compound	Paul Masson	Gallo	Nectarosé	Taylor
Cyclohexane	70	81	105	72
3-Methyl-1-butanol	883	789	401	851
Diethylene glycol	103	138	497	171
1-Hexanol	28	20	—	15
Methyl hexanol	28	31	33	—
Heptanoic acid	18	—	—	11
Hexadienoic acid	321	317	—	110
Benzeneethanol	188	266	697	37
Diethyl succinate	249	182	146	294
Caprylic acid	33	23	—	47
Ethyl caprylate	15	—	—	16
β-Phenylethyl isobutanoate	17	32	54	59
2,3-Butanediol	—	19	52	40
3-Methylthio + propanol	—	—	35	—

	Chablis			
Compound	Paul Masson	Chablis Fer Cru	Taylor	Almaden
Cyclohexane	81	94	T	85
2,2-Diemthylhexane	22	—	T	—
3-Methyl-1-butanol	956	1542	98	991
Diethylene glycol	106	146	18	108
1-Hexanol	32	48	T	17
Methyl hexanol	26	—	—	—
Heptanoic acid	63	55	T	67
Hexadienoic acid	295	—	32	331
Benzeneethanol	210	762	24	140
Diethyl succinate	118	425	17	196
Caprylic acid	36	—	T	38
Ethyl caprylate	24	33	T	23
β-Phenylethyl isobutanoate	25	38	—	35
2,3-Butanediol	—	—	T	—

	Burgundy			
Compound	Paul Masson	Taylor	Thomas Frères	Gallo
Cyclohexane	T	84	82	64
2,2-Dimethylhexane	T	17	17	26
3-Methyl-1-butanol	45	389	1081	174
Diethylene glycol	43	492	674	163
1-Hexanol	T	46	26	37
Methyl hexanol	T	57	54	68
Heptanoic acid	T	—	—	T
Hexadienoic acid	—	216	—	10
Benzeneethanol	43	418	353	334

Compound	Burgundy			
	Paul Masson	Thomas Taylor	Frères	Gallo
Diethyl succinate	11	68	T	155
Caprylic Acid	—	—	—	178
β-Phenylethyl isobutanoate	—	23	20	25
2,3-Butanediol	T	112	109	74
3-Methylthio + propanol	—	35	—	—

T = trace.

Table 1-12
Semivolatile Congeners in Selected Bourbons (mg/L)

Compound	Jim Beam	Jack Daniels	Weller
Cyclohexane	73	—	—
3-Methyl-1-butanol	569	61	849
Benzeneethanol	T	300	738
Ethyl caprylate	98	25	84
Ethylester of dodecanoic acid (mol wt 228)	42	—	40
Ethylester of dodecanoic acid (mol wt 220)	116	51	152
Diethoxy ethane	T	63	383
2-Methyl propanol	73	403	241
Urea	—	—	T
Furaldehyde	—	48	86

T = trace.

Table 1-13
Semivolatile Congeners in Tequila (mg/L)

Compound	Azteca	Cuervo
3-Methyl-1-butanol	2056	107
Benzeneethanol	105	—
Ethyl caprylate	51	T
Ethylester of dodecanoic acid (mol wt 228)	39	17
Ethylester of dodecanoic acid (mol wt 220)	173	27
Diethoxy ethane	33	—
2-Methyl propanol	66	—
Dimethoxy methane	435	—

T = trace.

Table 1-14
Semivolatile Congeners in Selected Gins (mg/L)

Compound	Tangueray	Beefeater	Gordon's	Gilbey's	Seagram's
Cyclohexane	—	—	—	T	—
3-Methyl-1-butanol	66	—	—	—	—
Benzeneethanol	86	111	90	T	137
Heptanoic acid	—	—	—	T	—
Ethyl caprylate	63	13	T	T	18
Ethylester of dodecanoic acid (mol wt 228)	—	—	—	T	—
Ethylester of dodecanoic acid (mol wt 220)	30	11	40	—	41
Diethoxy ethane	—	—	—	T	—
2-Methyl propanol	—	—	—	T	—
4-Carene (or similar terpine)	193	488	206	T	525

T = trace.

Table 1-15
Semivolatile Congeners in Selected Scotch Whiskies (mg/L)

Compound	Johnny Walker	Cutty Sark	J & B	Chivas Regal	Usher's
Cyclohexane	25	—	—	—	—
3-Methyl-1-butanol	504	1076	1796	906	1222
Benzeneethanol	112	128	278	86	108
Ethyl caprylate	166	106	123	76	85
Ethylester of dodecanoic acid (mol wt 228)	99	111	57	36	42
Ethylester of Dodecanoic acid (mol wt 220)	267	241	263	129	173
β-Methyl histamine	—	25	83	17	32
Diethoxy ethane	338	38	62	40	14
2-Methyl propanol	169	56	91	195	243
Pentyl ester of acetic acid	40	39	31	—	—

Table 1-16
Semivolatile Congeners in Selected Beers (mg/L)

Compound	Carta Blanca	Pilsner Urquell	Dos Equis	Budweiser	Michelob Lite	Guiness Stout	Heineken Dark	Heineken Light
3-Methyl-1-butanol	82	90	137	103	T	137	58	78
Benzeneethanol	98	51	T	78	—	T	98	68
β-Methyl histamine	—	—	T	T	—	T	—	T
Pentyl ester of acetic acid	—	T	T	T	—	T	—	T

T = trace.

REFERENCES

Anderson, B.M. Separation of alpha and beta and iso gamma acids in hop products and beer by high performance liquid chromatography. *J. Chromatogr.* 262:448–450, 1983.

Asmus, P.A., Landis, J.B., and Vila, C.L. Liquid chromatographic determination of lincomycin in fermentation beers. *J. Chromatogr.* 264:241–248, 1983.

Brown, D.G., and Clapperton, J.F. Discriminant analysis of sensory and instrumental data on beer. *J. Inst. Brewers* 84:318–323, 1978.

Carroll, R.B. Analysis of alcoholic beverages by gas-liquid chromatography. *Q. J. Stud. Alcohol* 5:6–19, 1970.

Chapman, L.F. Experimental induction of hangover, *Q. J. Stud. Alcohol* 5: 67–86, 1970.

Chatton, M.J., and Ullman, P.M. Nutrition; nutritional and metabolic disorders. In *Current Medical Diagnosis and Treatment*. (M.A. Krupp and M.J. Chatton, eds.), Lange Medical Publications, Los Altos, Calif., 1984, pp. 790–791.

Cleland, J.G. and Kingsbury, G.L. Multimedia environmental goals for environmental assessment. US Environmental Protection Agency publication No. 600/7–77–136b, Nov. 1977, pp. E29–450.

Gerhardt, R.E., Crecelius, E.A., and Hudson, J.B. Trace elements content of moonshine. *Arch. Environ. Health* 35:332–334, 1980.

Goth, A. *Medical Pharmacology;*, C.V. Mosby, St. Louis, 1978, pp. 103–104.

Greizerstein, H.B. Congener contents of alcoholic beverages. *J. Stud. Alcohol* 42:1030–1037, 1981.

Grossman, H.J., and Lembeck, H. *Grossman's Guide to Wines, Beers, and Spirits,* Charles Scribner's, New York, 1983.

Guthrie, H.A. *Introductory Nutrition*. C.V. Mosby, St. Louis, 1983, pp. 41–42.

Haag, H.G., Finnegan, J.K., Larson, P.S., et al. Studies on the acute toxicity and irritating properties of the congeners in whiskey. *Toxicol. Appl. Pharmacol.* 1:618–627, 1959.

Handson, P.D. Lead and arsenic levels in wines produced from vineyards where lead arsenate sprays are used for caterpillar control. *J. Sci. Food Agric.* 35:215–218, 1984.

Hoeft, H. and Obe, G. SCE-inducing congeners in alcoholic beverages. *Mutation Research*. 121:247–251, 1983.

Houser, W.C., and Vitek, R.K. Arsenic intoxication. *Postgrad. Med.* 66:225–226, 1979.

Konowalchuk, J., and Speirs, J.I. Virus inactivation by grapes and wines. *Appl. Environ. Microbiol.* 32:757–763, 1976.

Kupina, S.A., Kutschinski, J.L., Williams, R.D., et al. A refined gas chromatographic procedure for the measurement of acetic acid in wines and its comparison with the distillation method. *Am. J. Enol. Vitic.* 33:67–74, 1982.

Lehtonen, M. Gas-liquid chromatographic determination of volatile phenols in matured distilled alcoholic beverages. *J. Assoc. Off. Anal. Chem.* 66:62–70, 1983a.

Lehtonen, M. High performance liquid chromatographic determination of nonvolatile phenolic compounds in matured distilled alcoholic beverages. *J. Assoc. Off. Anal. Chem.* 66:71–78, 1983b.

Loquet, C., Toussaint, G., and Le Talaer, J.Y. Studies in mutagenic constituents of apple brandy and various alcoholic beverages collected in western

France, a high incidence area for oseophageal cancer. *Mutat. Res.* 88:155–164, 1981.

Lovenberg, W. Psycho- and vasoactive compounds in food substances. *J. Agric. Food Chem.* 22:23-26, 1974.

Marais, J., Van Rooyen, P.C., and Duplessis, C.S. Differentiation between wines originating from different red wine cultivars and wine regions by the application of stepwise discriminate analysis to gas chromatographic data. *S. Afr. J. Enol. Vitic.* 2:19–23, 1981.

Morrison, R.T., and Boyd, R.N. *Organic Chemistry*, Allyn & Bacon, Boston, 1983, pp. 463–464.

Obe, G. Mutagenic activity of ethanol. In *Animal Models in Alcohol Research.* (K. Eriksson, J.D. Sinclair, and K. Kiianmaa, eds.), Academic Press, New York, 1980, pp. 377–391.

Ondus, M.G., Wenzel, J., and Zimmerman, G.L. Sugar determination in foods with a radially compressed high performance liquid chromatography column. *J. Chem. Education* 60:776–778, 1983.

Otsuka, K., and Imai, S., *Agric. Biol. Chem.* 28:356–362, 1964.

Ough, C.S. Measurement of histamine in Claifornia wines. *J. Agric. Food Chem.* 19:241, 1971.

Parodi, A., Guarrera, M., and Rebora, A. Flushing in rosacea: An experimental approach. *Arch. Dermatol. Res.* 269:269–273, 1980.

Pirola, R.C. *Drug Metabolism and Alcohol.* University Park Press, Baltimore, 1978, pp. 123–129.

Proctor, N.H., and Hughes, J.P. *Chemical Hazards of the Work Place*. Lippincott, Philadelphia, 1978.

Robberecht, H., Van Schoor, O., and Deelstra, H. Selenium and chromium content of European beers as determined by AAS. *J. Food Sci.* 49:300–301, 1984.

Schreier, P. Flavor composition of wines: A review. *CRC Crit. Rev. Food Sci. Nutri.* 59–111, Nov. 1979.

Shinohara, T., and Watanabe, M. Gas chromatographic analysis of volatile esters of wines. *Agric. Biol. Chem.* 45:2903–2905, 1981.

Sonde, M.A., and Mandell, G.L. Miscellaneous antibacterial agents: Antifungal and antiviral agents. In *The Pharmacological Basis of Therapeutics*, 6th ed. (A.G. Gilman, L.S. Goodman, and A. Gilman, eds.), Macmillan, New York, 1980, p. 1225.

Stephany, R.W., and Schuller, P.L. Daily dietary intakes of nitrate, nitrite, and volatile *N*-nitrosamines in the Netherlands using the duplicate portion sampling technique. *Oncology* 37:203–210, 1980.

Trethewie, E.R. Wines and headaches. *Med. J. Aust.* 6:94–95, 1979.

Tyler, V.E., Brady, L.R., and Robbers, J.E. *Pharmacognosy*, Lea & Febiger, Philadelphia, 1981, pp. 103–472.

Van Vuuren, H.J.J, Kersters, K., Toerien, D.F., et al. The identification of Enterobacteriaceae from breweries: Combined use and comparison of API 20 E system, gel electrophoresis of proteins and gas chromatography of volatile metabolites. *J. Appl. Bacteriol.* 51:51–65, 1981.

Watt, B.K., and Merrill, A.L. *Composition of Foods*. Publication No. 8, Government Printing Office, 1963, pp. 75–76.

Weinstein, L. Miscellaneous antibacterial agents: Antifungal and antiviral agents. In *The Pharmacological Basis of Therapeutics*. (L.S. Goodman and A. Gilman, eds.), MacMillan, New York, 1975, ed. 5, pp. 1227–1228.

Zee, J.A., Szoghy, I.M., Simard, R.E., et al. Elemental analysis of Canadian,

European and American Wines by photon induced x-ray fluorescence. *Am. J. Enol. Vitic*. 34:152–156, 1983.

Committee on Dietary Allowances Food and Nutrition Board, *Recommended Dietary Allowances*, 9th edition, National Academy of Sciences, Washington, D.C., pp. 1–185, 1980.

Appendix

Method for Analysis of Alcoholic Beverages for Semivolatiles

1. Extraction
   - 1.1 30 mL of each beverage was placed in a 40-mL vial. Carbonated beverages were allowed to stand overnight to degas.
   - 1.2 3 mL of dichloromethane and 5 g of sodium chloride were added to each sample and the vial sealed with a Teflon cap.
   - 1.3 Samples were shaken for five minutes on an automatic shaker and the phases allowed to separate for 20 minutes.
   - 1.4 1 mL of the dichloromethane fraction was transferred to an autosampler vial and 40 μg of anthracene as an internal standard. The vial was then sealed with a crimp-on cap and stored at 0°C until analysis.
2. Chromatography
   - 2.1 Gas chromatographic separation was accomplished on a Hewlett-Packard 5840 GC under the following conditions:
     - 2.1.1 Column — HP fused silica = 30 m × 0.3 mm ID coated with 6% phemyl, 94% methyl bonded silozane phase.
     - 2.1.2 Carrier — Helium at 5 psi.
     - 2.1.3 Temperature program — 40°C for one minute. Program to 270°C at 5°/min for four min, 10°/min for five min, and 20°/min thereafter.
     - 2.1.4 Injector — 270° — split less for 0.2 minute.
     - 2.1.5 Detector — HP 5985B mass spectrometer.
     - 2.1.6 Injection — 3 μL.
3. Mass Spectrometry
   - 3.1 Hewlett-Packard 5985B mass spectrometer
   - 3.2 Mass spectrometer settings as follows:
     - 3.2.1 Ionization voltage — 70eV
     - 3.2.2 Source temperature — 200°C
     - 3.2.3 Mass range — 40 to 400
     - 3.2.4 Scan time — 1.2 seconds
     - 3.2.5 Run time — 30 minutes
     - 3.2.6 Threshold — 20
     - 3.2.7 Calibration — Auto tune on PFTBA
     - 3.2.8 Electron multiplier voltage — 400 above auto time
4. Treatment of Data
   - 4.1 Quantitation was based on area under each peak relative to 40 ppm internal standard without regard to relative response factors. Therefore quantitation is only valid when relating one sample to another.
   - 4.2 The total area under each peak was determined using the sum of all ions in each spectrum, not single ions.

2

Pharmacology of Ethyl Alcohol

James C. Garriott

Ethyl alcohol is such a pervasive agent in most societies that it is usually thought of as a social beverage and intoxicant, and we often lose track of the fact that it is a drug, comparable in many respects to more highly respected therapeutic and "recreational" drugs such as tranquilizers, narcotics, sedatives, and hypnotics. Since it is not controlled as a drug, but is available without restriction to all persons of legal age, it comes as a surprise to many that it has properties very similar to narcotic drugs such as morphine and heroin. Alcohol and narcotic drugs alike are euphorigenic, CNS and respiratory depressants, and induce tolerance and physical dependence. Probably the major distinctions between the two are the strong analgesic effects of narcotics versus the weak analgesic actions of alcohol, and the generally weaker potency of alcohol, requiring tens of grams for effectiveness rather than a few milligrams.

Due to the low potency of ethyl alcohol, high concentrations are present in the body when it is imbibed and consequently it affects virtually all organ and biochemical systems of the body.

This chapter consists primarily of an overview of the pharmacologic effects of alcohol with emphasis on the CNS effects, which are of most concern to forensic scientists.

SKIN

Alcohol in higher concentrations acts as a protein precipitant, as it dehydrates protoplasm, and is an irritant to denuded surfaces and mucous membranes. This is known as an astringent effect. Since it cools the skin as it evaporates and acts as a bactericidal agent, it may be used as a skin rubbing agent, especially in bedridden patients to prevent bedsores. Concentrations of about 70% are the most effective for antibacterial action (Ritchie, 1980).

Ingestion of alcohol in moderate doses induces a marked dilation of the blood vessels of the skin, resulting in a redness or flushing of the face and other parts of the body. Very large doses, resulting in high blood concentrations of alcohol, for example, greater than 0.30 to 0.40 g/dL, impair general circulation and the skin may be cold and pale.

GASTROINTESTINAL TRACT

The effects of ethyl alcohol on the gastrointestinal (GI) tract are influenced by many factors, such as the presence or absence of food, the types of food present, the degree of tolerance for alcohol, and the presence or absence of GI disease. As with other mucous membranes, alcohol acts as an irritant in higher concentrations (above 40%) and can cause hyperemia, gastritis, and erosion. It has been estimated that one out of three heavy drinkers suffers from chronic gastritis (Ritchie, 1980).

The presence of food in the stomach tends to dilute the alcohol, thus alleviating irritation, and delay absorption due to the mixing with alcohol and physical interactions with alcohol by some food types. In lower concentrations, alcohol stimulates gastric secretions, both by a direct action on the stomach and by reflex. Beverages with about 10% alcohol concentration result in a gastric secretion rich in acid, while the psychic reflex secretion is rich in pepsin. As the concentration rises above 20%, however, these secretions are inhibited and the stomach may secrete mucous as a protection against the irritation.

Although an indirect effect, alcohol regularly induces nausea and vomiting in nontolerant individuals. This is believed to be the result of a direct stimulation of the chemoreceptor trigger zone of the CNS. This action occurs when alcoholic beverages are consumed rapidly and when the blood concentration reaches about 0.12 g/dL. It also occurs when alcohol is administered intravenously (IV), thus proving it to be a central effect rather than a direct effect on the GI tract (Newman, 1954).

Continuous use of large amounts of alcohol causes a spectrum of deleterious effects on the GI and hepatic functions. Esophageal varices, resulting from impaired hepatic circulation in cirrhosis, and gastric lesions and ulceration are commonly seen in alcoholics. Acute and chronic pancreatitis occurs often in alcoholism, and may be due to a stimulation of pancreatic secretions combined with obstruction of pancreatic ducts (Ritchie, 1980).

Thus it appears that alcohol may have some beneficial effects on GI function in small or moderate doses and concentrations by stimulation of gastric digestive juices. Chronic or heavy alcohol consumption, however, is markedly detrimental — acutely by irritation, suppression of digestive functions, and nausea and vomiting; and after chronic heavy use by induction of severe organ system damage such as cirrhosis; esophageal varices, with risks of hemorrhaging; and acute or chronic pancreatitis.

CARDIOVASCULAR SYSTEM

Moderate doses of alcohol cause a slight increase in pulse rate and blood pressure. Moderate doses of alcohol also increase plasma high density lipoprotein (HDL) levels, often associated with lower coronary artery disease rates. Thus low to moderate alcohol consumption may have a beneficial effect on the heart. Several recent epidemiologic studies have demonstrated that the risk of coronary artery disease and myocardial infarction decreases with moderate alcohol consumption (Goldstein, 1983).

The most prominent effect with higher doses, however, is a depression of cardiovascular functions. This depression is probably a combination of central vasomotor and respiratory depression, and a direct depression of the heart muscle.

Chronic use of high doses of alcohol, as in chronic alcoholism, results in intracellular myocardial lesions, probably associated with congestive heart failure and hypertension (Regan, 1971; Ferrans, 1966). Alcoholic cardiomyopathy from excessive consumption of alcohol is a well-established syndrome. The damage to the heart muscle appears to be a direct toxic effect of alcohol. Fibrosis, edema, enlarged and distorted mitochondria, and lipid accumulation in the heart muscle cells are characteristic of alcoholic cardiomyopathy (Goldstein, 1983).

LIVER

Alcohol-induced liver disease is a very common condition. Cirrhosis ranks as the fourth most common cause of death in the United States, and chronic alcohol consumption is its most common cause. It is estimated that 8% to 20% of chronic alcoholics eventually develop cirrhosis. It is therefore apparent that factors other than alcohol consumption are involved in the etiology of cirrhosis, but these are as yet unknown (Mezey, 1979).

Fatty infiltration of the liver occurs readily after the ingestion of alcohol. This effect is due to an overloading of the liver's metabolic functions by alcohol, and the resultant storage of unmetabolized fatty acids (Goldstein, 1983). However, this is a reversible condition, and is not thought to result directly in cirrhosis. The deposition of excess collagen in the liver initiates hepatic fibrosis which becomes irreversible, developing into cirrhosis. The resultant progressive deterioration in liver function may culminate with liver failure, hepatic coma, and death. Alcoholic liver disease is unlikely with consumption of less than 80 g/d (about 6 oz of 100 proof whiskey or six beers), but increases dramatically when consumption exceeds 160 g/d, either regularly or in "binges" over a 10- to 15-year period (Marshall et al, 1979).

KIDNEY

The principal effect of ethyl alcohol on the kidney is that of a diuretic. This appears to be a direct effect, exerted by virtue of a decrease in renal tubular reabsorption of water. It is assumed that alcohol causes this diuresis by inhibiting the secretion of anti-diuretic hormone in the supraopticoneurohypophyseal system. The diuretic effect appears to be directly proportional to the blood alcohol concentration and occurs when the blood alcohol concentration is rising, but not when it is stable or falling (Ritchie, 1980; Goldstein, 1983).

No deleterious effect on the kidneys or renal function has been attributed to alcohol.

ENDOCRINE SYSTEM

Acute alcohol administration induces a stress effect on the adrenal cortex. Thus plasma levels of cortisol and other corticosteroids are increased in a dose-related response to alcohol. Ethanol essentially mimics the adrenocorticotropic hormone (ACTH) by stimulating the adrenal production of steroids (Goldstein, 1983).

In addition, alcohol produces an immediate increase in the excretion of epinephrine and norepinephrine. This release may be responsible for a transient hyperglycemia, pupillary dilatation, and a slight rise in blood pressure that occurs during early stages of alcohol intoxication (Ritchie, 1980).

Ethyl alcohol decreases plasma testosterone, and testicular synthesis of testosterone is inhibited. Hepatic androgen metabolism is stimulated, and the hypothalamic pituitary response to low levels of circulating testosterone is decreased (Goldstein, 1983). It has also been demonstrated that alcohol significantly decreases penile tumescence and vaginal pressure, thus decreasing sexual responsiveness in both men and women. Therefore, as Shakespeare wrote long ago, alcohol "provokes the desire, but it takes away the performance" (Ritchie, 1980).

A possible biochemical relationship between ethyl alcohol and opiate narcotics has been discovered. Epinephrine and norepinephrine may condense in the presence of acetaldehyde (the direct metabolite of ethyl alcohol) to form tetrahydroisoquinoline alkaloids. These are related to the alkaloids derived from opium, such as morphine. Thus, it has been proposed that the formation of these alkaloids in the presence of heavy alcohol consumption could provide a common mechanism for the addiction process in alcoholics and narcotic addicts (Cohen and Collins, 1970; Davis and Walsh, 1970; Collins et al, 1979).

CENTRAL NERVOUS SYSTEM

The central nervous system (CNS) is the bodily system most severely affected by alcohol, and since this system is the source of any behavioral aberrations due to alcohol, these effects are the most important to consider for medicolegal interpretation of alcohol-related situations.

The intensity of the CNS effects of alcohol is proportional to the concentration of alcohol in the blood. These general effects are outlined in relation to alcohol concentrations in Table 2-1 (Dubowski, 1985). However, the effects are considerably more pronounced when the blood

Table 2-1
Stages of Acute Alcoholic Influence/Intoxication

Blood-Alcohol Concentration g/100 mL	Stage of Alcoholic Influence	Clinical Signs/Symptoms
0.01–0.05	Subclinical	No apparent influence Behavior nearly normal by ordinary observation Slight changes detectable by special tests
0.03–0.12	Euphoria	Mild euphoria, sociability, talkativeness Increased self-confidence; decreased inhibitions Diminution of attention, judgment, and control Beginning of sensory-motor impairment Slowed information processing Loss of efficiency in finer performance tests
0.09–0.25	Excitement	Emotional instability; loss of critical judgment Impairment of perception, memory, and comprehension Decreased sensitory response; increased reaction time Reduced visual acuity, peripheral vision, and glare recovery Sensory-motor incoordination; impaired balance Drowsiness

Blood-Alcohol Concentration g/100 mL	Stage of Alcohol Influence	Clinical Signs/Symptoms
0.18–0.30	Confusion	Disorientation, mental confusion; dizziness Exaggerated emotional states (fear, rage, sorrow, etc) Disturbances of vision (diplopia, etc) and of perception of color, form, motion, dimensions Increased pain threshold Increased muscular incoordination; staggering gait; slurred speech Apathy, lethargy
0.25–0.40	Stupor	General inertia; approaching loss of motor functions Markedly decreased response to stimuli Marked muscular incoordination; inability to stand or walk Vomiting; incontinence of urine and feces Impaired consciousness; sleep or stupor
0.35–0.50	Coma	Complete unconsciousness; coma; anesthesia Depressed or abolished reflexes Subnormal temperature Incontinence of urine and feces Impairment of circulation and respiration Possible death
0.45+	Death	Death from respiratory arrest

Reprinted by permission of K.M. Dubowski, 1985.

level is rising than when falling. This is known as the Mellanby effect and is believed to result from so-called acute (functional) tolerance to alcohol, achieved during the course of the intoxication (Mellanby, 1919; Goldstein, 1983). It was previously proposed that a portion of this effect is due to the higher alcohol concentrations in the brain during the rising or absorptive phase of the blood alcohol curve due to rapid equilibration of the brain with arterial blood. Aside from this distributional artifact, however, it has been shown that rats are about twice as tolerant to a moderate alcohol dose at a given brain level 60 minutes after as compared to 10 minutes after the injection (LeBlanc et al, 1975). An extreme example of acute tolerance was reported in a human patient in whom a maximum blood alcohol level of 0.78 g/dL was found. When the patient reached a level of 0.30 g/dL, she was, by clinical observations, sober (Hammond et al, 1973).

The general CNS effects of alcohol and relation to locus of action are illustrated in Figure 2-1. The early effects of alcohol are often considered stimulant actions, mediated by depression of the reticular

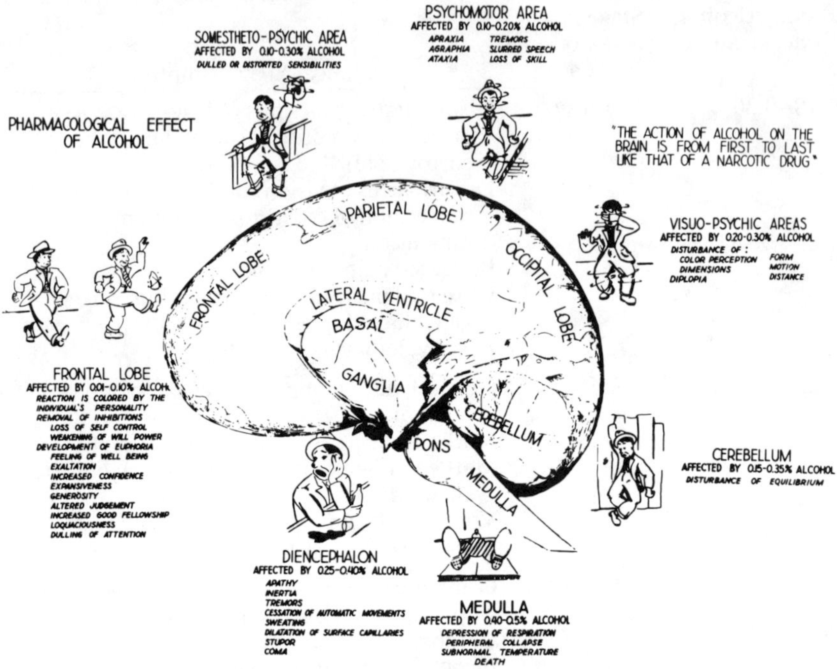

Figure 2-1 The effects of alcohol on CNS functioning at various blood alcohol concentrations (0.10% = 0.10 g/dL). (Reproduced by courtesy of S.R. Gerber, M.D., Coroner, Cuyahoga County, Cleveland.)

activating system, and thereby releasing the cortex from selective control and inhibition. Increased confidence, a more expansive and vivacious personality, mood swings, garrulousness, and increased social interactions are characteristic (Ritchie, 1980). These effects are actually due to depression of the inhibitory central mechanisms. Thus the intoxicated individual may act in ways or perform acts he would not ordinarily do. He may become more aggressive and even violent, due to pent-up hostilities, or express abnormal desires and drives normally kept under control. He may become overconfident and take dangerous risks he would not ordinarily take (eg, speeding and reckless driving).

First affected are processes that depend on previous training and experience and that govern self-restraint and inhibition. Memory, fine discrimination, and concentration functions are dulled as the blood alcohol level rises. All bodily functions and abilities governed by the brain are impaired progressively. With acute intoxication (blood levels in excess of 0.40 g/dL), even autonomic (automatic) functions are affected. At these levels, there is considerable risk of death from depression of the respiratory centers (Dubowski, 1985; Ritchie, 1980).

Impairment of Specific Functions Related to Driving Ability

Visual acuity A number of studies have been performed to test the effects of ethyl alcohol on vision, with conflicting results. Several early studies reported little or no effect, but doses were unusually low, in most cases ranging from 0.2 to approximately 0.7 g/kg (Marquis et al, 1957; Miles, 1924; Blomberg and Wassen, 1959). Mortimer (1963) reported only a 3% visual decrement at a blood alcohol concentration of 0.06 g/dL (Wallgren and Barry, 1970).

However, studies in which more substantial and socially realistic doses of alcohol were used have substantiated significant decrements of visual acuity after alcohol ingestion. With blood alcohol levels varying between 0.06 and 0.22 g/dL (average 0.115 g/dL), visual acuity was impaired in 54% of subjects with levels between 0.06 and 0.10 g/dL, and in 85% of the subjects with levels between 0.101 and 0.125 g/dL (Newman and Fletcher, 1941).

Some studies have shown that alcohol slows adaptation to both darkness and light, and lowers resistance to glare at blood alcohol levels ranging from 0.09 to 0.15 g/dL (Wallgren and Barry, 1970). Impairment of discrimination of colors has been observed after alcohol doses of 0.7 g/kg (Schmidt and Bingel, 1953; Wallgren and Barry, 1970).

Other studies have shown that alcohol may diminish the sensitivity, persistence, or speed of response to visual stimulation (Suzuki et al, 1957; Lewis et al, 1969; Idestrom and Cadenius, 1968).

Brecher showed the impairment of alcohol on binocular coordination by measuring fusion speed or focusing ability on two light sources. Decrements were seen with blood alcohol levels as low as 0.03 g/dL, and in up to 89% of subjects with levels of 0.18 g/dL (Brecher et al, 1955).

In a more recent study of alcohol effects on vision, tracking, and division of attention, it was found that when either visual or tracking functions were examined in complex situations requiring simultaneous visual and tracking responses, as occur in actual driving situations, large performance decrements occurred at low blood alcohol concentrations (Moskowitz, 1974).

In summary, studies performed to specifically measure the effects of alcohol on driving-related visual skills, in which more than simple visual skills were studied, showed that its effect is significant. Impairment may occur in some individuals at blood concentrations as low as 0.03 g/dL, and marked impairment occurs in nearly all individuals at concentrations greater than 0.08 g/dL (Honneger et al, 1970; Newman and Fletcher, 1941; Moskowitz, 1974; Mortimer, 1963).

Auditory discrimination The auditory sense seems to be more resistant to the effects of alcohol than most other senses. Auditory acuity is not generally affected in humans at low blood alcohol levels (less than 0.10 g/dL). Pihkanen and Kauko (1962) reported impairment in two out of three tests performed to measure auditory capability at average blood levels of 0.10 g/dL (Wallgren and Barry, 1970).

A large decrement in discrimination between volumes and intensity of sounds but a less clear effect on ability to detect faint sounds has been reported (Jellinik and McFarland, 1940).

Other sensory effects Olfactory and taste sensibilities are affected at low doses of alcohol (0.1–0.2 g/kg). These senses may be affected at blood levels of 0.04 g/dL or greater (Wallgren and Barry, 1970).

Reaction time Many studies have demonstrated that alcohol has a detrimental effect on reaction time. In general, blood levels in excess of 0.07 g/dL consistently impair reaction responses.

Blood levels of alcohol ranging from 0.012 to 0.12 g/dL increased reaction time by 5% to 17% (Blum et al, 1964; Boyd et al, 1962; Buffard 1959; Carlson et al, 1934). In other studies, blood levels of from 0.05 to 0.15 g/dL lengthened reaction time in 42% to 82% of subjects (Huber, 1955; Izard and Saby, 1962; Moureau, 1957).

An increase in reaction time of 40% to 55% was reported by Starck (1953) at blood levels of from 0.13 to 0.18 g/dL.

In slightly more complicated tasks, in which subjects perform more than one attentive task at one time, alcohol doses of 1.0 to 1.2 g/kg, giving alcohol levels averaging 0.11 g/dL, increased reaction time by more than 200% (Gruner, 1955; Gruner and Ptasnik, 1953). This situation may indicate more closely the effects of alcohol on driving skills, since the driver must control the speed and position of the vehicle, as well as monitor outside signals such as traffic lights and signs. The additional demands on the driver's attention and judgment appear to greatly enhance the detrimental effects of alcohol. Bjerver and Goldberg (1950) reported increased time required to perform certain driving skills ranging from 3% for a single task to 72% for a more complicated test of parking an automobile, at blood levels averaging 0.05 g/dL.

Many similar tests have demonstrated effects of alcohol at low to moderate blood levels detrimental to driving-related skills.

In summary, most testing for alcohol-related impairment of performance on driving-related skills shows distinct impairment at levels of 0.10 g/dL or even lower. Although few studies have examined the effects at higher levels (>0.15 g/dL), one can logically expect increases in reaction time of several hundred percent as blood concentrations exceed 0.2 and 0.3 g/dL, as well as drastic impairment of other driving-related senses and skills. Surveys of average blood alcohol levels in motor vehicle fatalities range from 0.16 g/dL upward (Cimbura et al, 1982; Garriott, 1977).

Effects of Alcohol in Combination with Other Drugs

Ethyl alcohol has some degree of interaction with a wide spectrum of other drugs. Classically, it exerts a potentiation or synergistic effect when ingested in the presence of other drugs having CNS depressant effects. When alcohol is ingested in the presence of other drugs having a depressant effect on the CNS, such as sedatives, hypnotics, anticonvulsants, antidepressants, tranquilizers, some analgesics, and opiates, a greatly enhanced depressant effect may occur. Pharmaceutical package inserts and other drug information circulars warn physicians of the dangers of concomitant use of drugs in the above classes and alcohol.

The enhanced intoxication effect can occur with low levels of alcohol. This effect can be profound, and numerous deaths have occurred resulting from "mixing alcohol and drugs." The severe intoxication that can occur in this manner also may be a significant factor in the incidence of motor vehicle accidents (Garriott and Latman, 1976; Garriott et al, 1977, Cimbura et al, 1982).

Chronic alcohol use also affects the body's disposition of other drugs. Many drug half-lives are significantly reduced in alcoholics, or by prior alcohol consumption, when compared with controls. The mean half-life of meprobamate was decreased by half after 4 weeks of ethanol consumption, from a mean control value of 16.7 to 8.1 hours (Rubin and Lieber, 1971). Other drugs similarly affected are pentobarbital, phenobarbital, phenytoin, warfarin, and probably many others (Kater et al, 1969; Iber, 1971; Mello and Mendelson, 1970). This effect results from an increase or hypertrophy of liver smooth endoplasmic reticulum, which contains a variety of drug-metabolizing enzymes. Thus a given dose of various drugs may have a reduced effect in drinking individuals as compared with nondrinkers (Lieber et al, 1971).

Alcohol may also interact with numerous drugs of other classes as well. These interactions may occur with agents including antidepressants, salicylates, antidiabetics (oral hypoglycemic agents), insulin, anticonvulsants and even certain food substances, such as mushrooms, among others (Iber, 1971; Wier and Tyler, 1960). These interactions may result in enhanced effects, reduced effects (antagonism), or severe toxic effects (Seixas, 1975).

Tricyclic Antidepressants

The tricyclic antidepressants potentiate sedation with alcohol, causing CNS depression and hypothermic coma in high doses. In addition, inhibition of intestinal movement and fatty changes in the liver may result from this interaction (Griffin and D'Arcy, 1975).

Driving skills are adversely affected if one ingests alcohol during therapy with tricyclic antidepressants. This effect may not persist after the first few days of therapy, and doxepin hydrochloride (Sinequan) plus alcohol may be less likely to impair driving performance than the other tricyclics (Landauer et al, 1969; Milner and Landauer, 1973; Lery et al, 1982). Tricyclic antidepressants are now a leading cause of deaths from drug overdose, and often these deaths involve alcohol as well.

Amphetamines

Amphetamines and other CNS stimulants may antagonize the depressant effect of alcohol to some degree, but do not effectively counteract the impaired motor function induced by alcohol (Martin, 1971).

Analgesics

Analgesics with CNS depressant properties may have this effect increased by alcohol. Thus narcotics such as codeine, morphine, propoxyphene, and other synthetic narcotics significantly act to enhance the depressant effects of alcohol. Salicylates (aspirin), when taken in the presence of alcohol, increase the probability of gastric hemorrhage (Martin, 1971).

Barbiturates

All barbiturates, but especially the rapid-acting ones, enhance the CNS depressant effects of alcohol, and vice versa, in a synergistic manner. Alcohol and barbiturates in combination have resulted in numerous deaths.

With even low doses of both agents, reaction time is lengthened and judgment is impaired.

An interesting paradoxical relationship exists between alcohol and barbiturates. A metabolic cross-tolerance occurs so that a chronic alcohol drinker can metabolize barbiturates faster than a nondrinker, and some barbiturates (eg, phenobarbital) appear to enhance the metabolism of alcohol, resulting in lowered blood levels. Yet, acute intoxication with alcohol inhibits the metabolism of barbiturates, resulting in higher barbiturate blood levels and therefore a greater combined effect. For example, the half-life of pentobarbital was doubled in the presence of alcohol (Hansten, 1976; Rubin and Lieber, 1971; Lery et al, 1982). The lethal combination of alcohol and barbiturate sleeping pills (most commonly secobarbital and amobarbital) has resulted in so many deaths in past years that these drugs are rarely prescribed today. As a result, combined barbiturate and alcohol deaths are rare today in most localities (Garriott et al, 1982).

Benzodiazepines

Although earlier studies using low doses of alcohol with chlordiazepoxide or diazepam demonstrated little or no enhancement of effects (Forney and Hughes, 1968), more recent observations have documented additive or synergistic detrimental effects of diazepam and alcohol (Linnoila and Hakkinen, 1974; Linnoila et al, 1974; Linnoila and Mattila, 1973; Lery et al, 1982). It is probable that moderate, therapeutic doses of benzodiazephines to which one is accustomed do not markedly add to the effect of low or moderate alcohol concentrations (Forney and Hughes, 1968). However, as the dosage of either or both drugs increases, the combined effect is more marked. Circumstantial evidence for this exists from observations of drivers arrested for "driving under the influence." In one study, 22% of drivers with drugs present had diazepam detected in their blood, and about half of these had benzodiazepines and alcohol in combination (Garriott and Latman, 1976).

A mechanism for synergism or enhanced effects with diazepam and alcohol may be the higher blood levels of diazepam when taken with alcohol. Peak blood levels were often twice as high when diazepam was ingested in an ethyl alcohol suspension than when ingested with water (Hayes et al, 1977). This phenomenon of enhanced and more rapid absorption of drugs from the GI tract may be applicable to many other drugs and may account for the increased lethality of other drugs, such as tricyclic antidepressants, when ingested with alcoholic beverages.

Caffeine

Since caffeine-containing beverages are often ingested to "sober up" after drinking, studies have been performed to determine if this drug can antagonize the effects of alcohol. No counteraction of alcohol effects could be demonstrated in animal or human experiments, and a few studies have demonstrated greater impairment when alcohol was combined with caffeine than with alcohol alone (Forney and Hughes, 1968).

A recent study investigating the effects of alcohol and caffeine, separately or in combination, on reaction time in human subjects reported a synergistic interaction of caffeine with alcohol (Osborne and Rogers, 1983). Thus the popular use of coffee to counteract the effects of alcohol may be ineffective for this purpose. The time taken to drink the coffee and the ingestion of nonalcoholic beverages after drinking alcohol may aid somewhat in the "sobering-up" of an intoxicated individual, however.

Disulfiram (Antabuse) and other acetaldehyde antagonists

The classic disulfiram-alcohol reaction results from the inhibition of metabolism of acetaldehyde by inhibiting the actions of acetaldehyde dehydrogenase. Thus acetaldehyde blood levels are increased, resulting in severe toxic effects. Even a few milliliters of ethanol can produce a reaction in a person taking disulfiram. Flushing, throbbing in the head and neck, throbbing headache, nausea, vomiting, sweating, palpitations, syncope, vertigo, blurred vision, and confusion may occur. Decreased blood pressure and respiratory depression can lead to shock and even death if the person is not treated (Ritchie, 1980).

A number of other agents can induce a similar reaction when consumed in the presence of alcohol. These include chloramphenicol, furazolidone, griseofulvin, quinacrine hydrochloride, metronidazole, procarbazine hydrochloride, sulfonylureas (oral antidiabetics), and some edible mushrooms, such as *Coprinus atramentarius* (inky cap) and *Clitocybe clavipes*, among others (Forney and Hughes, 1968; Griffin, 1975; Weir and Tyler, 1960).

Antagonists to Alcohol

Due to the frequent admission of acutely intoxicated alcohol drinkers to hospitals for treatment of injuries suffered as the result of alcohol-induced impairment or of alcoholic coma, an extensive search has long been under way for agents that may antagonize the effects of alcohol or accelerate the metabolism of alcohol. No effective "antidote" has yet been discovered, although caffeine and other respiratory stimulants are frequently used in hospitals. These may be mildly effective in counteracting some of the depressant actions of alcohol.

Fructose long ago was discovered to enhance the metabolism of alcohol. In some animal studies, the rate of disappearance was increased from 120% to 150%. However, doses of fructose must be high to be effective, and practical effectiveness in humans is questionable. In a double-blind study, intoxicated subjects were given IV 100 g of fructose or glucose in 1000 mL of water over a one-hour period. No differences in alcohol metabolism could be discerned between the two groups, and the authors recommended that fructose not be used for this purpose (Iber, 1977, Levy et al, 1977). This phenomenon is discussed further in chapter 3.

A dramatic reduction in lethality in mice was observed when dimethylsulfoxide (DMSO) was administered concomitantly with alcohol. In a limited human experiment, the alcohol was observed to be metabolized slightly faster with DMSO treatment, although psychomotor impairment was greater than with alcohol alone (Mallach and Etzler, 1965).

Naloxone hydrochloride (a commonly used narcotic antagonist) has been reported to arouse patients from alcoholic coma and to prevent the impairment of psychomotor performance induced by low levels of alcohol (MacKenzie, 1979; Jeffcoate et al, 1979; Sorensen and Mattison, 1978).

Tolerance

Drug tolerance may be defined as a diminution of effectiveness after a period of continuous or large-dose administration of the drug. This effect does not include individual variations in sensitivity to an agent, such as species, sex, age, genetic background, or other predetermined factors. Tolerance arises only after exposure to the drug or to a closely related drug. Tolerance occurring after exposure to another drug is known as cross-tolerance.

Tolerance may result from two separate mechanisms: dispositional (or metabolic) and functional. In *metabolic tolerance*, the drug is metabolized or inactivated at an increased rate after chronic administration. Thus a given dose produces lower blood levels after tolerance has developed. With *functional tolerance*, an actual change in the sensitivity of an organ or system to the drug occurs, so that with repeated administration, higher doses and higher blood levels are required to elicit the same effect.

Few studies have been performed to assess the actual ability of ethanol to stimulate its own metabolism. Well-controlled studies are difficult to perform in humans, due to the extreme variations in habits and genetics. However, what work has been done suggests that this form of tolerance to alcohol does occur. For example, in alcoholic volunteers and normal controls, alcohol metabolism rates increased 36% and 72%, respectively, after a period of chronic alcohol consumption (Mendelson et al, 1965). In one case report of an observation of an extremely high alcohol level in a presumed heavy drinker and subsequent metabolism, the subject had cleared alcohol from the blood at an average rate of about 53 mg/dL/h, over three times the rate considered to be average for metabolism in humans. This subject had been treated with IV fluids and diuresis, however, which could have enhanced urinary excretion (Hammond et al, 1973).

In comparisons of blood alcohol biological half-life between controls and still-drinking alcoholics, the drinking alcoholics' half-lives ranged from about 30 to 100 minutes versus nonalcoholic control half-lives of 80 to 250 minutes (Iber, 1971). Researchers comparing rates of blood alcohol elimination in nondrinkers, social drinkers, and alcoholics found marked differences in the three groups. The mean rates were: 12±4 mg/dL/h in nondrinkers; 15±4 mg/dL/h in social drinkers; and 30±9 mg/dL/h in alcoholics (Winek and Murphy, 1984). A group of 15 patients admitted to a treatment facility for alcohol dependency had serial blood alcohols performed on admission. The average initial blood alcohol concentration was 0.24 g/dL. The average rate of decline was 26.6 ± 7.0 mg/dL/h (range 15.9–43.0 mg/dL/h) (Clothier et al., 1985). These rates are considerably greater than the rates of 15 to 18 mg/dL/h, often considered as representing the "average" rate of alcohol metabolism (American Medical Association, 1968; Ritchie, 1980).

It has also been shown that the rate of metabolism varies in the individual according to the blood alcohol concentration. In 14 subjects, ethanol metabolism rates averaged 21.9±7.2 mg/dL/h for patients after acute alcohol intoxication with maximum concentrations of 336± 114 mg/dL. When doses leading to levels of 42±11 mg/dL were ingested at a later time, the rates were 14.6±4.8 mg/dL/h (Bogusz et al, 1977).

Functional or constitutional tolerance has been more easily demonstrated. Goldberg (1943) studied alcohol impairment in heavy drinkers, moderate drinkers, and abstainers. He found that the tolerance for alcohol was nearly twice that for habitual drinkers as compared to nondrinkers. In animal studies, tolerance to the effects of alcohol can be induced within 1 to 2 weeks; tolerance was lost within 2 weeks when exposure ceased (LeBlanc et al, 1975; Goldstein, 1983; Mello and Mendelson, 1970).

REFERENCES

American Medical Association, Committee on Medicolegal Problems. *Alcohol and the Impaired Driver*. American Medical Association, Chicago, 1968, pp. 21–22.

Bjerver, K., and Goldberg, L. Effect of alcohol ingestion on driving ability: Results of practical road tests and laboratory experiments. *Q. J. Stud. Alcohol* 11:1–30, 1950.

Blomberg, L.-H., and Wassen, A. Preliminary report on the effect of alcohol on dark adaptation determined by an objective method. *Acta Ophthalmol.* 37:2, 1959.

Blum, B., Stern, M.H., and Melville, K.I. A comparative evaluation of the actions of depressant and stimulant drugs on human performance. *Psychopharmacologia* 6:173–177, 1964.

Bogusz, M., Poch, J., and Stasko, W. Comparative studies on the rate of ethanol elimination in acute poisoning and in controlled conditions. *J. Forensic Sci.* 22:446–451, 1977.

Boyd, E.S., Morken, D.A., and Hodge, H.C. A psychomotor test to demonstrate a depressant action of alcohol. *Q. J. Stud. Alcohol* 23:34–39, 1962.

Brecher, G.A., Hartman, A.P., and Leonard, D.D. Effect of Alcohol on binocular vision. *Am. J. Ophthalmol.* 39:44–52, 1955.

Buffard, S. Study of the psychomotor reactions of 22 subjects after ingestion of a moderate quantity of alcohol. *Ann. Med. Leg.* 39:124–128, 1959.

Carlson, A.J., Kleitman, N., Muehlberger, C.W., et al. *Studies on the Possible Intoxicating Action of* 3.2 *Percent Beer.* University of Chicago Press, Chicago, 1934.

Cimbura, G., Lucas, D.M., Bennett, R.C., et al. Incidence and toxicological aspects of drugs detected in 484 fatally injured drivers and pedestrians in Ontario. *J. Forensic Sci.* 27:855–867, 1982.

Clothier, J., Kelly, J.T., Reed, K., et al. Varying rates of alcohol metabolism in relation to detoxification medication. *Alcohol* 2:443–445, 1985.

Cohen, G., and Collins, M. Alkaloids from catecholamines in adrenal tissue: possible role in alcoholism. *Science* 167:1749–1751, 1970.

Collins, M.A., Num, W.P., Borge, G.F., et al. Dopamine-related tetrahydroisoquinolines: significant urinary excretion by alcoholics after alcohol consumption. *Science* 208:1184–1186, 1979.

Davis, V.E., and Walsh, M.J. Alcohol, amines, and alkaloids: A possible biochemical basis for alcohol addiction. *Science* 167:1005–7, 1970.

Dubowski, K.M. *Stages of Acute Alcoholic Influence/Intoxication*, The University of Oklahoma College of Medicine, Oklahoma City.

Ferrans, V.J. Alcoholic cardiomyopathy. *Am. J. Med. Sci.* 252:89–104, 1966.

Forney, R.B., and Harger, R.N. Toxicology of ethanol. *Annu. Rev. Pharmacol.* 9:379–392, 1969.

Forney, R.B., and Hughes, F.W. *Combined Effects of Alcohol and Other Drugs.* Charles C Thomas, Springfield, Ill. 1968.

Garriott, J.C., and Latman, N. Drug detection in cases of "driving under the influence." *J. Forensic Sci.* 21:398–415, 1976.

Garriott, J.C., Di Maio, V.J.M., and Petty, C.S. Death by poisoning: a ten-year survey of Dallas County. *J. Forensic Sci.* 27:868–879, 1982.

Garriott, J.C., Di Maio, V.J.M., Zumwalt, R.E., et al. Incidence of drugs and alcohol in fatally injured motor vehicle drivers. *J. Forensic Sci.* 22:383–389, 1977.

Goldberg, L. Quantitative studies on alcohol tolerance in man. *Acta Physiol. Scand.* 5 (suppl. 16):1–128, 1943.

Goldstein, D.B. *Pharmacology of Alcohol.* Oxford University Press, New York, 1983, p. 80.

Griffin, J.P., and D'Arcy, P.F. *A Manual of Adverse Drug Interactions.* John Wright & Sons, Bristol, England, 1975, p. 57.

Gruner, O. Alkohol und Aufmerksamkeit. Ihre Bedeutung im motorisierten Verkehr. *Dtsch. Z. Ges. Gerichtl. Med.* 44:187–195, 1955.

Gruner, O., and Ptasnik, H. Zur Frage der Beeinflussung alkoholbedingten Leistungsabfalles durch Laevulosegaben. *MMW* 95:931–933, 1953.

Hammond, K.B., Rumack, B.H., and Rodgerson, D.O. Blood ethanol: A report of unusually high levels in a living patient. *JAMA* 226:63–64, 1973.

Hansten, P.D. *Drug Interactions*, 3d ed. Lea & Febiger, Philadelphia, 1976, pp. 156–161.

Hayes, S.L., Pablo, G., Radomsky, T., et al. Ethanol and oral diazepam absorption. *N. Engl. J. Med.* 296:186–189, 1977.

Honneger, H., Kampschulte, R., and Klein, H. Störung der Sehschärfe für bewegte Objekte durch Alkohol. *Blutalkohol* 7:31–44, 1970.

Huber, O. Untersuchungen über die Veränderung der Fahrtüchtigkeit von Kraftradfahrern nach mässigem Alkoholgenuss. *Dutsch. Z. Ges. Gerichtl. Med.* 44:559–577, 1955.

Iber, F.L. Increased drug metabolism in alcoholics. In *Advances in Mental Science*, vol. 3 *Biological Aspects of Alcohol*. (M.K. Roach. W.M. McIsaac, and P.J. Creaven, eds.) University of Texas Press, Austin, 1971, pp. 94–110.

Iber, F.L. The effect of fructose on alcohol metabolism. *Arch. Intern. Med.* 137:1121,1977.

Idestrom, C.-M., and Cadenius, B. Time relations of the effects of alcohol compared to placebo. *Psychopharmacologia* 13:189–200, 1968.

Izard, A., and Saby, G. Contribution a l'étude du comportement psychomoteur de l'homme après absorption de doses moyennes d'alcool. *Arch. Mal. Prof.* 23, 854–858, 1962.

Jeffcoate, W.J., Herbert, M., Cullen, M.H., et al. Prevention of effects of alcohol intoxication by naloxone. *Lancet*, 2:1157–1159, 1979.

Jellinek, E.M., and McFarland, R.A. Analysis of psychological experiments on the effects of alcohol. *Q. J. Stud. Alcohol* 1:272–371, 1940.

Kater, R.M., Carulli, N., and Iber, F.L. Differences in the rate of ethanol metabolism in recently drinking alcoholic and non-drinking subjects. *Am. J. Clin. Nutr.* 22:1608–1617, 1969.

Landauer, A.A., Milner, G., and Patman, J. Alcohol and amitriptyline effects on skills related to driving behavior. *Science* 163:1467–1468, 1969.

LeBlanc, A.E., Kalant, H., and Gibbins, R.J. Acute tolerance to ethanol in the rat. *Psychopharmacologia* 41:43–46, 1975.

Lery, N., Rouzioux, M.N., Roussot, J.F., et al. Interactions between alcohol and drugs. *Vet. Hum. Toxicol.* 24:427–443, 1982.

Levy, R., Elo, T., and Hanenson, I.B. Intravenous fructose treatment of acute alcohol intoxication. *Arch. Intern. Med.* 137:1175–1177, 1977.

Lewis, E.G., Dustman, R.E., and Beck, E.C. The effect of alcohol on sensory phenomena and cognitive and motor tasks. *Q. J. Stud. Alcohol* 30:618–633, 1969.

Lieber, C.S., Rubin, E., and deCarli, L.M. Interactions of ethanol, drug, and lipid metabolism: Adaptive changes after ethanol consumption. In *Advances in Mental Science*, vol. 3. *Biological Aspects of Alcohol*, (M.K. Roach, W.M. McIsaac, and P.J. Creavan, eds.) University of Texas Press, Austin, 1971, pp. 138–167.

Linnoila, M., and Hakkinen, S. Effects of diazepam and codeine, alone and in combination with alcohol, on simulated driving. *Clin. Pharmacol. Ther.* 15:368, 1974.

Linnoila, M., and Mattila, M.J. Drug interaction on psychomotor skills related to driving: diazepam and alcohol. *Eur. J. Clin. Pharmacol.* 5:186–194, 1973.

Linnoila, M., Saario, I., and Maki, M. Effect of treatment with diazepam or lithium and alcohol on psychomotor skills related to driving. *Eur. J. Clin. Pharmacol.* 7:337–342, 1974.

MacKenzie, A.I. Naloxone in alcohol intoxication. *Lancet* 2:733–734, 1979.

Mallach, H.J., and Etzler, K. Tierexperimentelle Untersuchungen über die gemeinsame Wirkung von Dimethylsufoxid und Aethylalkohol. *Arzneimittelforsch.* 15:1305–1308, 1965.

Marquis, D.G., Kelly, E.L., Miller, J.G., et al. Experimental studies of behavioral effects of meprobamate in normal subjects. *Ann. N.Y. Acad. Sci.* 67:701–711, 1957.

Marshall, J.P., Parker, T.H., Roberts, R.K., et al. Biochemistry of hepatic coma in alcohol-induced liver diseases and other types of hepatic dysfuntion. In *Biochemistry and Pharmacology of Ethanol.* (E. Majchrowicz and E.P. Noble, eds.) Plenum Press, New York, 1979, vol. 1, pp. 479–499.

Martin, E.W. Table of Drug Interactions. In *Hazards of Medication.* (S.F. Alexander, W.E. Hassan, and D.J. Farage, eds). J.B. Lippincott, Philadelphia, p. 415, pp. 430–437, 1971.

Mehar, G.S., Parker, J.M., and Tubas, T. Interaction between alcohol, minor tranquilizers and morphine. *Int. J. Clin. Pharmacol.* 9:70–74, 1974.

Mellanby, E. *Alcohol: Its Absorption into and Disappearance from the Blood Under Different Conditions.* Medical Research Committee, Special Report Series, No. 31, 1919.

Mello, N.K., and Mendelson, J.H. Experimentally induced intoxication in alcoholics. A comparison between programmed and spontaneous drinking. *J. Pharmacol. Exp. Ther.*, 173:101–116, 1970.

Mendelson, J.H., Stein, S., and Mello, N.K. Effects of experimentally induced intoxication on metabolism of ethanol-1-C^{14} in alcoholic subjects. *Metab. Clin. Exp.* 14:1255–1266, 1965.

Mezey, E. Ethanol and hepatic fibrogenesis. In *Biochemistry and Pharmacology of Ethanol.* (E. Majchrowicz and E.P. Noble, eds.), Plenum Press, New York, 1979, vol. 1, pp. 459–479.

Miles, W.R. *Alcohol and Human Efficiency.* Carnegie Institute publication No. 333, Pittsburgh, 1924.

Milner, G., and Landauer, A.A. The effects of doxepin, alone and together with alcohol, in relation to driving safety. *Med. J. Aust.* 1:837, 1973.

Mortimer, R.G. Effect of low blood alcohol concentrations in simulated day and night driving. *Percept. Mot. Skills* 17:399–408, 1963.

Moskowitz, H. Alcohol influences upon sensory motor function, visual perception, and attention. In *Alcohol, Drugs, and Driving.* National Highway Traffic Safety Administration, U.S. Dept. of Transportation publication No. (HSM) 80–1096, Mar. 1974, pp. 49–69.

Moureau, P. Tendances de la legislation belge en ce qui concerne l'intoxication alcoolique et les accidents de roulage. *Rev. Alcoolisme* 4:178–180, 1957.

Newman, H.W., and Fletcher, E. The effect of alcohol on vision. *Am. J. Med. Sci.* 202:723–731, 1941.

Newman, H.W. Emetic action of ethyl alcohol. *Arch. Intern. Med.* 94:417–419, 1954.

Osborne, D.J., and Rogers, Y. Interactions of alcohol and caffeine on human reaction time. *Aviat. Space Environ. Med.* 54:528–534, 1983.

Pihkanen, T.A. and Kauko, O., The effects of alcohol on the perception of musical stimuli. *Ann. Med. Exp. Fenn.* 40:275–285, 1962.

Regan, T.J. Ethyl alcohol and the heart. *Circulation* 44:957–963, 1971.

Ritchie, J.M. The aliphatic alcohols. In *The Pharmacological Basis of Therapeutics*, 6th ed. (A.G. Gilman, L.S. Goodman, and A. Gilman, eds.) MacMillan New York, 1980, p. 72, pp. 376–390.

Rubin, E., and Lieber, C.S. Alcoholism, alcohol, and drugs. *Science* 172:1097–1102, 1971.

Schmidt, I., and Bingel, A.G.A. *Effect of Oxygen Deficiency and Various Other*

Factors on Color Saturation Thresholds. U.S.A.F. School of Aviation Medicine Project Reports: Project No. 21–31–002, 1953.

Seixas, F.A. Alcohol and its drug interactions. *Ann. Intern. Med.* 83:86–92, 1975.

Sorensen, S.C., and Mattison, K.W. Naloxone as an antagonist in severe alcohol intoxication. *Lancet* 2:688–689, 1978.

Starck, H.J. Untersuchungen über die Verkehrssicherheit alkoholgewohnter Kraftfahrer bei Blutalkoholwerten um 1.5 g-°/00. *Dtsch. Z. Ges. Gerichtl. Med.* 42:155–161, 1953.

Suzuki, K., Umetsu, J., Kobayashi, M., et al. Effects of injection of analgetics and alcohol drinking on values of electric flicker. *Tohoku J. Exp. Med.* 66: 327–331, 1957.

Wallgren, H., and Barry, H. III. *Actions of Alcohol, Vol. I. Biochemical Physiological, and Psychological Effects*. Elsevier, New York, 1970, pp. 287–292.

Wier, J.K., and Tyler, V.E. An investigation of *Coprinus atramentarius* for the presence of disulfiram. *J. Am. Pharmacol. Assoc.* 49:426–429, 1960.

Winek, C.L., and Murphy, K.L. The rate and kinetic order of ethanol elimination. *Forensic Sci. Int.* 25:159–166, 1984.

3

Disposition of Alcohol in Man

Randall C. Baselt
Ivan E. Danhof

The passage of ethyl alcohol through the human body may be described by a series of steps that includes absorption from the gastrointestinal (GI) tract, distribution to the various tissues, metabolism by hepatic enzyme systems, and excretion of unchanged alcohol and its metabolites from the body. A thorough understanding of each of these steps is necessary to the forensic scientist, who is often required to relate an alcohol concentration in a biological specimen to the dose of alcohol consumed, to the period of time over which it was consumed, and to alcohol concentrations in other specimens or in the same specimen at a different time. This chapter reviews current knowledge regarding the disposition of orally ingested alcohol in man.

ABSORPTION

General Features

Alcohol is absorbed from all the mucosal surfaces of the GI tract at a rate that is best described by simple diffusion. Fick's law states that this rate is proportional to the concentration gradient of alcohol across the membrane and to a diffusion coefficient that is a constant for ethyl alcohol and the specific membrane being studied. The extent of absorption of alcohol by a discrete area of the GI tract, then, will depend on the concentration of alcohol presented to the membranes, the length of time the alcohol remains in contact with the membranes, the blood flow to the region, and the surface area available for absorption. Although alcohol comes into contact with the mucosa of the mouth and esophagus, the period of contact is relatively brief and the blood supply to these regions is relatively poor. In the stomach, a single dose of alcohol may be present for up to several hours, the regional blood flow is high, and there is substantial surface area available. By comparison, however, the small intestine, 2.8 m in length and 300 m^2 in surface area, is the most efficient region of the GI tract for alcohol absorption. The colon is also capable of absorbing alcohol, but due to the efficiency of the small intestine it is unlikely that a significant portion of a dose is ever presented to this region in a normal, healthy individual.

Estimates of the percentage of a dose of alcohol absorbed by each region are difficult to make due to the variability in gastric and intestinal motility, gastric emptying time, and regional blood flow in different individuals and in different situations. Studies involving isolated anatomical regions of the GI tract in experimental animals often yield exaggerated results due to the artificial nature of the situation. Various authorities seem to agree, however, that fasting individuals absorb 20% to 25% of a dose from the stomach and 75% to 80% from the small intestine proximal to the pyloric sphincter. Negligible amounts are absorbed from the mouth and colon (Schwar, 1979).

The process of absorption is never complete in the sense that 100% of the administered dose is removed from the GI tract. Rather, absorption is complete when the concentration gradient of alcohol across the intestinal mucosa approaches unity. As long as alcohol is present in the body, the intestinal contents will contain alcohol in proportion to the water contained therein, and a small fraction of the dose may be eliminated from the body in the feces. It should be noted that about 1 to 2 g of alcohol is formed endogenously in man daily, probably by microbial fermentation in the intestine, leading to a normal blood alcohol concentration of about 0.0002 g/dL. This very low level is below the detectability limit of most forensic analytical procedures, however (Lester, 1962; Blomstrand, 1971).

Factors Affecting Absorption

FOOD The fact that food taken along with alcohol results in a lower, delayed blood alcohol concentration was first reported by Mellanby in 1920. In 1931, Widmark (1981) reasoned that this effect was due to a slowing of the absorption rate as well as to another factor that he believed may have involved esterification of alcohol with fatty acids during the digestive process. More recently, the reduction in area under the blood alcohol concentration–time curve that occurs with food intake has been shown to be the result of two factors, contributing in nearly equal amounts: (1) the reduction in efficiency of absorption of alcohol due to prolonged gastric emptying time, and (2) the Michaelis-Menten kinetic behavior of alcohol elimination, such that lower amounts of alcohol in the body are metabolized at a proportionately higher rate (Lin et al, 1976; Wilkinson et al, 1977).

Figure 3-1 illustrates the relative shapes of blood alcohol curves when alcohol is consumed on an empty or full stomach. In this experiment, the peak blood alcohol concentration in trial A (empty stomach) occurred at 1.3 hours after the end of the consumption period, while the peak in trial B (full stomach) occurred at 2.0 hours. The blood concentrations achieved in trial A are very similar to the theoretical values (dashed line) calculated using the Widmark formula, while those in trial B are approximately 20% lower than theoretical.

Although the peak blood alcohol concentration is not exactly coincidental with the completion of absorption, Schwar (1979) suggested that it is useful as a practical estimation of the time at which most of an

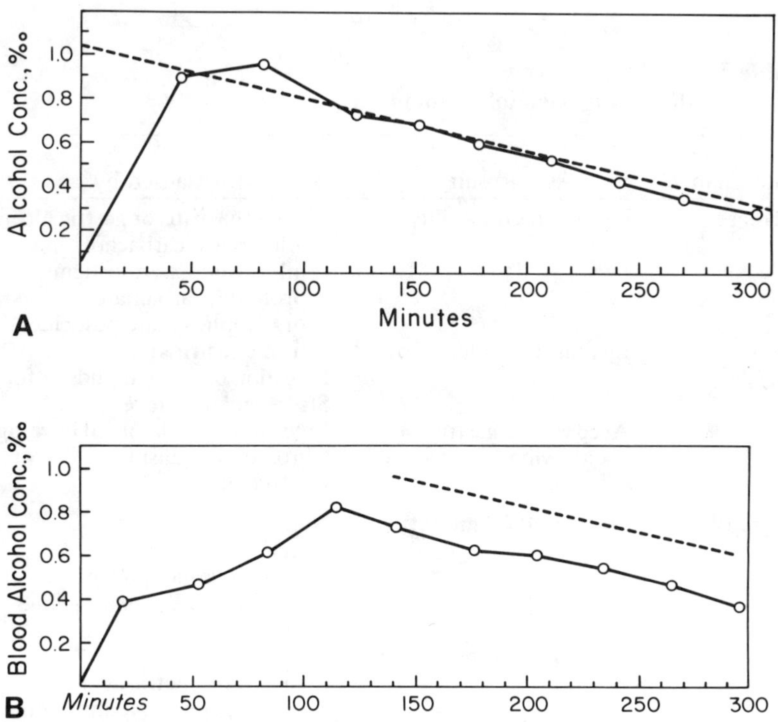

Figure 3-1 **A** A 78-kg female consumed 56 g alcohol on an empty stomach. The actual blood alcohol concentration is shown by the solid line, while the theoretical concentration is shown by the dashed line. **B** A 77-kg male consumed 63 g alcohol after a full meal. (Reproduced with permission from Widmark, 1981.)

alcohol dose has been absorbed. Various authors, employing several hundred experimental subjects, have shown that fasting subjects exhibit peak blood alcohol concentrations within 0.5 to 2.0 hours (average 0.75–1.35 hours, depending on dose and time of last meal), while non-fasting subjects exhibit peak levels within 1.0 to 6.0 hours (average 1.06–2.12 hours). Such studies have shown that the type of food (carbohydrate, fat, protein) has relatively little influence, but the extent of effect is directly proportional to the size of the meal and inversely proportional to the elapsed time between food and alcohol consumption. The reduction of peak blood alcohol concentration by food in these studies ranged on average from 9% to 23% (Abele and Kropp, 1958; Herbich and Prokop, 1963; Krauland et al, 1967).

Pathophysiologic status Changes in the motility, blood supply, or morphology of the GI tract, whether induced by internal or external factors, may result in a significant change in the rate of absorption of ethanol. Table 3-1 lists a number of the important factors that ought to

Table 3-1
Factors Influencing Alcohol Absorption

Absorption Rate Change	As a Result of	Caused by
Increase	Increased GI motility	Chronic gastritis or gastric ulcers Cholinergics (carbachol, pilocarpine, pyridostigmine bromide, carbamate, organophosphate pesticides)
	Increased GI blood flow	Chronic gastritis Ingestion of warm liquids or food Stress, anxiety, fever
	Accelerated gastric emptying	Ingestion of carbonated beverages Chronic alcoholism Gastrectomy
Decrease	Decreased GI motility	Nausea Shock Anticholinergics (atropine, dicyclomine, propantheline bromide)
	Decreased GI blood flow	Fear, pain Sympathomimetric agents (amphetamine, fenfluramine Stimulants (caffeine, nicotine) Exercise
	Delayed gastric emptying	Emotional disturbances Gastric fibrosis or carcinomatosis

Derived from Schwar (1979).

be considered in a medicolegal situation. The effect of alcohol itself is discussed below.

Continuous monitoring of the venous blood alcohol concentration has shown that the blood alcohol curve is not smooth and continuous but is wavy and sometimes jagged, with several peaks of approximately equal magnitude possible over a one- to two-hour period (Leithoff, 1964). This phenomenon, referred to as "spiking," is probably due to the erratic emptying of the stomach contents and the resultant rapid absorption of the released alcohol by the small intestine. Spiking is especially important in regard to the large differences in arterial-venous blood alcohol concentrations that may arise (see below).

Concentration and dose of alcohol Most authors agree that alcohol is most rapidly absorbed when the concentration of the ingested solution is between 10% and 30%. More dilute solutions result in a lower concentration gradient across the absorbing membrane and, because of the larger volume involved, may also delay gastric emptying. More concentrated solutions are irritating to the gastric mucosa and to the pyloric sphincter, causing increased secretion of mucus and delayed gastric emptying (Kalant, 1971; Schwar, 1979).

A tripling of the dose, from 0.4 to 1.2 g/kg of alcohol, produced a 79% increase in the time required to achieve the peak blood alcohol concentration in fasting subjects and a 61% increase in nonfasting subjects (Krauland et al, 1967). In most social drinking situations, however, the total dose of alcohol would be administered over a much longer period of time than under experimental conditions and it is less likely that the size of the dose would be a significant factor.

Some investigators have noted differences in the rate of absorption of alcohol when different beverages are compared, that is, wine, vodka, Scotch, etc, even when the alcohol concentration and dose are normalized. These differences tend to be demonstrated only in the first 30 minutes after consumption, however, and other investigators have not confirmed such differences (Schwar, 1979).

DISTRIBUTION

General Features

Alcohol is very hydrophilic and is therefore present in any body tissue or fluid as a function of the water content of that tissue or fluid. The blood concentration that is produced at time zero (Cp) after instantaneous equilibration of a dose of alcohol (D) within an individual of body weight W may be estimated using the standard pharmacokinetic equation:

$$Cp(g/L) = \frac{D(g)}{Vd(L/kg) \times W(kg)}$$

where Vd is the volume of distribution for that individual. Since alcohol distributes through body water, then Vd for alcohol in an individual is also an expression of total body water. Widmark (1981) expressed this relationship using the formula:

$$c = \frac{A}{rp}$$

where c is the blood concentration, A is the alcohol dose, r is the volume of distribution, and p the body weight. Since Widmark expressed blood alcohol concentrations in units of mass/mass, his r value also had units of mass/mass rather than volume/mass as does Vd. Direct comparisons of Widmark's values with modern data therefore involve an error of about 6%, due to the specific gravity of blood, which averages 1.06 (Schwar, 1979).

Summarizing the results of numerous authors, Schwar (1979) concluded that the Vd of alcohol for adult males has been found to average 0.62 to 0.79 (range 0.59–0.90) and for adult females, 0.55 to 0.66 (range 0.46–0.86). Schwar himself used average values of 0.70 and 0.60 for males and females, respectively, in calculations of amount of alcohol consumed from known blood alcohol concentrations (for comparison, Widmark's average values, obtained some 40 years earlier, were 0.68 and 0.55, respectively). For individuals of the same sex and similar body weight, differences in Vd (which may be considerable) are largely due to differences in adiposity. This is so because alcohol is to a great degree excluded from adipose tissue, the fat-water partition coefficient being 0.018 (Kalant, 1971). Age is another important factor, since total body water, and therefore the Vd of alcohol, decreases with increasing age; total body water decreases from an average of 61% of body weight in males aged 18 to 40 years to 52% in those over 60 years, and from 51% in females aged 18 to 40 years to 46% in those over 60 years (Schwar, 1979).

Blood

Distribution within the vascular system As long as alcohol is still being absorbed from the site of administration, blood alcohol concentrations at different points in the vascular system may differ considerably. Once administration has ceased and absorption is complete, an equilibrium occurs such that blood at all points in the system contains approximately the same concentration of alcohol. The greatest differences occur between arterial and venous blood. This phenomenon can give rise to a large disparity in living subjects between breath alcohol, representing arterial blood alcohol, and blood alcohol measured in a specimen from the customary site, the cubital vein. In postmortem toxicology, the traditional site of sampling, the heart, provides a specimen of either arterial or pooled central venous blood, a large proportion of which is portal vein blood, rich in alcohol in subjects for whom absorption is not yet complete.

Forney et al (1964) studied two living subjects who consumed 1.0 g/kg of alcohol in 30 minutes. One subject, who achieved his peak venous blood alcohol concentration at 15 minutes after consumption, showed a 26% elevation of arterial blood alcohol over venous blood alcohol immediately after consumption, declining to 8% by 15 minutes. The other subject, who did not reach his peak venous blood alcohol concentration until 75 minutes after consumption, demonstrated a 66% elevation of arterial over venous blood alcohol both immediately and 15 minutes after consumption, a 41% elevation by 30 minutes, and a 23% elevation by 45 minutes.

In some countries, finger-tip capillary blood has been used to establish blood alcohol concentrations in automobile drivers. Capillary blood is generally considered to be more representative of arterial than venous blood in terms of alcohol concentration during alcohol absorption. Sedman et al (1976) showed capillary-venous blood differences of as much as +36% at ten minutes after the administration of 30 mL of absolute alcohol in one subject and +40% at 20 minutes in another.

Positive postmortem blood alcohol differences, attributed to recent drinking, of from 1% to 48% were reported between heart blood and femoral vein blood in 69% of over 50 cases studied by Turkel and Gifford (1957). Such differences could be minimized by drawing the heart blood specimen using a syringe rather than allowing blood to flow into the collection container from an incision, according to Plueckhahn (1967), who felt that pericardial sac fluid contributed to the discrepancies noted by Turkel and Gifford. Still, arterial-venous differences of up to 14% were admitted by this author even using his refined collection technique, and such differences should be recognized when interpreting a postmortem heart blood alcohol concentration based on a legal standard of 0.10% that pertains to venous blood.

Distribution within blood The usual forensic specimen for determination of alcohol content is whole blood, whereas it is more likely in clinical practice that a serum or plasma specimen will be obtained by allowing blood to clot upon exposure to air or by centrifuging anticoagulated blood, respectively.

Payne et al (1968), working with heparinized samples from 20 subjects, found that plasma–whole blood alcohol concentration ratios ranged from 1.10 to 1.35 and averaged 1.18. Other authors have reported similar values for the serum–whole blood ratio (Schwar, 1979). These differences can be accounted for by the relative water content of these three fluids. Normal variations, within an individual and from one individual to the next, in the percentage of whole blood volume occupied by the red cells (Hct) make it difficult to apply a uniform correction factor when attempting to convert a serum or plasma alcohol concentration to a whole blood concentration.

Brain

Since brain tissue is lower (76%) in water content than blood (81%), it is to be expected that at equilibrium brain will contain slightly less alcohol than whole blood. The data of Backer et al (1980) are in general agreement with earlier data from other authors in that human brain–blood alcohol concentration ratios averaged 0.86, with a range of 0.64 to 1.20 for 33 cases. The equilibrium of brain tissue alcohol content with that of blood is felt to be relatively rapidly achieved and it has been shown that alcohol has an extraction ratio of at least 0.90 during a single passage through cerebral capillaries. Uniform distribution of alcohol within the gray matter occurs within five minutes of an intravenous (IV) dose in cats, but requires 76 minutes to become uniform in the less highly vascularized white matter (Kalant, 1971). While cerebrospinal fluid is, at equilibrium, higher in alcohol content than blood, averaging 14% higher (Backer et al, 1980), it achieves equilibrium relatively slowly and therefore tends to lag behind blood during alcohol absorption (Schwar, 1979).

Breath

We have discussed two of the factors that give rise to variations in the blood-breath alcohol ratio, namely the arterial-venous difference that is observed during alcohol absorption and the unpredictability of hematocrit in a given individual. Widmark, in 1931, was one of the first to recognize that, during the absorptive period, "the values from air analysis and blood analysis often do not agree." The type of discrepancy that is often observed between blood and breath following alcohol consumption is shown in Figure 3-2. Other factors affecting the blood-breath partition ratio, including body temperature, pulmonary disease, contamination from mouth or GI tract alcohol, and breathing techniques, have been recently discussed by Hlastala (1985) and Cohen (1986). While the figure of 2100 is utilized as a "standard" partition ratio in

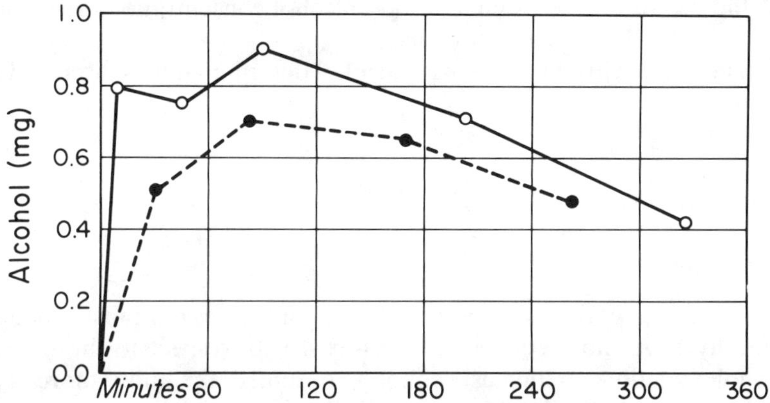

Figure 3-2 Blood (dashed line, mg/cm^3) and breath (solid line, mg/2L) alcohol concentrations after oral administration of alcohol to a subject (Reproduced with permission from Widmark, 1981.)

most evidentiary breath alcohol devices, the blood-breath ratio for individual subjects has been shown to vary from about 900 to about 3400 (Alobaidi et al., 1976; Mason and Dubowski, 1976; Yamamoto and Ueda, 1972). Although Dubowski and O'Neill (1979) pointed out that the actual average partition ratio in subjects known to be postabsorptive may be closer to 2280, he also indicated (Mason and Dubowski, 1974) that "when a blood test is allowable, an administered breath test is discriminatory, because in law-enforcement practice the status of absorption is always uncertain."

Further discussion of breath alcohol considerations is presented in chapters 6 and 7.

Other Tissues or Fluids

Saliva has been shown to equilibrate rapidly with blood in terms of its alcohol content, being slightly higher on average than whole blood. Saliva–whole blood ethanol concentration ratios were found to average 1.08 for 48 male subjects within the first six hours after drinking, with an overall range of 0.84 to 1.36 (Jones, 1979). Recently, a colorimetric test strip has been devised for semiquantitative estimation of saliva alcohol and it has received limited use as a screening device for drinking drivers.

Bile has been used as a body fluid for alcohol determination in order to substantiate a blood alcohol result or in the absence of an adequate blood specimen. In a study of 78 paired postmortem specimens, Stone and Rooney (1984) found blood-bile alcohol ratios to average 0.92, with a standard deviation of 0.22. The authors concluded that the use of bile to estimate blood alcohol concentrations was most reliable at levels in excess of 0.10%.

The use of vitreous humor for alcohol determination is discussed in chapters 4 and 5.

METABOLISM

Mechanism

The major portion of ingested alcohol undergoes biotransformation in the liver. As no feedback controls exist with respect to the rate of ethanol oxidation, so long as alcohol is consumed, the body is forced to handle it metabolically (Morgan, 1979). Biotransformation occurs in three steps:

1. Alcohol → acetaldehyde
2. Acetaldehyde → acetic acid
3. Acetic acid → CO_2 and H_2O

The transformation to acetaldehyde can be accomplished by three systems: (1) alcohol dehydrogenase; (2) catalase; and (3) microsomal ethanol-oxidizing system (MEOS). Of these mechanisms, alcohol dehydrogenase (and its several isozymes) is by far the most important (Goldstein, 1983). The rate-limiting factor in this reaction is the regeneration of nicotine adenine dinucleotide (NAD), as follows:

$$CH_3CH_2OH + NAD^+ \rightarrow CH_3CHO + NADH + H^+$$

An ethanol load imposed on the liver causes practically all metabolic dynamics to be directed toward the metabolic handling of alcohol, causing a marked diminution and "shortchanging" of other hepatic metabolic functions to the extent that fatty acids coming to the liver are stored, but remain unmetabolized, and produce fatty infiltration (Goldstein, 1983; Tottmar et al, 1973).

Catalase abounds in the liver as a protection against hydrogen peroxide (H_2O_2) formed by various oxidases. Catalase, acting as a peroxidase, uses H_2O_2 to oxidize other substances. Ethanol has been shown to serve as a substrate for this reaction (Goldstein, 1983; Keilin and Hartree, 1945).

Microsomal fractions of liver can oxidize ethanol in the presence of molecular oxygen and reduced nicotinamide adenine dinucleotide phosphate (NADPH), a mixed-function oxygenase system, which metabolically handles a variety of exogenous compounds (Goldstein, 1983).

There are differences in the way alcoholics and social drinkers metabolize alcohol. In the latter group, the metabolic conversion of ethanol to acetaldehyde is accomplished at a tremendously rapid rate, whereas the oxidative transformation of acetaldehyde to acetic acid is not conducted at a comparable rate (Watterlond, 1983). Acetic acid may be converted to CO_2 and H_2O in skeletal muscle (Watterlond, 1983), or alternatively, may be handled in the citric acid cycle and converted to fatty acids, which accelerate the accumulation of fats in the liver where ethanol-metabolizing pathways predominate to the exclusion of other metabolic functions (Morgan, 1979). Thus fatty metamorphosis seen early in ethanol ingestion excess is a combination of:

1. Predominance of metabolic pathways devoted to the handling of alcohol
2. Marked limitation in hepatic handling of fatty acids normally in dynamic translocation from adipose tissues
3. Acceleration of fatty acid formation by biotransformation of ethanol-derived acetic acid through the citric acid cycle to fatty acids

An additional factor, but of limited quantitative significance, is the alcohol metabolized by the gastric and small intestinal mucosae. Alcohol dehydrogenase has been demonstrated to be present in the mucosa of the stomach, jejunum, and ileum, but only in small concentrations. The amount of alcohol metabolized in the digestive tract lining is also limited because the affinity for alcohol is lower for the intestinal than hepatic dehydrogenases. It is possible that some triglyceride synthesis may be linked to mucosal metabolism of alcohol (Mezey, 1983).

Behavioral signs of acute intoxication correlate with blood levels of alcohol, not with the levels of acetaldehyde, even though small amounts of acetaldehyde escape to the circulation because the aldehyde dehydrogenases in the liver are incapable of keeping abreast of acetaldehyde production (Tottmar et al, 1973). Acetaldehyde does not enter the brain tissue because of the efficient aldehyde-metabolizing enzymes in the cerebral endothelium. Further, the administration of pyrazole, which limits the production of acetaldehyde by inhibiting alcohol dehydrogenase, does not prevent signs of intoxication (Goldstein, 1983).

Kinetics

The vast majority (95%) of ingested alcohol is metabolized in the liver. This metabolic removal begins as soon as the alcohol contained in the blood reaches the liver. The rate of accessibility of alcohol to the circulatory system is of major importance. If a drink is sipped with sufficient slowness, the liver may be able to metabolize the alcohol at a rate at which the alcohol enters the circulation. Under these circumstances, the blood alcohol concentration (BAC) would theoretically remain near zero and show no typical incremental-decremental curve. Further, spacing of alcoholic beverages allows for hepatic elimination rather than corporal accumulation of the alcohol.

The decline in blood alcohol concentrations resulting from metabolism and excretion is generally considered to represent a zero-order (linear) process, at least at midrange concentrations. Dubowski (1976) has shown this rate of decline to average 0.015 g/dL/h (range 0.011–0.022) for 25 males and 0.018 g/dL/h (range 0.011–0.022) for 15 females. More recently, Shajani and Dinn (1985) reported an average of 0.018 g/dL/h (range 0.013–0.023) for eight males and 0.020 g/dL/h (range 0.017–0.026) for eight females. Thus normal healthy adult females appear to eliminate alcohol at a slightly higher rate than normal healthy adult males.

At very low blood alcohol concentrations (0.02 g/dL or less), Wagner et al (1976) showed that first-order kinetics (nonlinear) predominate and that the aforementioned rates of decline can no longer be applied. Other authors (Hammond et al, 1973; Bogusz et al, 1977) have published evidence that first-order kinetics also apply at very high blood alcohol concentrations (over 0.30 g/dL), and that a more rapid rate of decline than normally expected would be observed, at least until blood concentrations fall into the range where zero-order kinetics would again be observed.

Factors Influencing Rate

A number of investigators have reported higher alcohol elimination rates in chronic consumers of alcohol, apparently due to induction of the liver enzymes that metabolize this chemical. Clothier et al (1985), for example, reported an average rate of decline of 0.027 g/dL/h (range 0.016–0.043) for 15 alcoholic subjects (sex not indicated), while Misra et al (1971) reported an increase of up to 72% in the rate of alcohol disappearance from the blood of naive subjects following alcohol pretreatment. Other authors, however, have not been able to reproduce these results (Holtzman et al, 1985) or have found that the effect is not consistent in all subjects (Vesell et al, 1971). More discussion on this topic is presented in chapter 2.

Various reports have been published that Eskimos, American Indians, and Orientals exhibit significantly different rates of alcohol elimination than whites, presumably due to a genetic difference in metabolic capacity (Fenna et al, 1971; Reed et al, 1976), but other authors indicate that such differences are either insignificant or can be explained on the basis of morphometric variations (Bennion and Li, 1976; Wilson and Erwin, 1983).

Increasing age affects total body water in man, but is considered to be a negligible factor in women. With increasing age, hepatic metabolic capacity decreases somewhat and, together with decremental changes in total body water, may result in a lowered tolerance to alcohol in the aged.

Disease states may alter the ability to metabolize alcohol efficiently. Any process that directly or indirectly decreases the blood supply to the liver is likely to decrease the rate of alcohol metabolism. Malnourishment also impairs metabolic handling of alcohol. Diseases that alter total body water, such as cardiac and renal diseases, may also influence BACs and the time course of BAC curves (Rix, 1983c). Cardiac output, stroke volume, and heart rate all increased in a dose-response manner in 14 healthy male volunteers given varying amounts of alcohol. Peripheral resistance, however, was significantly reduced. These hemodynamic alterations were thought to be due to cerebral or central nervous reflex mechanisms due to central actions of alcohol (Juchems and Klobe, 1969).

The disappearance curve of alcohol from the body can be enhanced by concomitant administration of fructose, glycine, or alanine.

The fact that coadministration of fructose and alcohol hastens the elimination of alcohol by the liver has been known for nearly 50 years. Table 3-2 reflects some of the studies corroborating this fact. A variety of effects have been observed with the infusion of alcohol and fructose. Liver blood flow increased about 30%. Liver biochemical changes included a 60% increase in oxygen uptake, a 60% decrease in lactate and pyruvate production, and a 200% increase in the hepatic output of glucose. With alcohol alone, about 80% of the uptake of oxygen was used to transform alcohol to acetate; with alcohol and fructose, the percentage of oxygen required to transform alcohol to acetate was reduced even though the amount of alcohol converted to acetate showed a twofold increase. The suggestion was made that some of the degradation products of fructose serve as hydrogen acceptors in the dehydrogenation of part of the ethanol, circumventing the limiting step in the transformation of alcohol to acetaldehyde, namely, the dissociation of the complex alcohol dehydrogenase and reduced nicotinamide adenine dinucleotide (Forney and Harger, 1969; Lowenstein et al, 1970).

The amino acids glycine and alanine also may increase the elimination rate of alcohol. Experiments performed in 12 fasting cats showed that glycine and alanine increased the splanchnic elimination of alcohol

Table 3-2
Fructose Acceleration of Blood Alcohol Elimination

Observation	Reference
1. 30–60 g fructose in human subjects given 10–20 mL alcohol shortened the alcohol disappearance period to about two thirds of that of the controls.	Carpenter and Lee, 1937
2. 0.9–1.9 g/kg fructose caused an increase of 48%–68% in the β_{60} of human subjects given 0.9–1.0 g/kg alcohol; this large dose of fructose caused severe epigastric pain	Pletscher et al, 1952a
3. 1–2 g/kg fructose increased the β_{60} of dogs 80%	Pletscher et al, 1952b
4. 100 g fructose in normal human subjects increased the β_{60} by an average of 24%	Bernstein et al, 1955
5. Fructose increased the β_{60} for alcohol in dogs by about 50%	Clark and Hulpieu, 1958
6. Human subjects ingested 0.5 g/kg of alcohol, and, beginning 2 h later, ate 22 g of fructose at half-hour intervals; four of five subjects showed increased β_{60} of 28% to 56%; the fifth subject showed only a 2% increase in β_{60}.	Lundquist and Wolthers, 1958
7. Delineated the possible mechanism of action of fructose	Tygstrup et al, 1965
8. In human subjects, fructose infusion lowered blood alcohol levels by 43%	Lowenstein et al, 1970
9. Fructose was shown to be ineffective in preventing delerium tremens	Friend et al, 1971
10. Both sucrose and fructose in chronic alcoholic volunteers speeded alcohol disappearance	Soterakis and Iber, 1973

and the consumption of oxygen. The latter phenomenon was correlated with a change in the mitochondrial redox state toward increased oxidation levels; no change was observed in cytoplasmic redox state. The discrepancy between the amino acid–induced effect on the mitochondrial and cytoplasmic redox levels may be related to the increase in alcohol elimination, which increases the production of reducing equivalents in the hepatic mitochondria, whereas the cytoplasmic redox state is maintained at the control level (Krarup and Larsen, 1974).

EXCRETION

General Features

It is estimated that less than 5% of an alcohol dose is eliminated unchanged in man, but this may be as high as 10% during periods of diuresis, profuse sweating, or hyperventilation. The percentage is also higher with large doses, since the elimination processes are first-order (dose-dependent), while the metabolic process is essentially zero-order (Kalant, 1971). Excretion of alcohol can occur via the expired air, urine, sweat, feces, milk, and saliva. Only the urine will be discussed in any detail due to its forensic interest.

Urine

Urine is accepted as a specimen for the forensic determination of alcohol content in some jurisdictions in the United States, although a technical manual published by the US Department of Transportation cautions against its use (Dubowski, 1977). In California, for instance, a specimen may be collected from the driver of an automobile suspected of being under the influence of alcohol by first asking the individual to void his bladder and then collecting a fresh specimen after at least 20 minutes have passed. The alcohol content of this specimen is divided by 1.3 (assumed average urine-blood concentration ratio) and expressed as a blood alcohol concentration equivalent.

As seen in Figure 3-3, urine alcohol concentrations generally lag behind blood concentration until the blood value reaches its peak, and then remain somewhat higher than the blood values during the declining phase of blood alcohol concentrations. Purely on the basis of the average water content of urine (98%) relative to that of blood (80%), we would expect the average urine-blood alcohol ratio to be approximately 1.23.

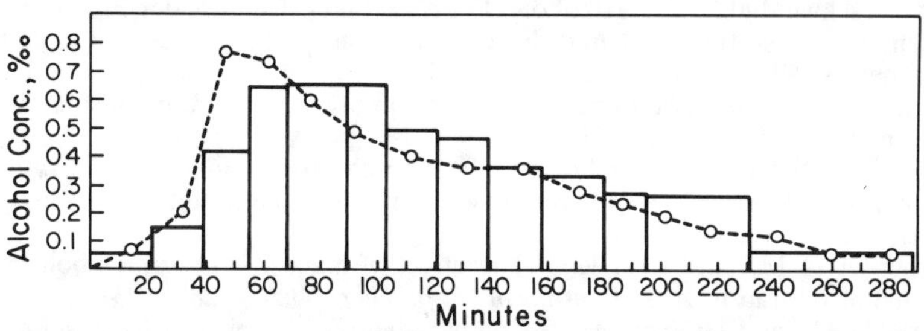

Figure 3-3 Relationship between venous blood alcohol concentration (dashed line) and urine alcohol concentration (solid lines) over a five-hour period (Reproduced with permission from Widmark, 1981.)

However, variations in Hct and urinary solute concentration, and perhaps short-term fluctuations in blood alcohol concentration or renal function, undoubtedly lead to significant interindividual differences in this ratio.

Payne et al (1967) found urine-blood alcohol concentrations ranging from 1.10 to 2.44 in 35 subjects, with an average of 1.44. The authors concluded that the use of the 1.33 urine-blood ratio for medicolegal purposes could "lead to miscarriages of justice." Dunnet and Kimber (1968) reported a range of 0.94 to 1.40 in their study of nine subjects. In a report by Flanagan et al (1977) on 40 subjects, ratios of 0.32 to 1.34 were observed.

In view of the above findings and after consideration of the physiology of urine formation, it is apparent that a pooled urine specimen does not accurately reflect the blood alcohol concentration at any single point in time. Rather, it represents an average urine concentration over the period of time that the urine was produced, and is related to the alcohol concentration in blood by a number of uncontrollable factors that vary from one individual to the next and even within an individual over time. Thus Schwar (1979) concluded that a "urine analysis should not be used as a substitute for blood alcohol analyses."

REFERENCES

Abele, G., and Kropp, R. Der Anstieg der Blutalkoholkonzentration nach dem Trinken von Schnaps (38–40 Vol.%). *Dtsch. Z. Ges. Gerichtl. Med.* 48: 68–72, 1958.

Alobaidi, T.A.A., Hill, D.W., and Payne, J.P. Significance of variations in blood:breath partition coefficient of alcohol. *Br. Med. J.* 2:1479–1481, 1976.

Backer, R.C., Pisano, R.V., and Sopher, I.M., The comparison of alcohol concentrations in postmortem fluids and tissues. *J. Forensic Sci.* 25:327–331, 1980.

Bennion, L.J., and Li, T.K. Alcohol metabolism in American Indians and whites. *N. Engl. J. Med.* 294:9–13, 1976.

Bernstein, A., Pletscher, A., and Renschler, H. Zur Beeinflussung der Umsatzgeschwindigkeit des Alkohols. IV. Mitteilung. Einfluss der Fructose auf den Alkoholstoffwechsel und die Umsatzgeschwindigkeit des Alkohols bei Hepatitis. *Klin. Wchschr.* 33:488–491, 1955.

Blomstrand, R. Observations on the formation of ethanol in the intestinal tract in man. *Life Sci.* 10:575–582, 1971.

Bogusz, M., Pach, J., and Stasko, W. Comparative studies on the rate of ethanol elimination in acute poisoning and in controlled conditions. *J. Forensic Sci.* 22:446–451, 1977.

Carpenter, T.M., and Lee, R.C. The effect of glucose on the metabolism of ethyl alcohol in man. *J. Pharmacol. Exp. Ther.* 60:264–285, 1937.

Clark, W.C., and Hulpieu, H.R. Comparative effectiveness of fructose, dextrose, pyruvic acid and insulin in accelerating the disappearance of ethanol from dogs. *Q. J. Stud. Alcohol* 19: 47–53, 1958.

Clothier, J., Kelley, J.T., Reed, K., et al. Varying rates of alcohol metabolism in relation to detoxification medication. *Alcohol* 2:443–445, 1985.

Cohen, H.M. Limitations of the current alcohol-testing procedures. *D.W.I. J.* 1:55–90, 1986.

Dubowski, K.M. Human pharmacokinetics of alcohol. *Alcohol Tech. Rep.* 5: 55–63, 1976.

Dubowski, K.M. *Manual for Analysis of Ethanol in Biological Liquids*. U.S. Dept. of Transportation, Report No. DOT-TSC-NHTSA-76-4. 1977, pp. 5–7.

Dubowski, K.M., and O'Neill, B. The blood/breath ratio of ethanol. *Clin. Chem.* 25:1144, 1979.

Dunnett, N., and Kimber, K.J. Urine-blood alcohol ratio. *J. Forensic Sci. Soc.* 8:15–24, 1968.

Fenna, D., Mix, L., Schaefer, O., et al. Ethanol metabolism in various racial groups. *Can. Med. Assoc. J.* 105:472–475, 1971.

Flanagan, N.G., Goff, D.K., Butt, W., et al. Further observations on the validity of urine alcohol levels in road traffic offenses. *Med. Sci. Law* 17: 269–272, 1977.

Forney, R.B., and Harger, R.N. Toxicology of ethanol. *Annu. Rev. Pharmacol.* 9:379–392, 1969.

Forney, R.B., Hughes, F.W., Harger, R.N., et al. Alcohol distribution in the vascular system. *Q. J. Stud. Alcohol* 25:205–217, 1964.

Friend, W.G., Sardesai, V.M., Pitt, J.J. et al. Effect of fructose on delerium tremens. *JAMA* 217:474–475, 1971.

Absorption, distribution, and elimination of ethanol. In *Pharmacology of Alcohol*, D.B. Goldstein (ed.). Oxford University Press, New York, 1983, pp. 3–17.

Hammond, K.B., Rumack, B.H., and Rodgerson, D.O. Blood ethanol. *JAMA* 226:63–64, 1973.

Herbich, J., and Prokop, L. Untersuchungen über den Einfluss von Nahrungs- und Flüssigkeitsaufnahme auf den Blutalkoholspiegel. *Wien Klin. Wchnschr.* 75:421–427, 1963.

Hlastala, M.P. Physiological errors associated with alcohol breath testing. *Champion*, July 1985, pp. 16–39.

Holtzman, J.L., Gebhard, R.L., Eckfeldt, J.H., et al. The effects of several weeks of ethanol consumption on ethanol kinetics in normal men and women. *Clin. Pharmacol. Ther.* 38:157–163, 1985.

Jones, A.J. Inter- and intra-individual variations in the saliva/blood alcohol ratio during ethanol metabolism in man. *Clin. Chem.* 25: 1394–1398, 1979.

Juchems, R., and Klobe, R. Hemodynamic effects of ethyl alcohol in man. *Am. Heart J.* 78:133–134, 1969.

Kalant, H. Absorption, diffusion, distribution, and elimination of ethanol: effects on biological membranes. In *The Biology of Alcoholism* (B. Kissin and H. Begleiter, eds.), Plenum Press, New York, 1971, vol. 1, pp. 1–62.

Keilin, D., and Hartree, E.F. Properties of catalase. Catalysis of coupled oxidation of alcohols. *Biochem. J.* 39:293–301, 1945.

Krarup, N., and Larsen, J.A. Relation between splanchnic ethanol elimination and oxygen consumption. *Acta Physiol. Scand.* (*Suppl.*) 87:43A-44A, 1974.

Krauland, W., Wojahn, H., and Glass, F. Trinkmenge und Blutalkoholkonzentration. In *Forschungsergebnisse der gerichtlichen Medizin* (F. Schleyer, ed.), Verlag Max Schmidt-Romhild, Lübeck, West Germany, 1967, pp. 162–182.

Leithoff, H. Die Aufstellung von Blutalkoholkurven im Trinkversuch mit einer neuen Methode der kontinuierlichen Blutalkoholbestimmung. *Blutalkohol* 2:541–550, 1964.

Lester, D. The concentration of apparent endogenous ethanol. *Q. J. Stud. Alcohol* 23:17–25, 1962.

Lin, Y.J., Weidler, D.J., Garg, D.C., et al. Effects of solid food on blood levels of alcohol in man. *Res. Comm. Chem. Path. Pharmacol.* 13:713:922, 1976.

Lowenstein, L.M., Simone, R., Boulter, P., et al. Effect of fructose on alcohol concentration in the blood of man. *JAMA* 213:1899–1901, 1970.

Lundquist, F., and Wolthers, H. The influence of fructose on the kinetics of alcohol elimination in man. *Acta Pharmacol. Toxicol.* 14:290–294, 1958.

Mason, M.F., and Dubowski, K.M. Alcohol, traffic, and chemical testing in the United States: a resume and some remaining problems. *Clin. Chem.* 20: 126–140, 1974.

Mason, M.F., and Dubowski, K.M. Breath-alcohol analysis: uses, methods and some forensic problems — review and opinion. *J. Forensic Sci.* 21:9–41, 1976.

Mellanby, E. Alcohol and alcoholic intoxication. *Br. J. Inebriety* 17:157–178, 1920.

Mezey, E. Gastrointestinal complications of alcoholism. *Pract. Gastroenterol.* 7:7–17, 1983.

Misra, P.S., LeFevre, A., Ishii, H., et al. Increase of ethanol, meprobamate and pentobarbital metabolism after chronic ethanol administration in man and in rats. *Am. J. Med.* 51:346–351, 1971.

Morgan, M.Y. Alcohol and the liver. *J. Hum. Nutr.* 33:350–356, 1979.

Payne, J.P., Foster, D.V., Hill, D.W., et al. Observations on interpretation of blood alcohol levels derived from analysis of urine. *Br. Med. J.* 3:819–823, 1967.

Payne, J.P., Hill, D.W., and Wood, D.G.L., Distribution of ethanol between plasma and erythrocytes in whole blood. *Nature* 217: 963–964, 1968.

Pletscher, A., Bernstein, A., and Staub, H. Beschleunigung des Alkoholabbaus durch Fruktose beim Menschen. *Experientia* 8:307–308, 1952a.

Pletscher, A., Bernstein, A., and Staub, H. Zur Beeinflussung der Umsatzgeschwindigkeit des Alkohols. I. Mitteilung. Die Beschleunigung des oxydativen Alkoholabbaus durch Fructose. *Helv. Physiol. Acta* 10:74–83, 1952b.

Pleuckhahan, V.D. The evaluation of autopsy blood alcohol levels. *Med. Sci. Law* 8:168–176, 1967.

Reed, T.E., Kalant, H., Gibbins, R.J., et al. Alcohol and acetaldehyde metabolism in Caucasians, Chinese and Amerinds. *Can. Med. Assoc. J.* 115: 851–855, 1976.

Ritchie, J.M. The aliphatic alcohols. In *The Pharmacologic Basis of Therapeutics*, 6th ed. (A.G. Gilman, L.K. Goodman, and A. Gilman, eds.), MacMillan, New York, 1980, pp. 376–390.

Rix, K. Predicting blood concentrations. 1. The theory. *Nurs. Times* 79:55–56, 1983a.

Rix, K. Predicting blood alcohol concentrations. 2. Taking metabolism into account. *Nurs. Times* 79:67–68, 1983b.

Rix, K. Predicting blood alcohol concentrations. 3. The effect of food, illness and age. *Nurs. Times* 79:68–69, 1983c.

Schwar, T.G. *Alcohol, Drugs and Road Traffic* (W.E. Cooper, T.G. Schwar, and L.S. Smith, eds.), Juta & Co., Capetown, 1979.

Sedman, A.J., Wilkinson, P.K. and Wagner, J.G. Concentrations of ethanol in two segments of the vascular system. *J. Forensic Sci.* 21:315–322, 1976.

Shajani, N.K., and Dinn, H.M. Blood alcohol concentrations reached in human subjects after consumption of alcoholic beverages in a social setting. *Can. Soc. Forensic Sci. J.* 18:38–48, 1985.

Soterakis, J., and Iber, F.L. Increased rate of alcohol removed from blood with oral fructose and sucrose. *Gastroenterology* 64:805, 1973.

Stone, B.E., and Rooney, P.A. A study using body fluids to determine blood alcohol. *J. Anal. Toxicol.* 8:95–96, 1984.

Tottmar, S.O.C., Pettersson, H., and Kiessling, K.H. The subcellular distribution and properties of aldehyde dehydrogenase in rat liver. *Biochem. J.* 135:557–586, 1973.

Turkel, H.W., and Gifford, H. Erroneous blood alcohol findings at autopsy. *JAMA* 164:1077–1079, 1957.

Tygstrup, N., Winkler, K., and Lundquist, F. The mechanism of the fructose effect on the ethanol metabolism of the human liver. *J. Clin. Invest.* 44: 817–830, 1965.

Vessel, E.S., Page, J.G., and Passananti, G.T. Genetic and environmental factors affecting ethanol metabolism in man. *Clin. Pharmacol. Ther.* 12: 192–201, 1971.

Wagner, J.G., Wilkinson, P.K., Sedman, A.J., et al. Elimination of alcohol from human blood. *J. Pharmacol. Sci.* 65:152–154, 1976.

Watterlond, M. The telltale metabolism of alcoholics. *Science* 83:72–76, 1983.

Widmark, E.M.P. *Principles and Applications of Medicolegal Alcohol Determination.* Biomedical Publications, Davis, Calif., 1981. Translated from German by Scitrans Inc., Santa Barbara, Calif., 1932.

Wilkinson, P.K., Sedman, A.J., Sakmar, E., et al. Fasting and nonfasting blood ethanol concentrations following repeated oral administration of ethanol to one adult male subject. *J. Pharmacokinet. Biopharm.* 5:41:52, 1977.

Wilson, J.R., and Erwin, V.G. Rate of alcohol metabolism; do not correct the β_{-60} estimate for comparisons among ethnic groups. *J. Stud. Alcohol* 44: 1093–1096, 1983.

Yamamoto, K., and Ueda, M. Studies on breath alcohol analysis for the estimation of blood alcohol levels. *Forensic Sci.* 1:207–224, 1972.

4

Blood, Urine, and Other Fluid and Tissue Specimens for Alcohol Analyses

Yale H. Caplan

BLOOD

General Considerations

Undoubtedly, the determination of alcohol is the most widely requested analysis in analytical toxicology. These requests may be on a living subject, where knowledge of the role of alcohol in a particular situation is required, or on a deceased person, where alcohol may have contributed to that person's death or to the death of another. In either case, a decision as to the type of specimen to be analyzed is important to facilitate proper interpretation of the results. Since alcohol affects the brain, a specimen that is reflective of the alcohol content of the brain is most useful. Because the blood compartment is in equilibrium with the brain, the blood alcohol concentration is expected to best reflect the effects of alcohol on the brain. In view of the fact that the majority of tests will be conducted on living subjects, blood or a constituent of blood is most commonly used. In postmortem cases, the brain itself, among other specimens, becomes available; however, blood is commonly used since comparison to antemortem situations is often required. Blood, available with equal ease from living or deceased persons becomes the more practical specimen; hence the first step in the alcohol analysis is to obtain the proper blood samples.

The average person contains approximately 5 L of blood constituting about 8% of the total body weight. There are two principal components of blood: the plasma and the cells. The plasma is the liquid portion and contains the lipids, proteins, ions, vitamins, and other constituents. There are two principal types of blood cells; the red blood cells and the white blood cells. Red blood cells, or erythrocytes, contain hemoglobin which binds oxygen and facilitates oxygen transport throughout the body. White blood cells, or leukocytes, are responsible for the cell-mediated immune responses to foreign organisms. There are approximately 500 times more erythrocytes than leukocytes. The ratio that indicates the relative volume of the plasma and cells is the hematocrit (Hct), which is defined as the volume of red cells divided by the total blood volume. An average Hct is between 40% and 50%. A low Hct would imply a greater water content of the blood. Alcohol distributes in the body's total water; therefore, its concentration would vary according to whether whole blood or a component of blood is selected for testing.

Although chapter 9 deals in more detail with the question of storage and stability of alcohol in blood, a few words must be included here. Ordinarily, days or even weeks may pass between the sampling and analysis of a blood specimen. Since the interest of the analyst is in the blood alcohol concentration at the time that the specimen was drawn, it is important that the integrity of the sample remain intact over this time period. Specifically, the degradation of the blood by normal biological events and changes in the original ethanol concentration must be avoided.

Many reports in the literature have shown that there may be decreases as well as increases in ethanol concentration with time. Improperly sealed containers, microorganism oxidation of ethanol, and a temperature-dependent conversion of ethanol to acetaldehyde have resulted in decreases in ethanol concentration (Brown et al, 1973; Smalldon and Brown, 1973; Chang et al, 1984) while increases in ethanol concentration have been attributed to microbial conversion of glucose to alcohol. To prevent these changes, blood samples should be well sealed and stored at low temperatures. Anticoagulants such as oxalate salts, citrate salts, or heparin should be added to prevent clotting. Microorganism growth can be inhibited by adding fluoride salts, mercuric salts, or azide salts. Postmortem blood samples are ordinarily obtained without using sterile technique, and therefore have an increased likelihood of bacterial contamination and may require a greater amount of fluoride to prevent in vitro ethanol formation. A combination of potassium oxalate at a concentration of 5 mg/mL of blood, and sodium fluoride at 1 mg/mL of blood is frequently used, along with storage of the blood at 4°C or −20°C.

It is important that the blood sample, once drawn, be properly handled until it reaches the location for analysis. Samples should be labeled with the subject's name, the time of drawing, the location site from which the sample was drawn and the name of the person who withdrew the blood. The time of blood withdrawal is especially important in living subjects because the blood alcohol concentration determined may be used in estimation of the blood concentration at an earlier time. The tube should be sealed by the person drawing the blood and a chain of custody must be established from the time of withdrawal until the time of analysis. When samples are mailed in from an outside source, the US Postal Service has been determined by the courts to be an acceptable link in the chain.

Several studies (Heise, 1959; Dubowski, 1977; Kaye, 1980) using living subjects have demonstrated that externally applied alcohol can produce false-positive results. Although one study suggests that this is not a problem when isopropanol-containing antiseptics are used (Goldfinger and Schaber, 1982), it seems reasonable to use a nonalcohol-containing antiseptic during the venipuncture procedure. For postmortem cases, such antiseptics are not used; however, care must still be exercised in obtaining the specimen. The sample should be drawn from an exposed area to ensure that the sample is, in fact, blood. For instance, in trauma cases, it is possible for the blood to be mixed with the stomach contents and if alcohol were present in the stomach contents, an artificially elevated blood alcohol concentration could result.

Sources of Specimens

The location from which the blood specimen is obtained in the body is important. For the most part, alcohol is absorbed from the gastrointestinal (GI) tract and enters the portal circulation; during the early absorption process, the portal blood contains the highest concentration of alcohol. This suggests that portal blood would not be a good blood specimen to obtain in postmortem cases. Past the liver, the portal blood passes into the heart. At this point, the alcohol concentration is diluted by blood from other sources. From the heart, the alcohol is distributed to the rest of the tissues.

During the absorption phase, alcohol concentrations in blood from different parts of the body may vary (Haggard et al, 1940). Numerous studies have reported on the length of time required for alcohol to equilibrate throughout the body (Harger et al, 1956; McCallum and Scroggie, 1960; Forney et al, 1964; Dundee et al, 1971; Sedman et al, 1976). For instance, in one study (Forney et al, 1964) five subjects were administered a fixed dose per weight of alcohol and at subsequent time intervals, blood samples from the cubital vein and the finger tip were drawn for alcohol analysis. Blood from the finger tip represented capillary blood, which was assumed to be equivalent to arterial blood. At the end of the drinking period, the alcohol concentration in the finger tip blood exceeded that in the cubital vein in each case, ranging from a 12% to 40% difference. At 30 minutes, differences were still observed, but for the remainder of the two-hour period, no further differences between the two blood sites were noted. Blood from the foot vein had a much lower alcohol concentration than that of the cubital vein.

Another report (Sedman et al, 1976) indicated that it may take somewhat longer for the equilibrium between capillary blood and venous blood to occur. Following equilibrium, a point is reached where the venous blood slightly exceeds the capillary blood concentration. Ideally, arterial blood should be used because arterial blood alcohol concentrations correlate best with CNS impairment (Mason and Dubowski, 1974). However, the analysis of arterial blood requires arterial puncture, which is more painful, presents greater medical risk, and requires specially trained personnel to draw the blood. Therefore, the more easily and safely obtained venous blood is regularly used. The proper interpretation of the results may require knowledge as to whether or not the blood was drawn in the postabsorptive period, when it can be assumed that the venous blood alcohol concentration is approximately equal to the arterial blood concentration.

In postmortem cases the medical examiner or coroner is able to obtain a blood sample directly from the heart. As mentioned previously, it is important that the blood specimen not be mixed with other bodily fluids, for this may increase or decrease the alcohol concentration. It is also recommended that a second blood sample from an alternate site, such as the femoral vein or other peripheral site, be obtained at autopsy. The two blood samples can provide some information as to whether the subject was in the postabsorptive state. More importantly, in those cases where the heart blood may have been contaminated, the alternative specimen can be used to provide a blood alcohol concentration.

Serum and Plasma

In clinical laboratories, analyses for alcohol are commonly performed on serum or plasma, rather than on whole blood. Therefore, it is important to understand the relationship between blood alcohol and serum or plasma alcohol concentrations. Since alcohol distributes according to the water content of the tissue or fluid and since there is about 10% to 12% more water in a volume of plasma than in a corresponding volume of whole blood, one would expect that serum or plasma would have a higher alcohol concentration than the corresponding whole blood. Further, by using the Hct of the blood sample, one can calculate the expected serum-blood ratio of alcohol concentrations. Several reports (Grumer, 1957; Illchmann-Christ, 1959; Dotzauer et al, 1952) have determined experimentally serum-blood and plasma-blood ratios. Serum-blood ratios vary from 1.12 to 1.17 whereas plasma-blood ratios ranged from 1.10 to 1.35, with an average of about 1.18 (Payne et al., 1968). Thus there appears to be no significant difference between plasma-blood and serum-blood ratios.

URINE

Aside from breath and blood, a widely used specimen for determining alcohol intoxication has been urine. Urine is the end product of the physiology involving the kidney, which is responsible for the removal of waste products from the body. Each minute, the kidneys receive 1200 mL of blood, which is approximately one fourth of the cardiac output. This renal blood flow corresponds to a renal plasma flow of 650 mL/min. About one fifth, or 130 mL/min, is filtered at the glomeruli. This means that 180 L of protein-free filtrate is generated each day. However, only about 1.5 L are excreted as urine. The remainder is reabsorbed by the renal tubules. Un-ionized chemicals are more likely to be absorbed while more polar, or water-soluble, compounds remain in the filtrate.

Intrinsically, urine has some advantages over blood. Since it can be obtained without invading the body, it does not require specialized personnel or equipment. Because of this, many studies have been undertaken to correlate urine alcohol concentrations with blood alcohol concentrations. The majority of these studies suggest that the average urine-blood ratio is about 1.3. However, there is tremendous variation in the ratios determined. For example, in one study (Payne et al, 1967), blood and urine samples of 35 drivers suspected of drunk driving were analyzed; urine-blood ratios were found to vary from 1.10 to 2.44. In postmortem samples, Kaye and Cardona (1969) obtained blood and urine samples for alcohol analysis in 148 autopsied cases and found that the urine-blood ratio averaged 1.28, but ranged from 0.21 to 2.66. Using the average ratio, they calculated a blood alcohol concentration from the urine alcohol concentration and compared it to the actual blood concentration. They found that in 21.5% of the cases, the calculated blood alcohol concentration exceeded the actual value while in 34.5% of the cases, the calculated value underestimated the actual blood alcohol concentration.

Another study (Backer et al, 1980) found urine-blood alcohol ratios ranging from 0.53 to 2.17 in postmortem specimens. Jones (1980) studied 21 healthy males by collecting blood and urine samples at different time intervals for seven hours after drinking. He determined that the urine-blood ratio could be divided into two phases: an absorptive phase when the ratio is less than 1.0 and a postabsorptive phase when the ratio is greater than 1.3 and may even exceed 2.0. This suggests that although urine alcohol concentrations by themselves are not useful in determining blood alcohol concentrations, when they are used in conjunction with blood alcohol concentrations, some information can be inferred regarding the time frame of the individual's drinking. A low urine-blood alcohol ratio suggests that little time has passed between drinking and sampling such that absorption is still occurring. A higher ratio implies absorption has been completed and the individual is in the elimination phase.

In addition to pharmacokinetic considerations, there are other explanations for such a wide variation in urine-blood alcohol ratios. Alcohol has a diuretic effect, resulting from inhibition of the release of antidiuretic hormone (ADH). There are great individual differences in sensitivity to this effect. An individual producing a more dilute urine would be expected to have a lower urine-blood ratio than one producing a more concentrated urine. A related factor is the frequency of urination between alcohol ingestion and urine collection. To diminish these problems, the following procedure has been used: The bladder is emptied and the urine is discarded. After a 20- to 30-minute wait, a second urine specimen is obtained and this is used for the analysis. The alcohol concentration in the second urine sample reflects more accurately the blood alcohol concentration at that time.

SALIVA

Although blood and urine are the two most popular fluids for alcohol analysis, saliva has been used as an alternate specimen. Although it has the advantage of urine in being obtainable by noninvasive techniques, it also has the limitation of urine in that it is a highly variable specimen. Saliva is composed of secretions from three major salivary gland sources: the parotid, the submaxillary, and the sublingual glands. The degree to which each gland contributes to the make-up of the saliva depends on numerous factors: type, duration, intensity of stimulation, time of day, diet, age, sex, and disease state (Danhof and Breimer, 1978). Furthermore, the pH of saliva shows greater inter- and intra-individual variation (Mucklow, 1982). Fortunately, this is not a problem with alcohol since, unlike other drugs, alcohol distributes according to the water content of a fluid and is independent of pH. Also, there are many techniques that can be used to collect saliva, with each method producing saliva of different composition.

In spite of these pitfalls, numerous researchers have tried to use saliva alcohol concentrations as an estimate of blood alcohol concentrations. Coldwell and Smith (1959) found a good correlation between blood and saliva alcohol concentrations. Jones (1980) found that after 30 minutes of alcohol ingestion, the saliva-blood alcohol ratio remained constant at 1.10 throughout a seven-hour period. This value was lower than expected when considering the expected water content. However, Jones's experiments were carried out on 21 healthy men under controlled laboratory conditions and a single method was used for obtaining the saliva.

BRAIN AND CEREBROSPINAL FLUID

In postmortem cases, of course, a greater variety of specimens can be subjected to alcohol analysis. It could be assumed that since brain is available, it would be the specimen of choice. However, brain-blood alcohol concentration ratios have also shown a great variability, ranging from 0.31 to 8.00 (Hine, 1951; Freireich, 1960; Budd, 1983). This is not surprising in view of the heterogenous make-up of the brain. Different parts of the brain have different water contents and what is generally reported is an average of all of these parts.

Cerebrospinal fluid (CSF) is another specimen that can be used for alcohol analysis. Intuitively, CSF appears to be useful because it might more closely indicate the ethanol concentration in the CNS. Gettler and Freireich (1931) reported an average ratio of 1.08 for 15 subjects. Harger et al (1937) found a lumbar CSF-blood alcohol ratio of 1.14 in 46 samples. Hebold (1959) reported a range of 0.93 to 1.40 in 22 subjects. Although no concentrations were published, Marcellini (1961) administered alcohol orally to ten fasting nonalcoholic patients and obtained blood and CSF fluid every half-hour for six hours after drinking. The maximum blood alcohol concentration was reached within 90 minutes in eight of the ten patients, but the maximum CSF concentration was not reached until three hours after drinking in nine of the ten subjects. Moreover, during the elimination phase, the concentration in the CSF exceeded that in the blood. In more recent studies, average ratios of 1.1 and 0.9 were reported in two sets of postmortem cases (Backer et al, 1980; Budd, 1982).

VITREOUS HUMOR

Over the past few years, the use of vitreous humor as a specimen for alcohol analysis in postmortem cases has increased. Vitreous humor is a relatively easy specimen for the medical examiner to obtain and is a relatively stable postmortem specimen. Since the vitreous humor is in a peripheral body compartment, there is a delay in alcohol uptake and removal in vitreous in comparison to blood. Sturner and Coumbis (1966) were the first to show a close correlation between vitreous humor and blood alcohol concentrations in postmortem specimens; an average vitreous-blood ratio of 1.10 was reported. Coe and Sherman (1970) studied 174 cases; the average vitreous-blood alcohol ratio was 1.12. Other studies (Backer et al, 1980; Leahy et al, 1968; Felby and Olsen, 1969; Scott et al, 1974; Budd, 1982) have produced average ratios of between 0.90 and 1.38.

Scott et al (1974) illustrated the potential of using vitreous humor to determine alcohol involvement in those cases where the body has been embalmed. In eight cases in which the blood was positive for alcohol, preembalmed and postembalmed vitreous samples were obtained and analyzed. The average preembalmed vitreous-blood alcohol ratio was 0.91, while the postembalmed ratio was 0.81. This indicates that vitreous humor can be a useful specimen to analyze for alcohol in embalmed cases. Furthermore, Zumwalt et al (1982) studied vitreous humor in relation to bacterial infiltration in decomposed bodies after assessing the degree of putrefaction based on eight physical changes. They found that even in moderately decomposed bodies, few bacteria were detected in the vitreous humor, suggesting that postmortem formation of alcohol in vitreous humor would be negligible under these circumstances. Therefore any alcohol found in the vitreous humor could be presumed to be of exogenous origin.

The interpretation of alcohol concentrations in decomposed specimens without vitreous humor can be a difficult process since concentrations can increase or decrease in biological fluids with time and other factors. Realizing that this information is needed in many cases, it is suggested that a negative alcohol result probably means that no alcohol was present at death while a very high blood alcohol concentration was probably not caused by alcohol neoformation alone. Blood alcohol concentrations exceeding 0.10 g/dL in postmortem cases are likely the result of true alcohol ingestion when the analysis is conducted by gas chromatography.

OTHER SPECIMENS

Little has been published regarding the distribution of alcohol into the central body compartments, such as liver and kidney. This is surprising because liver is a frequently analyzed specimen for most other drugs. Presumably, since these organs have a rich blood supply, these tissues reach equilibrium with the blood quite rapidly after absorption. This has been confirmed in animal studies. Harger et al (1937), in dog studies, found no change in liver-blood ratios from five minutes to 12 hours, with a ratio of 0.78. Christopoulos et al (1973) conducted distribution studies of alcohol in various body tissues and fluids obtained from 13 postmortem cases involving a violent death with a positive blood alcohol concentration. Liver-blood ratios averaged 0.63 ± 0.10 with a range of 0.51 to 0.83. In ten cases of acute alcohol intoxication

(>0.49%) the average liver-blood ratio was 0.60±0.056 with a range of 0.54 to 0.72; the average kidney-blood ratio was 0.66±0.058 with a range of 0.57 to 0.76.

Besides the analysis of the more common toxicologic specimens for alcohol, many attempts have been made to correlate blood alcohol concentrations with alcohol concentrations in unusual specimens. Isokoski et al (1968) analyzed blood and femur bone marrow for alcohol in 12 postmortem cases. These specimens were analyzed using both the Widmark and ADH methods. The marrow-blood ratios ranged from 0.21 to 0.67 in ten of the cases with an average ratio of 0.34±0.14. Of the remaining two cases, one had a ratio of 1.75, whereas the other had a negative blood and a positive marrow alcohol. The authors concluded that due to the great individual variations in the ratios, it was impossible to determine the exact blood alcohol concentration from a given marrow alcohol concentration.

Winek and Jones (1980) performed similar studies, but instead of using femur marrow, they used rib marrow, and found an average marrow-blood ratio of 0.47±0.066, ranging from 0.34 to 0.61. They postulated that this wide range may be due to differences in the lipid content of the marrow, and in a subsequent study from their laboratory (Winek and Esposito, 1981), an attempt was made to correct for the differences in lipid content in the bone marrow. A weighed amount of marrow was extracted with ether and after centrifugation and separation, the ether layer was evaporated to dryness. The resulting residue

Table 4-1
Ratio of Various Specimens to Blood Alcohol Concentrations

Specimen	Study	No.	Average	Range
Serum or plasma	Grumer, 1957		1.16	1.13–1.17
	Illchmann-Christ, 1959		1.17±.06	
	Dotzauer et al, 1952		1.12±.006	
	Payne et al, 1968		1.18	
Urine	Jetter, 1938	372	1.23	1.00–2.30
	Bavis, 1940	66	1.17	0.81–1.65
	Mozes and Katonak, 1941	100	1.16	0.63–1.65
	Ellenbrook and Van Gaazbeek, 1943	76	1.26	0.69–1.71
	Prag, 1953	75	1.31	1.00–1.64
	Coldwell and Smith, 1959	91	1.24±0.08	
	Lundquist, 1961	55	1.35	1.12–1.51
	Morgan, 1965	518	1.38	0.9 –2.4
	Heise, 1967	20	1.40±0.84	1.29–1.58
	Payne et al, 1967	35	1.44	1.10–2.44
	Kaye and Cardona, 1969	148	1.28	0.21–2.66

Specimen	Study	No.	Average	Range
	Christopoulos et al, 1973[a]	9	1.01 ± 0.15	0.79–1.16
	Backer et al, 1980	92	1.16	0.53–2.17
	Budd, 1982	109	1.5	
	Stone and Rooney, 1984	88	1.29	
Saliva	Friedeman et al, 1938	13	1.10	0.97–1.31
	Prag, 1953	6	1.20±0.13	1.10–1.40
	Coldwell and Smith, 1959	244	1.12	
	Jones, 1980	21	1.10	
CSF	Gettler and Freireich, 1931	15	1.08	0.42–12.5
	Harger et al, 1937	46	1.18±0.09	
	Christopoulos et al, 1973	7	0.92±0.058	0.84–1.01
	Backer et al, 1980	54	1.14	0.79–1.64
	Budd et al, 1982	5	0.9 ±0.4	
Vitreous humor	Sturner and Coumbis, 1966	38	0.99±0.22	0.46–1.40
	Leahy et al, 1968	20	1.08±0.078	0.89–1.23
	Felby and Olsen, 1969	27	1.34±0.29	0.52–1.82
	Coe and Sherman, 1970	174	1.12	
	Scott et al, 1974	8	0.91±0.17	0.67–1.13
	Backer et al, 1980	110	1.05	0.48–1.72
	Budd, 1982	15	1.3 ±0.60	
	Stone and Rooney, 1984		1.34	
Brain	Gettler and Freireich, 1931	12	0.96	0.63–1.47
	Ellenbrook and Van Gaasbeek, 1943	19	0.92	0.76–1.13
	Van Hecke et al, 1957	47	0.69	0.37–1.35
	Hine, 1951	100	0.65	0.31–2.00
	Freireich et al, 1960	82	0.94	0.69–1.47
	Herold and Prokop, 1960	35	0.69	0.38–1.30
	Christopoulos et al, 1973	10	0.62 (acute alcohol death)	0.51–0.76
	Backer et al, 1980	33	0.86	0.64–1.20
	Budd, 1982	51	1.24	0.31–8.00
Liver	Christopoulos et al, 1973.		0.63±0.10 (violent death)	0.51–0.83
			0.60±0.056 (acute alcohol death)	0.54–0.72
Kidney	Christopoulos et al, 1973		0.66±0.058 (acute alcohol death)	0.57–0.76
Bone marrow	Isokoski et al, 1968	10	0.34±0.14	0.21–0.67
	Winek and Jones, 1980	18	0.47±0.066	0.34–0.61
	Winek and Esposito, 1981	36	0.53 (actual)	0.31–0.77
			0.79 (corrected)	0.60–1.03

*All deaths were acute alcohol fatalities.

was weighed and it was assumed that this fraction of the total weight was the lipid fraction while the remaining weight was the aqueous fraction. This "corrected" marrow concentration was equal to the observed marrow concentration divided by the aqueous fraction. Without the correction, the average marrow-blood ratio was 0.53 with a range of 0.31 to 0.77; with the correction, the average ratio was 0.79 with a range of 0.60 to 1.03.

Skeletal muscle is another unusual specimen studied. Felby and Olsen (1969) determined leg muscle–blood and arm muscle–blood alcohol ratios from 15 postmortem cases; the average ratios were 0.89 and 0.90, respectively. This was in agreement with the ratio later found by Krauland et al (1980) of 0.91.

All ratios of the various specimens to blood alcohol concentrations in human studies are summarized in Table 4-1.

REFERENCES

Backer, R.C., Pisano, R.V., and Sopher, I.M. The comparison of alcohol concentrations in postmortem fluids and tissues. *J. Forensic Sci.* 25:327–331, 1980.

Bavis, D.F. 145 drunken drivers: A blood alcohol study. *J. Lab. Clin. Med.* 25:223–273, 1940.

Brown, G.A., Neyland, D., Reynolds, W.J., et al. The stability of ethanol in stored blood: Part I. Important variables and interpretation of results. *Anal. Chim. Acta* 66:271–283, 1973.

Budd, R. Ethanol levels in postmortem body fluids. *J. Chromatogr.* 252: 315–318, 1982.

Budd, R. Postmortem brain alcohol levels. *J. Chromatogr.* 259:353–355, 1983.

Chang, R.B., Smith, W.A., Walkin, E., et al. The stability of ethyl alcohol in forensic blood specimens. *J. Anal. Toxicol.* 8:66–67, 1984.

Christopoulos, G., Kirch, E.R., and Gearrien, J.E. Determination of ethanol in fresh and putrefied postmortem tissues. *J. Chromatogr.* 87:455–472, 1973.

Coe, J.E., and Sherman, R.E. Comparative study of postmortem vitreous humor and blood alcohol. *J. Forensic Sci.* 15:185–190, 1970.

Coldwell, B.B., and Smith, H.W. Alcohol levels in body fluids after ingestion of distilled spirits. *Can. J. Biochem. Physiol.* 37:43–52, 1959.

Danhof, M., and Breimer, D.D. Therapeutic drug monitoring in saliva. *Clin. Pharmacokinet.* 3:39–57, 1978.

Dotzauer, G., Redetzki, H., Johannsmeier, K., et al. Erprobung einer spezifischer Fermentmethode zur Mikrobestimmung von Äthylalkohol. *Dtsch. Z. Ges. Gerichtl. Med.* 41:15, 1952.

Dubowski, K. *Manual for Analysis of Ethanol in Biological Liquids*. U.S. Dept. of Transportation Report No. DOT-TSC-NHTSA0-76-4, 1977, pp. 5–7.

Dundee, J.W., Isaac, M., and Taggart, J. Blood ethanol levels following rapid intravenous infusion. *Q. J. Stud. Alcohol* 32:741–747, 1971.

Ellenbrook, L.D., and Van Gaasbeek, C.B. The reliability of chemical tests for alcoholic intoxications. *JAMA*. 122:996–1002, 1943.

Felby, S., and Olsen, J. Comparative studies of postmortem ethyl alcohol in vitreous humor, blood, and muscle. *J. Forensic Sci.* 14:93–101, 1969.

Forney, R.B., Hughes, F.W., Harger, R.N., et al. Alcohol distribution in the vascular system: Concentration of orally administered alcohol in blood from various parts in the vascular system and in rebreathed air during absorption. *Q. J. Stud. Alcohol* 25:205–217, 1964.

Freireich, A.W., Landau, D.P., and Lukash, L. A comparison of alcohol levels in brain, heart blood, and peripheral blood. Read to the Second International Meeting on Forensic Pathology and Medicine, New York University Medical Center, New York, 1960, abstract 10–1, p. 49.

Friedemann, T.E., Motel, W.G., and Necheles, H. The excretion of ingested alcohol in saliva. *J. Lab. Clin. Med.* 23:1007–1014, 1938.

Gettler, A.O., and Freireich, A.W. Determination of alcoholic intoxication during life by spinal fluid analysis. *J. Biol. Chem.* 92:199–209, 1931.

Goldfinger, T.M., and Schaber, D. A comparison of blood alcohol concentration using non-alcohol and alcohol-containing skin antiseptics. *Ann. Emerg. Med.* 11:665–667, 1982.

Grumer, O. The distribution of alcohol in the blood. *Dtsch. Z. Ges. Gerichtl. Med.* 46:10, 1957.

Haggard, H.W., Greenberg, L.A., and Rakietin, N. Studies on the absorption, distribution, and elimination of alcohol. VI. The principles governing the concentration of alcohol in the blood and the concentration causing respiratory failure. *J. Pharmacol. Exp. Ther.* 69:252–265, 1940.

Harger, R.N., Forney, R.B., and Baker, R.S. Estimation of the level of blood alcohol from analysis of breath: II. Use of rebreathed air. *Q. J. Stud. Alcohol* 17:1–18, 1956.

Harger, R.N., Hulpieu, H.R., and Lamb, E.B. The speed with which various parts of the body reach equilibrium in the storage of ethyl alcohol. *J. Biol. Chem.* 120:684–704, 1937.

Hebold, G. Evaluation of alcohol findings in the CSF; studies on 68 cadavers. *Dtsch. Z. Ges. Gerichtl. Med.* 48:257, 1959.

Heise, H.A. How extraneous alcohol affects the blood test for alcohol. *Am. J. Clin. Pathol.* 32:160–170, 1959.

Heise, H.A. Concentrations of alcohol in samples of blood and urine taken at the same time. *J. Forensic Sci.* 12:454–462, 1967.

Herold, K., and Prokop, O. Postmortem alcohol distribution differences in brain. *Dtsch. Z. Ges. Gerichtl. Med.*50:1, 1960.

Hine, C.H. Blood/brain distribution in 100 postmortem cases. *Proc. Am. Acad. Forensic Sci.* 1:161, 1951.

Illchmann-Christ, A. Research on the relation of blood clot–total blood (serum) alcohol values with a contribution to the conversion of serum alcohol to total blood concentrations. *Dtsch. Z. Ges. Gerichtl. Med.* 49:113, 1959.

Isokoski, M., Alha, A., and Laiho, K. Bone marrow alcohol content in cadavers. *J. Forensic Med.* 15:9–11, 1968.

Jetter, W.W. Studies in alcohol: I. The diagnosis of acute alcoholic intoxication by a correlation of clinical and chemical findings. *Am. J. Med. Sci.* 196:475–487, 1938.

Jones, A.W. Quantitative relationships among ethanol concentrations in blood, breath, saliva, and urine during ethanol metabolism in man. Proceedings of the Eighth International Conference on Alcohol, Drugs, and Traffic Safety, Stockholm, Sweden, June 15–19, 1980, pp. 550–569.

Kaye, S. The collection and handling of the blood alcohol specimen. *Am. J. Clin. Pathol.* 74:743–746, 1980.

Kaye, S., and Cardona, E. Errors of converting a urine alcohol value into a blood alcohol level. *Am. J. Clin. Pathol.* 52:577–584, 1969.

Krauland, W., Klug, E., and Toffel, P. Determination of alcohol concentrations in organs of human corpses. *Blutalkohol* 17:198–206, 1980.

Leahy, M.S., Farber, E.R., and Meadows, T.R. Quantitation of ethyl alcohol in the postmortem vitreous humor. *J. Forensic Sci.* 13:498–502, 1968.

Lundquist, F. The urinary excretion of ethanol by man. *Acta Pharmacol. Toxicol.* 18:231–238, 1961.

Marcellini, D. Blood alcohol and spinal fluid alcohol. *Q. J. Stud. Alcohol* 22: 145–146, 1961.

Mason, M.F., and Dubowski, K.M. Alcohol, traffic, and chemical testing in the United States: A resume and some remaining problems. *Clin. Chem.* 20: 126–140, 1974.

McCallum, N.E.W., and Scroggie, J.G. Some aspects of alcohol in body fluids: III. Study of alcohol in different parts of the body. *Med. J. Aust.* 2:1031, 1960.

Morgan, W.H.D. Concentrations of alcohol in samples of blood and urine taken at the same time. *J. Forensic Sci. Soc.* 5:15–21, 1965.

Mozes, E.B., and Katonak, L.J. One hundred drunken drivers. *Ohio State Med. J.* 37:21–24, 1941.

Mucklow, J.C. The use of saliva in therapeutic drug monitoring. *Ther. Drug Monit.* 4:229–247, 1982.

Payne, J.P., Foster, D.V., Hill, D.W., et al. Observations on interpretation of blood alcohol levels derived from analysis of urine. *Br. Med. J.* 3:819–823, 1967.

Payne, J.P., Hill, D.W., and Wood, D.G.L. Distribution of ethanol between plasma and erythrocytes in whole blood. *Nature* 217:963–964, 1968.

Prag, J.J. The chemical and the clinical diagnosis of driving under the influence of alcohol and the use of chemical tests in traffic law enforcement. *S. Afr. J. Clin. Sci.* 4:289–325, 1953.

Scott, W., Root, I., and Sanborn, B. The use of vitreous humor for determination of ethyl alcohol in previously embalmed bodies. *J. Forensic Sci.* 19:913–916, 1974.

Sedman, A.J., Wilkinson, P.K., and Wagner, I.G. Concentrations of ethanol in two segments of the vascular system. *J. Forensic Sci.* 21:315–322, 1976.

Smalldon, K.W., and Brown, G.A. The stability of ethanol in stored blood. Part II. The mechanism of ethanol oxidation. *Anal. Chim. Acta* 66:285–290, 1973.

Stone, R.E., and Rooney, P.A. A study using body fluids to determine blood alcohol. *J. Anal. Toxicol.* 8:95–96, 1984.

Sturner, W.Q., and Coumbis, R.J. The quantitation of ethyl alcohol in vitreous humor by blood gas chromatography. *Am. J. Clin. Pathol.* 46:349–351, 1966.

Van Hecke, W., Handovsy, H., and Thomas, F. Analyse statistique de 597 dosages d'alcool éthylique practiques dans le sanq, les humeurs et les organes d'un total de 93 cadavres: Signification physiologique et intérèt médico-légal. *Ann. Med. Legale*, 31:291, 1957.

Winek, C.L., and Esposito, F.M. Comparative study of ethanol levels in blood versus bone marrow, vitreous humor, bile, and urine. *Forensic Sci. Int.* 17: 27–36, 1981.

Winek, C.L., and Jones, T. Blood versus bone marrow ethanol concentrations in rabbits and humans. *Forensic Sci. Int.* 16:101–109, 1980.

Zumwalt, R.E., Bost, R.O., and Sunshine, I. Evaluation of ethanol concentrations in decomposed bodies. *J. Forensic Sci.* 27:549–554, 1982.

5

Analysis for Alcohol in Postmortem Specimens

James C. Garriott

Analysis for ethyl alcohol is the most frequent determination required of laboratories performing toxicology for medical examiners and coroners. Studies have shown that alcohol is the commonest drug found in persons dying of all causes, but with highest incidences in deaths from violent circumstances (Norton et al, 1982; Baselt and Cravey, 1980).

Ethyl alcohol is also one of the leading causes of acute overdose deaths, ranking with carbon monoxide and heroin (Garriott et al, 1982; Taylor and Hudson, 1977).

It is therefore of great importance in forensic autopsy investigations to perform accurate analyses for alcohol, using the optimal specimens for this purpose, and to know the significance (and limitations) of alcohol findings in these specimens.

ANALYTICAL CONSIDERATIONS

The blood or other fluids or tissues taken at a postmortem examination for alcohol analysis are more likely to be contaminated with volatile substances that could potentially interfere with alcohol analysis as compared with specimens from living subjects.

These interfering substances include methanol and formaldehyde from embalming processes; low boiling decomposition products, such as other alcohols; and abnormal metabolic products, such as acetone (eg, as is formed in deaths resulting from malnutrition or starvation, or in diabetic ketoacidosis). Alcoholics may ingest liquids that contain rubbing alcohol (isopropanol), wood alcohol (methanol), antifreeze (ethylene glycol), or various other volatile solvents.

Therefore it is even more essential when analyzing postmortem samples for alcohol to utilize a completely specific technique. These interfering components would interfere most with the nonspecific oxidation techniques, and least with gas chromatographic procedures, which are designed to separate all low-boiling compounds eluting in the same range as ethyl alcohol (see chapter 8).

An advantage in analysis of postmortem cases is that a greater choice of specimens is available. Whether or not decomposition is present, it may be desirable to analyze additional specimens for optimal interpretation.

DISTRIBUTION OF ALCOHOL IN THE BODY

Blood

Blood is the most important of autopsy specimens to analyze for alcohol, and other specimens analyzed are usually related to blood concentrations. The blood itself is subject to variation, depending on site of sampling, collection technique, and other factors to be discussed. In living subjects, venous blood is sampled, usually from the anterior cubital vein of the arm. After death, peripheral blood is much more difficult to obtain, and sampling is usually from the heart or major vessels. Arterial blood is up to 40% higher in alcohol concentration than venous blood in the absorptive phase, whereas there is little difference between the two specimens in the postabsorptive phase (see chapter 4 for a more detailed discussion of arterial-venous differences). Thus blood from the heart or other large blood vessels may differ from venous blood in alcohol concentration just prior to death (Forney et al, 1950; Martin et al, 1984). This difference was demonstrated by comparing heart blood with femoral blood in 51 cases, 35 of which had higher cardiac blood alcohol concentrations, the greatest difference observed being 0.09 g/dL (Turkel and Gifford, 1957).

It is for this reason that it is often desirable to analyze several specimens comparatively, to optimally relate the alcohol concentrations found in a deceased individual to those that would have been found at the time of death.

Other Body Tissues

Alcohol is distributed primarily in the body water. Consequently, the alcohol concentration in various organs or body fluids is dependent on the water content of that specimen. Harger et al (1937), after administering alcohol to dogs, reported that when equilibrium is reached (after two to three hours), the brain, liver, muscle, stomach tissue, upper intestine, and lower intestine store practically the same amount of alcohol per gram of water. Their calculated distribution ratios after equilibrium, based on brain as 1.00, were: blood 1.18±0.08; liver 0.94±0.04; muscle 1.01±0.04; stomach contents 1.13±0.08; stomach tissue 0.93±0.06; upper intestine 0.97±0.03, and lower intestine: 0.99±0.05. Spinal fluid–blood ratios in 46 human subjects averaged 1.18±0.09.

Since blood is today the most commonly utilized specimen for alcohol analysis (both living and postmortem) the values of Harger et al. may be converted to tissue- or fluid-blood ratios for more useful comparisons (Table 5-1).

A recent study reported the skeletal muscle–blood ratio in rats to be 0.97 two hours after alcohol dosing using femoral muscle (Nanikawa et al, 1982). Harger et al (1937) stated that muscle lagged about four hours behind the other tissues in the time required to reach equilibrium and reported a femoral muscle–blood ratio of 0.856. The reason for the difference in the ratios reported for the two species is not apparent, and equilibrium times are not known for humans. In the studies of Harger et al all tissues were in equilibrium at three hours, at which time only 1% of the alcohol dose remained unabsorbed in the stomach. At 30 minutes the unabsorbed alcohol was dependent on the dose; 6.2% and 49.1%, respectively, remained after 0.5- and 6.0-g/kg doses.

Luvoni and Marozzi (1968) studied tissue distribution of alcohol in 59 human autopsies, and found that they could be divided into two groups: those with tissue concentrations of alcohol lower than those in the blood, and those with tissue concentrations higher than those in the blood. Those with lower tissue concentrations were presumed to have been in the preabsorption phase after alcohol ingestion, while those

Table 5-1
Alcohol Distribution Ratios in Various Organs and Body Fluids After Equilibrium

	Distribution Ratio	Water Content (%)
Whole blood	1.00	78.6
Brain-Blood	0.847	76.3
Liver-Blood	0.797	73.2
Femoral Muscle-Blood	0.856	70.6
Stomach Contents-Blood	0.958	92.5
Stomach Tissue-Blood	0.788	79.9
Upper Intestine-Blood	0.788	55.7
Lower Intestine-Blood	0.876	77.4
CSF-Blood	1.18	92.7

Based on data from Harger et al (1937).

with higher concentrations were in the postabsorptive phase. They concluded that only when the individual was in the postabsorptive phase at death, could be blood alcohol concentrations be predicted from concentrations of the tissues.

Brain alcohol concentrations appear to be subject to regional differences. Meyer (1959) reported the following brain-blood distribution ratios after administering a 3-g/kg dose to rats and permitting equilibrium to be established: telencephalon 0.689; diencephalon and mesencephalon 0.546; cerebellum 0.55; and medulla oblongata 0.426. He suggested that brain distribution depends more on blood supply than on water content. These ratios are considerably lower than those reported by some other authors, however.

In a more recent study of human autopsy tissue, brain-blood ethanol ratios varied from 0.29 to 8.00, with 82% of the values between 0.80 and 1.50. The mean ratio was 1.24, with a standard deviation of 1.01. If one eliminates the single 8.00 observation (occurring with a blood alcohol of only 0.01%) the range of ratios would be 0.29 to 2.00 (Budd, 1983). From these observations, it would seem unwise to attempt to extrapolate brain alcohol concentrations to those of blood unless one were careful to analyze a sample representative of the whole brain. The study of Harger et al (1937) used the whole brain.

The organ-blood ratios are relatively consistent, provided the subject was in the postabsorption phase of alcohol distribution. Postabsorption means after that point in time when all ingested alcohol has been absorbed from the gastrointestinal (GI) tract. In dogs, Harger et al (1937) found that three hours after a single dose, virtually all alcohol had been absorbed. In the interim, the alcohol is present in irregular proportions in various organs, and no good extrapolation can be made.

In order to determine this postabsorptive condition, it has been suggested that an analysis for ethyl alcohol be performed on the gastric contents (Backer et al, 1980). If the concentration is greater than 0.5 g/100 mL, the subject has most likely ingested alcohol recently, and is in the preabsorptive state, whereas if the level is less than 0.5 g/dL, the individual can be considered to be in the postabsorptive phase. In a study of 60 autopsy cases using these criteria, Backer et al obtained good agreement between the theoretical ratios and the actual ratios for brain, bile, spinal fluid, and urine in 37 autopsy cases with stomach alcohol concentrations less than 0.5 g/dL. They found that the bile-blood ratio was the least variable and that bile could be used more reliably than other tissues to predict the blood alcohol concentration both in the preabsorptive and the postabsorptive phases. Average tissue-blood ratios obtained from 37 human autopsy cases with stomach alcohols less than 0.5 g/dL were: bile 0.99; brain 0.91; spinal fluid 1.16; vitreous humor 1.19; and urine 1.32.

Vitreous Humor

The vitreous humor of the eye has been used extensively for toxicological analyses in recent years, and found to be an extremely useful specimen for postmortem alcohol determinations. The advantages of its use are that it is readily available and easily collected, there is less chance of bacterial contamination than in blood and other organs, and alcohol enters the vitreous and establishes equilibrium about as fast or faster than in other body compartments. Approximately 2.0 mL of vitreous fluid can be collected from each eye, which is sufficient for alcohol analysis and often for other toxicologic procedures.

The ratio of alcohol concentration in the blood and vitreous humor is dependent upon the time after ingestion, as is that of other body organs and fluids. However, the time required for establishment of equilibrium values is not as lengthy as for most other organs and fluids. In experiments reported by Hentsch and Müller (1965), and Garriott (1976), alcohol was given orally to rabbits in a single dose, after which the animals were sacrificed periodically, and vitreous alcohol concentrations were measured. Prior to one hour, the alcohol concentrations were higher in the blood by about 0.05 g/dL but at about one hour, the two specimens equilibrated, and the concentrations were approximately the same for a short period. After this period, the vitreous humor concentration reached a higher value than blood, and remained so until complete disappearance (Figure 5-1).

Since the average water contents of blood and vitreous humor are

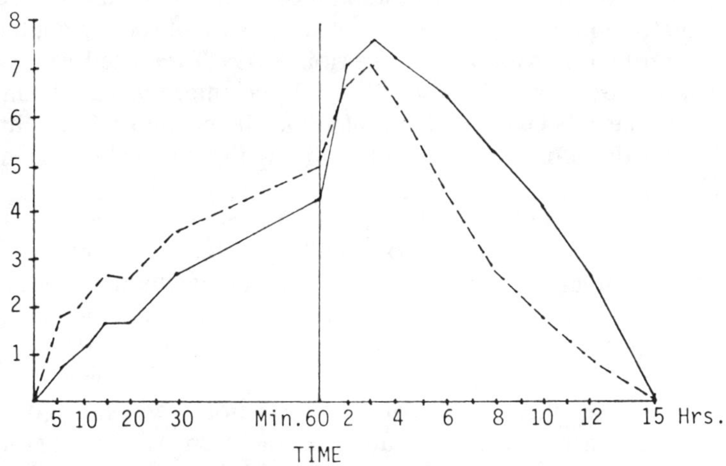

Figure 5-1 Comparative blood (dotted line) and vitreous humor (solid line) alcohol concentrations after oral dosing in rabbits (reproduced with permission from Hentsch and Müller, 1965).

78% and 99%, respectively, the average vitreous-blood ratio should be about 1.27, when distribution is complete.

A number of investigators have performed blood and vitreous humor analyses for alcohol in human autopsy specimens. In 174 cases, Coe and Sherman (1970) found an average vitreous-blood ratio of 1.12. Felby and Olsen (1969) found an average ratio of 1.37 in 31 cadavers. They pointed out that hemoconcentration could account for a higher ratio, and that those dying before diffusion equilibrium is reached (with vitreous-blood ratio of less than 1.0) will have lower ratios.

Backer et al (1980) reported an average ratio of 1.19 (range 0.86–1.72) in 37 cases with stomach alcohol concentrations less than 0.5 g/dL. When the stomach concentrations were greater than 0.5 g/dL, indicating recent ingestion, the average ratio was 0.89 (range 0.48–2.00). Sturner and Coumbis (1966) found an average ratio of 1.12 in 38 cases, the ratios varying from 0.46 to 5.4. They reported a wider range between the two specimens in cases with higher blood alcohol levels. Of course, the comparison of blood and vitreous humor alcohol concentrations in postmortem cases depends on the time between ingestion and death. In postmortem cases this is rarely established, so a wide variation can be expected.

The general relationship between the vitreous humor and blood alcohol after a single-dose ingestion is shown in Figure 5-1. One could estimate the blood alcohol concentration from the vitreous humor reasonably accurately if it could be assumed that death occurred at least two hours after ingestion of any alcohol. If based on the water contents of the two fluids as exists premortem, the ratio for conversion would be, as mentioned above, 1.27. This estimate could in fact be more accurate than actual blood analysis, due to the more variable water content of postmortem blood. Audrlicky and Pribilla (1971) reported water contents varying from 68.2% to 90.1% in 20 postmortem blood samples taken from the subclavian or femoral vein. The postmortem pooling of blood could therefore lead to artificially high or low values for blood alcohol.

These aberrations are probably due to variations in the hematocrit values (cell volume) resulting from pooling of the blood, but are probably not significant in most cases since the fluctuation should be within the difference between the alcohol concentration in whole blood (1.0) and that in plasma (1.12) (Mason and Dubowski, 1974). However, the nearer the bottom of the "pool" from which one takes the sample, the lower the alcohol concentration would be expected to be, due to the increased cell volume and thus the decreased water content. These variations can usually be avoided by taking as nearly a homogeneous blood sample as possible for analysis or by analyzing more than one sample.

POSTMORTEM EFFECTS ON BLOOD ALCOHOL CONCENTRATIONS

Diffusion

One of the factors potentially affecting postmortem alcohol determinations is contamination of the specimen by diffusion from another body organ. If one should die shortly after drinking alcoholic beverages, so that the stomach or upper intestine has a high concentration of alcohol, this would continue to diffuse after death into surrounding organs and blood, causing falsely high alcohol concentrations.

It was shown that alcohol present in the stomach at death may diffuse into the pericardial sac and pleural cavity after death. In 20 autopsies in which 500 mL of 10% ethyl alcohol was instilled into the stomach, false readings greater than 0.15 g/dL were found in the pericardial sacs in six cases. However, blood samples taken from the intact heart chambers or the femoral blood vessels showed no contamination (Plueckhahn and Ballard, 1967; Plueckhahn, 1968). Samples of autopsy blood taken from pooled blood in the pericardial sac or pleural cavities are most liable to contamination by diffusion of stomach alcohol, when present.

It has also been observed that the stomach is unlikely to contain much alcohol at the time of death. After analysis of numerous autopsies for alcohol distribution, Sunshine (1957) stated that "people simply do not die with a bellyful of strong liquor." He also concluded that heart blood is not liable to contamination from stomach alcohol. Backer et al (1980), in a study of 37 autopsy cases with stomach concentrations less than 0.5 g/dL and 23 cases greater than 0.5 g/dL, did not report actual concentrations of stomach alcohols, but observed that only a few stomach alcohol levels actually exceeded 5 g/dL. They concluded that the alcohol diffuses rapidly from the stomach, and that concentrations greater than 0.5 g/dL indicate very recent ingestion.

Although alcohol is absorbed from the stomach rapidly, a larger quantity is absorbed from the small intestine. Thus postmortem diffusion into the abdominal cavity could contaminate any abdominal cavity fluid, and surrounding organs. In general, any cavity fluid or blood should be avoided. A combination of heart, femoral, or subclavian blood, vitreous humor and urine, if available, should be used for alcohol analysis.

Postmortem Decomposition

It is well known that decomposing tissues in the body can produce alcohol. The mechanisms and details of this phenomenon are discussed in chapter 9.

A major problem in forensic alcohol analysis lies in attempting to determine if the alcohol found was from antemortem ingestion or if all or a portion of the alcohol was produced postmortem. The object is to determine if the subject was intoxicated at the time of his death and, if so, what blood alcohol concentration had been present. Ethyl alcohol formed by postmortem decomposition is the same ethyl alcohol that is ingested in alcoholic beverages. Therefore one cannot determine analytically ingested alcohol versus alcohol formed postmortem.

Many factors have to be considered in making this interpretation. One of the most important considerations is the distribution of alcohol in the body at postmortem. One can generally utilize the distribution ratios determined in antemortem studies to interpret postmortem values.

The vitreous humor and urine are of utmost value in this determination since glucose (the major substrate for alcohol formation) is usually of very low concentration. Of course, in advanced decomposition, neither these fluids nor blood are usually available. However, in most postmortem cases, vitreous humor is present. Urine is less reliably available due simply to the normal periodic emptying of the bladder. In a study of 130 decomposing bodies, vitreous humor was obtained in 70% of cases, while urine was available in only 35%. Vitreous humor was reported to be present until advanced decomposition (Zumwalt et al, 1982).

In the mild to moderately decomposed body, the eye chamber is intact, and vitreous humor can be obtained for alcohol analysis, for comparison with blood or urine. If the vitreous humor contains no alcohol, any alcohol found in blood or other body specimens can be assumed to have been formed postmortem. Vitreous humor is generally protected from bacterial contamination and has not been reported to produce ethanol endogenously.

In the intact, decomposing body, ethyl alcohol is usually not formed rapidly, and rarely reaches high levels in postmortem blood. In one study, 24 (80%) of 30 mildly decomposing bodies contained no ethanol. Only one of those found positive could be presumed to have been from postmortem formation. Of 33 mild to moderately decomposed bodies, 18 (55%) contained no ethanol. Endogenous production was presumed in nine (27%) of the 33 cases. Endogenous ethanol was present in eight (19%) of 42 moderately decomposed bodies, while no ethanol was found in 12 (29%).

In 23 severely decomposed bodies, three (13%) exhibited endogenously formed alcohol, no alcohol was found in three (13%), while exogenous alcohol was found in seven (30%). No determination could be reached in the remaining ten cases.

Twenty-three (17%) of the 130 cases studied had presumed production of alcohol postmortem. Of the 23 cases in which presumed endogenous alcohol was found in blood, 19 (83%) had levels of 0.070 mg/dL or less. Four cases had 0.110, 0.120, 0.130, and 0.220 mg/dL, respectively. The vitreous humor and urine were used as the criteria for determining the presence of endogenously formed alcohol (Zumwalt et al, 1982).

In the "fresh" body, refrigerated within four hours of death, no endogenous alcohol was found, even in the presence of bacterial contamination (Clark and Jones, 1982).

In the more severely decomposed body, when no vitreous humor, urine, or even blood may be available, the interpretation of alcohol levels is much more difficult. All body tissues can form alcohol, and the amounts formed in organs are usually greater than those in blood. A good indication of putrefactive processes in tissue is the presence of other alcohols and putrefactive products. *N*-propanol production was found to agree closely with ethyl alcohol production in muscle and blood of rat corpses. The *n*-propanol concentrations were generally greater than 10% of the ethyl alcohol concentration in muscle, and greater than 5% of the alcohol concentration in blood. The postmortem production of ethanol was always greater in blood than in muscle. The authors suggest that a concomitant determination of *n*-propanol in blood or tissues can distinguish between cases in which alcohol was formed postmortem, and those in which it was present antemortem (Nanikawa et al, 1982). In a similar study with dog corpses, stored up to 14 days, *n*-propanol was reported to be present in all cases, and in concentrations up to 32% of those of ethanol. Traces of amyl alcohol also were present in some cases (Mebs et al, 1978).

There is currently no proven method for determining how much of the alcohol might have been formed postmortem, and how much was present antemortem in cases with advanced putrefaction, but further research on other putrefaction products, such as *n*-propanol, or butanol, might lead to at least a partial answer to this question.

Effects of Embalming

The embalmed body has had much of the blood replaced by embalming fluid. Embalming fluids generally contain formalin as the major active component, but also may contain methanol, other alcohols, various odorants, salts, etc. Table 5-2 shows some typical mixtures of embalming fluids (Rendon, 1971).

The most universal contaminants in embalming fluids are formaldehyde and methanol. Although ethanol may be present in some cavity fluids, it is not a standard component of embalming fluids, and would not be expected to contaminate the vitreous humor. Usually, in the embalmed body, vitreous humor will contain a low concentration of

Table 5-2
General Formulations of Embalming Preparations

Ingredient	Composition
Type I (nonformaldehyde)	
EDTA	3.0%
Monosodium phosphate	1.0%
Sodium citrate	1.0%
Sorbitol	10.0%
Methanol	10.0%
Water	74.0%
Nonionic surfactant	1.0%
Type II (primary fluid)	
Borax	4.2%
Boric acid	2.5%
Glycerin	16.8%
Water	47.0%
Methanol	17.5%
Formalin	11.0%
Anionic or nonionic surfactant	0.6%
Reodorant and coloring agents, as desired	0.4%
Type III (arterial fluid)	
Glutaraldehyde	8%–12%
Formalin	8%–25%
Water	27%–42%
Glycerin	6%–12%
Borax	2%–6%
Methanol	15%–26%
Tetrahydrofurfuryl alcohol	5%–10%
Alkyl aryl sodium sulfonate	0.5%–1.0%
Reodorant and coloring agents, as desired	
Type IV (arterial fluid)	
Glycerin	20 lb
Polyarcylic acid (Carbopol 934)	4 lb
Sulfonated naphthenic mineral oil (Atlantic Soluble Oil No. 1)	25 lb
Formaldehyde (46% solution in methanol)	516 lb
P-dichlorobenzene	20 lb
O-dichlorobenzene	42 lb
Pine oil	20 lb
Rhodamine B (2% aqueous solution)	2000 mL
Bismarck Brown (3% aqueous solution)	2500 mL
Sodium hydroxide (crystals)	38 oz
Water	528 lb
Methanol	53 lb
Type V (arterial fluid; diluted to 1 pt [473 mL] with water)	
Trimethylolnitromethane	200 g
Potassium carbonate	5 g
Anionic surfactant (a phosphated, higher alcohol)	5 g
Sulfanilimide	1 g
Eosin dye and perfume, as desired	
Type VI (cavity fluid)	
Formalin	70.0%
Alcohol (methanol, ethanol, or isopropyl alcohol)	29.5%
Wetting agent (Triton X-100 or equivalent)	0.5%

Reproduced with permission from Rendon (1971).

methyl alcohol and/or formaldehyde. Any ethyl alcohol present in the vitreous humor in fresh or embalmed bodies, other than trace amounts, is most likely the result of antemortem ingestion.

ACUTE ETHYL ALCOHOL FATALITIES

Acute alcoholism or death from overdose of alcohol is a frequent phenomenon. In one 10-year study of a major metropolitan area, 91 cases of acute alcohol overdose were diagnosed, which amounted to 0.3% of all deaths seen, and 8% of all deaths resulting from drugs or toxic agents. These deaths were more frequent than those from any other agent, excepting carbon monoxide and narcotics (Garriott et al, 1982). In another comparable survey, 157 acute alcoholism deaths occurred over a 6-year period. These amounted to 9.1% of all deaths due to drugs or other toxic agents. This compared with 13.4% of the cases resulting from acute narcotics overdose (Caplan et al, 1985).

In another study, 2.5% of all deaths certified in North Carolina over a 24-month period were determined to be from acute alcohol overdose (Taylor and Hudson, 1979).

The diagnosis of death from acute ethanol poisoning is usually made on the basis of a high blood ethanol level, combined with circumstances consistent with overdose of alcohol. The usually accepted minimum lethal concentration for alcohol in blood is 0.40 g/dL. Lower concentrations are not necessarily inconsistent with death from alcohol overdose, however. Stress from pre-existent disease, individual tolerance to alcohol, and many other factors may result in lower lethal blood alcohol concentrations at death.

While ethanol levels in excess of 0.30 g/dL indicate severe alcohol intoxication with concomitant respiratory depression, there have been numerous observations of individuals driving a motor vehicle with blood alcohol concentrations greater than 0.30 and occasionally greater than 0.40 g/dL, indicating the wide variation in individual tolerance (Garriott et al, 1977; Taylor and Hudson, 1977; Cimbura et al, 1982).

The acute alcohol fatality usually will have blood ethanol greater than 0.30 g/dL with a vitreous humor level considerably higher. In 213 cases of acute ethanol deaths examined by Taylor and Hudson, 62% of the cases had blood levels greater than 0.40 g/100 mL, while the remaining 38% had levels between 0.30 and 0.40 g/100 mL.

Of 39 ethanol fatalities in another study, a mean postmortem blood alcohol of 0.416 g/dL was found. Levels ranged from 0.237 to 0.592 g/dL (Garriott et al, 1982; Garriott, unpublished data, 1986). Six of the cases had blood levels less than 0.30 g/dL. In these cases, it is usually assumed that the subject may have had a "lethal" blood alcohol concentration some hours before death, and that death was from the resultant brain

Table 5-3
Alcohol Concentration in Acute Fatalities (g/dL)

Age/Race/Sex	Blood (Bl)	Vitreous Humor (V)	V/Bl Ratio
30 W/M	0.59	0.47	0.79
60 W/M	0.41	0.43	1.05
45 B/M	0.35	0.48	1.39
43 B/M	0.24	0.38	1.58
31 W/M	0.24	0.37	1.57
48 W/M	0.52	0.54	1.04
30 W/M	0.33	0.46	1.39
45 W/F	0.39	0.45	1.15
51 W/M	0.50	0.59	1.18
54 W/F	0.35	0.46	1.31
20 B/M	0.53	0.48	0.91
40 B/M	0.56	0.59	1.05
24 W/M	0.59	0.66	1.12
43 W/F	0.36	0.46	1.28
65 W/F	0.54	0.31	0.57
41 W/M	0.38	0.47	1.23
48 W/M	0.37	0.42	1.14
37 W/M	0.40	0.51	1.20
49 W/M	0.45	0.53	1.18
37 W/M	0.64	0.77	1.20
17 W/M	0.35	0.39	1.12

damage, even though the subject survived to metabolize a significant proportion of the alcohol. In such cases, urine and vitreous humor are of great value in supporting the previously higher alcohol levels. Blood and vitreous alcohol concentrations in ethanol fatalities are compared in Table 5-3.

REFERENCES

Audrlicky, I., and Pribilla, O. Vergleichende Untersuchung der Alkoholkonzentration im Blut, der Glaskörperflüssigkeit, der Synovialflüssigkeit und im Harn. *Blutalkohol* 8:116–121, 1971.

Backer, R.C., Pisano, R.V., and Sopher, I.M. The comparison of alcohol concentrations in postmortem fluids and tissues. *J. Forensic Sci.* 25:327–331, 1980.

Baselt, R.C., and Cravey, R.H. Forensic toxicology. In *Toxicology, the Basic Science of Poisons*, 2nd ed. (J. Doull, C. Klassen, and M. Amdur, eds.) MacMillan, New York 1980, p. 663.

Budd, R.D. Postmortem brain alcohol levels. *J. Chromatogr.* 259:353–355, 1983.

Caplan, Y.H., Ottinger, W.E., Park, J., et al. Drug and chemical related deaths: Incidences in the state of Maryland, 1975–1980. *J. Forensic Sci.* 30: 1012–1021, 1985.

Cimbura, G., Lucas, D.M., Bennett, R.C., et al. Incidence and toxicological aspects of drugs detected in 489 fatally injured drivers and pedestrians in Ontario. *J. Forensic Sci.* 27:855–867, 1982.

Clark, M.A., and Jones, W.D. Studies on putrefactive ethanol production. 1. Lack of spontaneous ethanol production in intact human bodies. *J. Forensic Sci.* 27:366–371, 1982.

Coe, J.I., and Sherman, R.E. Comparative study of postmortem vitreous humor and blood alcohol. *J. Forensic Sci.* 15:185–190, 1970.

Felby, S., and Olsen, J. Comparative studies of postmortem ethyl alcohol in vitreous humor, blood, and muscle. *J. Forensic Sci.* 14:93–101, 1969.

Forney, R.B., Hulpieu, H.R., and Harger, R.N. The levels of alcohol in brain, peripheral blood and heart blood ten minutes after oral administration. *J. Pharmacol. Exp. Ther.* 98:8–9, 1950.

Garriott, J.C. Relationship of vitreous humor and blood alcohol concentrations in rabbits. *Forensic Sci. Gaz.* 7:4–5, 1976.

Garriott, J.C., Di Maio, V.J.M., and Petty, C.S. Death by poisoning: a ten-year survey of Dallas County. *J. Forensic Sci.* 27:868–879, 1982.

Garriott, J.C., Di Maio, V.J.M., Zumwalt, R.E., et al. Incidence of drugs and alcohol in fatally injured motor vehicle drivers. *J. Forensic Sci.* 22:383–389, 1977.

Harger, R.N., Hulpieu, R.H., and Lamb, E.B. The speed with which various parts of the body reach equilibrium in the storage of ethyl alcohol. *J. Biol. Chem.* 120:689–704, 1937.

Hentsch, R., and Müller, H.P. Tierexperimentelle Untersuchungen über die Konzentration von peroral zugeführtem Äthanol in Blut und Glaskörper. *Albrecht Von Graefes Arch. Klin. Exp. Ophthalmol.* 168:330–334, 1965.

Luvoni, R., and Marozzi, E. Ethyl alcohol distribution in the various organs and fluids of cadavers. *J. Forensic Med.* 15:67, 1968.

Martin, E., Moll, W., Schmid, P., et al. The pharmacokinetics of alcohol in human breath, venous and arterial blood after oral ingestions. *Eur. J. Clin. Pharmacol.* 26:619–626, 1984.

Mason, M.F., and Dubowski, K.M. Alcohol, Traffic, and chemical testing in the United States: A resume and some remaining problems. *Clin. Chem.* 20:126–170, 1974.

Mebs, D., Schmidt, K., and Gerchow, J. Experimental studies on postmortem alcohol formation. *Blutalkohol* 15:145–150, 1978.

Meyer, K.H. Experimentelle Untersuchung über das Verhältnis des Blutalkohols zum Alkoholgehalt des Gehirns, abstracted from dissertation. *Q. J. Stud. Alcohol* 20:785, 1959.

Nanikawa, R., Ameno, A., Hashimoto, Y., et al. Medico-legal studies on alcohol detected in dead bodies — alcohol levels in skeletal muscle. *Forensic Sci. Int.* 20:133–140, 1982.

Norton, L.E., Garriott, J.C., and Di Maio, V.J.M. Drug detection at autopsy: a prospective study of 247 cases. *J. Forensic Sci.* 27:66–71, 1982.

Plueckhahn, V.D. The evaluation of autopsy blood alcohol levels. *Med. Sci. Law* 8:168–176, 1968.

Plueckhahn, V.D., and Ballard, B. Diffusion of stomach alcohol and heart blood alcohol concentration at autopsy. *J. Forensic Sci.* 12:463–470, 1967.

Rendon, L. Embalming chemicals. In *Encyclopedia of Industrial Chemical Analysis.* (F.D. Snell and L.S. Ettre, eds.), Interscience Publishers, New

York, 1971, pp. 162–164.

Sturner, W.Q., and Coumbis, M.S. The quantitation of ethyl alcohol in vitreous humor and blood by gas chromatography. *Am. J. Clin. Pathol.* 46:349–351, 1966.

Sunshine, I. Postmortem distribution of ethyl alcohol. Presented at the American Academy of Forensic Sciences, Chicago, Feb. 1957.

Taylor, H.L., and Hudson, R.P. Acute ethanol poisoning: a two-year study of deaths in North Carolina. *J. Forensic Sci.* 22:639–653, 1977.

Turkel, H.W., and Gifford, H. Erroneous blood alcohol findings at autopsy, avoidance by proper sampling technique. *JAMA* 164:1077–1079, 1957.

Zumwalt, R.E., Bost, R.O., and Sunshine, I. Evaluation of ethanol concentrations in decomposed bodies. *J. Forensic Sci.* 27:549–554, 1982.

6

Breath as a Specimen for Analysis for Ethanol and Other Low Molecular Weight Alcohols

Morton F. Mason
Kurt M. Dubowski

The use of breath analysis for alcohol in traffic law enforcement arose in order to avoid the involvement of a physician or a nurse in the process of arrest, charge, and trial of a subject suspected of DWI (driving while intoxicated).* Their participation was required because to obtain blood as a specimen the body must be entered. Although urine could be collected by police officers, it was generally recognized that, for a number of reasons, its concentration of ethanol might vary widely from that in the blood at the time of arrest. The need to use medical personnel often lengthened the time between apprehension and actual drawing of blood and, in addition, the final report on its analysis might be excluded from trial if the physician or nurse were not present to testify, or if there were defects in the record of the chain of custody of the specimen. Further, the specimen, in most instances, was venous blood and thus, except after absorption and distribution had been completed, did not reflect, precisely, the concentration of ethanol in the blood supply of the brain, whereas the ethanol in alveolar (deep lung) air is in equilibrium with that of arterial blood plasma which *is* the concentration to which the brain is exposed.

To shorten maximally the interval between apprehension and procuring of a specimen of breath requires the use of an instrument or device suitable for being carried in patrol vehicles. Some of the larger

*Unless otherwise specified, the term "alcohol" will refer to ethanol. For convenience the terms will often be used interchangeably.

instruments, eg, the Breathalyzer, are stationed at police headquarters or substations so that the interval may be variably prolonged, depending upon distance and traffic density, in which to reach the test site.

For many years the concentration of ethanol found in breath was converted by *calculation* to a presumed blood concentration which was the quantity reported and upon which any charge of violation of law was based. Not only was the calculation difficult for a jury to understand, but "in actual law-enforcement practice, when a breath-sample is analyzed for alcohol, the quantity found cannot be used to calculate the simultaneously existing actual blood concentration without making assumptions having uncertain validities in any given case because they have not been assessed" (Mason and Dubowski, 1974; Mason and Dubowski, 1976). This view was supported and documented by the unacceptable lack of agreement of found and calculated concentrations in numerous blood-breath correlation studies and in the discordant values reported for the blood-breath concentration ratio for alcohol, which varied considerably from the value of 2100:1 which, essentially arbitrarily, was employed for many years (Mason and Dubowski, 1974; Borkenstein et al, 1972).

In the United States these matters have been, it is hoped, recently resolved by acceptance of recommendations of the Committee on Alcohol and Other Drugs of the National Safety Council (National Safety Council, 1979) and by the action of the National Committee on Uniform Traffic Laws and Ordinances (1979) to amend section 11-902.1a of the Uniform Vehicle Code (UVC) (1980) to read that "Alcohol concentration shall mean either grams of alcohol per 100 milliliters of blood or grams of alcohol per 210 liters of breath."

Thus the offense of DWI is defined, not only in respect to concentration of alcohol in the blood, but also in terms of exceeding a specified concentration of alcohol, *analytically determined*, in a specimen of breath. (It should be noted that alveolar [deep lung] air is not required. Inasmuch as in an otherwise correctly performed breath test, failure to obtain air *only* of alveolar composition gives a nearly proportionately lower result and is without prejudice to the defendant, the question of the specimen being entirely alveolar in origin need not arise.)

HISTORY OF BREATH ALCOHOL ANALYSIS

Reports of detection of alcohol in breath and subsequent development of methods for breath analysis considerably preceded forensic applications, eg, the demonstration of alcohol in human breath after consumption of wine in 1847 and analyses for alcohol in rabbit breath (Bouchardat and Sandras, 1847; Subbotin, 1891). The earliest English-language publication is that of Anstie in 1874 (Anstie, 1874). Since then many methods and instruments have been described and references to them may be found in several sources; (Harger et al 1950; American Medical Association, 1959; Dubowski, 1973; Forrester, 1960; American Medical Association, 1970; Dubowski, 1970; Mason and Dubowski, 1974; Mason and Dubowski, 1976).

Although presently most breath alcohol analyses are for forensic purposes related to traffic law enforcement, some are done for diagnostic purposes and in evaluation of subjects upon admission to a hospital to determine whether observed symptoms, signs, or other immediate causes for need for medical help are alcohol-related. Examples include unexplained coma, signs of cirrhosis of the liver, trauma from unexpected workplace accidents, and, especially, injuries caused by violence such as gunshot, stabbing, blunt weapon trauma, vehicular accidents, etc. Any of these occurrences can lead to later civil litigation or criminal prosecution.

Other applications of breath analysis than for alcohol have considerably expanded as technologies for vapor-phase analysis have further developed. Thus, by 1974, 135 compounds had been identified in breath and two to three times as many had been separated (ie, detected) (Ellin et al, 1973; Ellin et al, 1974; Pauling et al, 1971, 1976). Dubowski (1974) listed applications that might be encountered in a clinical chemistry laboratory. The list included nine methods or devices for determination of ethanol, four for diagnosis, seven for physiologic and metabolic studies, three for therapeutic monitoring, two for occupational health monitoring, and only two primarily for other forensic purposes. Since that time the number of other clinical applications has greatly increased (Manolis, 1983). For the years 1976 to 1978 a National Library of Medicine literature search revealed 49 clinical applications (including several which involved industrial monitoring and could have forensic uses) and only eight with clear-cut relevance to the forensic purposes of breath analysis. The scope of the expanded clinical applications is revealed by (Perman et al, 1978; Schneider et al, 1978; Haines et al, 1977; Schoeller et al, 1977; Lauterburg, 1978).

During the 1920s there were rapid increases in the number of vehicles and miles driven, and irregular increases in traffic density along with increases in vehicular speeds and accelerations attainable. There was an accompanying rise in death and injury from accidents involving drivers, passengers, and pedestrians. After repeal of prohibition in 1933, a sharp rise in alcohol-related deaths and injuries became apparent, resulting in a demand for statutory control of alcohol in relation to traffic.

A number of states passed legislation requiring a driver "to have command of the normal use of his mental and physical faculties in order to legally operate a motor vehicle." It soon appeared that statutory definition of "normal use" in terms of concentration of alcohol in the blood was desirable, but this required guidelines for specification of the relation between blood alcohol concentration (BAC) and degree of impairment. On the basis of scanty experimental evidence available at the time, the Committee on Tests for Intoxication (now the Committee on Alcohol and Other Drugs) of the National Safety Council (1938) and a committee report approved by the House of Delegates of the American Medical Association in 1939 presented such guidelines which provided the basis for statutory law in a number of states, Indiana in 1939 being the first. These guidelines were to the effect that any individual having a blood alcohol concentration in excess of 0.15% wt/vol (1.5 g/L or 150 mg/dL) was to be considered under the influence of alcohol and that if values between 0.05% wt/vol and 0.15% wt/vol were found he might or might not be under the influence, with the decision to rest upon other evidence. If the concentration found was less than 0.05% wt/vol, he was not to be prosecuted for driving while under the influence of alcohol (American Medical Association, 1939). As experimental information on these matters accumulated, these guidelines were modified over the next three decades (Mason and Dubowski, 1976).

The significant changes which took place during this period in the utilization of breath alcohol analysis have been reviewed in detail (Mason and Dubowski, 1974; Mason and Dubowski, 1976). It was soon recognized that estimating the volume of alveolar air in a breath specimen on the basis of the weight of carbon dioxide present was fraught with error and abandonment of this practice was urged by the Committee on Alcohol and Drugs of the National Safety Council, followed by extensive documentation of its position (National Safety Council, 1967, 1968; Dubowski, 1975).

In 1960, the National Safety Council Committee on Alcohol and Drugs recommended that the presumptive definition of alcoholic impairment of drivers be lowered to 0.10% wt/vol (National Safety Council, 1979). Although this was not uniformly accepted by the various states in statutory law and enforcement, it resulted in more vigorous scrutiny of breath test results in courts, and with this, airing of such matters as the magnitude of discrepancies in the results of blood-breath studies. Further, there was lack of agreement on the value of the blood-breath ratio for alcohol which was used to convert a breath concentration finding to a presumed blood concentration. At the same time, there was general recognition of the evidence relating driving impairment to BAC and that about 40% of vehicular injuries and deaths were alcohol-related. In one notable study of vehicular deaths where driver responsibility could be certainly fixed, 73% were alcohol-related (McCarroll and Haddon, 1962).

Federal intervention into traffic matters followed to assure uniformity of traffic laws and procedures, including the reliability of the latter. In 1966, Congress established the Department of Transportation with one of its units being the National Highway Safety Agency (later designated the National Highway Safety Bureau [NHSB] and, in 1970, as the National Highway Traffic Safety Administration [NHTSA]), charged to study motorized vehicle traffic and to develop program standards for the states to reduce its hazards.

In anticipation of what in 1968 became volume 8 of the Highway Safety Program Manual, *Alcohol in Relation to Highway Safety* and its "Appendix A, Highway Safety Program Standard 4.4.8," the Committee on Alcohol and Drugs of the National Safety Council had prepared the document, *A Model Program for the Control of Alcohol for Traffic Safety* (National Safety Council, 1967). Most of its elements were incorporated into the program manual presented in 1968, including limiting breath testing instruments to those designed to collect only "substantially alveolar air" and specific requirements for training of breath test operators, administration of tests with use of necessary scientific safeguards, and periodic inspection of instruments (National Highway Safety Bureau, 1968).

A number of breath alcohol analyses of uncertain capability appeared briefly. Following a recommendation by the Committee on Alcohol and Drugs of the National Safety Council, the NHTSA required quantitative evidential breath testers purchased with federal funds to meet federal performance standards developed in cooperation with the National Bureau of Standards (National Safety Council, 1971; *Federal Register*, 1973). Comments and recommendations on these were made by the National Safety Council and were accepted (National Safety Council, 1974). A qualified products list for devices found to meet these standards first appeared in the *Federal Register* in 1974. The list was amended in 1979 and again in 1980 and 1986 (*Federal Register*, 1979, 1980, 1986). The last list includes 17 instruments meeting all then existing performance requirements for Mobile Evidential Breath Testers, and four devices meeting all existing requirements excluding those for Mobile Evidential Breath Testers, ie, the devices are suitable for evidential testing only at fixed test sites. For analysis of alcohol in remotely collected specimens of breath, nonspecialized gas chromatographs can be used (Dubowski and Essary, 1982). The several remote sampling devices have not as yet had performance standards specified.

SAMPLING

The physiologic and physiochemical considerations involved in the relationship between the alcohol in substantially alveolar air and in pulmonary arterial blood have been summarized by Dubowski (1970, 1974, 1975). The practical application of these by a breath test operator include procedural matters common to all types of instrumentation.

The prime objective in sampling is to procure a specimen of substantially alveolar air, free from contamination proximal to the larynx which could contribute to the amount of alcohol subsequently found by analysis, and which is protected from loss of alcohol by condensation prior to reaching the final measuring device; eg, an oxidizing solution, an optical path, a gas chromatographic detector, etc.

While not presently (1986) a statutory requirement, the collected air should have a temperature of "close" (±0.5°C) to 34.5°C. Hyperthermia will increase the partial pressure of alcohol in the vapor phase from blood and hypothermia will have the opposite effect. It seems likely that instrumental measurement of the delivered breath temperature from which a sample is taken for analysis will be a required feature of evidential breath testers in the future.

Contamination of a delivered breath specimen can result from residual alcoholic beverage in the mouth, by the presence of residual vomitus containing alcohol in the mouth, by the regurgitation of stomach contents, or by eructation of gas having a significant component of alcohol. These can be avoided by careful and constant observation of the subject for 15 minutes to assure that nothing enters his mouth prior to sampling (Dubowski, 1970; National Safety Council, 1968; *Federal Register*, 1979). Salivary flow, reflex swallowing, and absorption into mucous membranes remove the alcohol rapidly and completely from residual beverage and other contaminating materials. Alternatively, and perhaps advisably in the case of denture wearers, the mouth can be rinsed with water at body temperature; but in order to have the residual water come to equilibrium with alcohol in the salivary and mucous membrane secretions, breath sampling must be delayed for at least six minutes during which the subject must be closely observed (Dubowski, 1960; Dubowski, 1970; Dubowski, 1975; Smith et al, 1969). Immediate sampling would give a falsely low result.

Losses by condensation are prevented by performing the test in a room (or closed squad car) with the air and instrument parts leading to the volume-measuring device or light path presenting a minimal surface at an initial temperature of not less than 35°C. Under these circumstances significant loss by condensation, if any, is restricted to the initial portion of the breath which is discarded (see below).

Delivery of the breath can be made from the sitting or standing position into an inlet equipped with a mouthpiece or saliva trap to prevent aqueous droplets from entering whatever volume or optical path-measuring device is employed, which in turn depends upon which instrument is being used. In any event, at least the first two thirds of the delivered breath should be discarded before taking the actual "last phase" expiratory portion to be analyzed which has now reached an alveolar plateau, that is, it is now "substantially expired alveolar air" (Dubowski, 1975).

Difficulty in obtaining a suitable breath specimen is occasionally encountered in intoxicated subjects or subjects who have severe broncho-pulmonary disorders. In most instances, a sufficient amount of less than substantially alveolar air can be obtained in which it is likely that an alcohol concentration in excess of the statutory threshold will be found if the subject is indeed intoxicated.

The concentration of alcohol appearing in alveolar air at a given concentration in the pulmonary blood is independent of the barometric pressure, provided a measured volume of the air is *obtained and analyzed* at existing ambient pressure (Mason, 1974). Following remote sampling, differences in barometric pressure at the time of collection and analysis may be ignored as long as the collected specimen is not reconverted to a volume.

Other suggested safeguards related to sampling include the analysis of at least two breath specimens from a subject (ie, duplicate, but separate, analyses) even though this may not be a statutory requirement. The results should agree within the limits of 0.02 g/210 L, with the lower or the mean value to the second decimal place being reported. Thus values of 0.130 and 0.139 g/210 L would average 0.1345 g/210 L and would be reported as 0.13 g/210 L. Values of 0.175 g/210 L and 0.170 g/210 L would average 0.1725 g/210 L and would be reported as 0.17 g/210 liters, etc.

For vapor from aqueous reference standards or controls of 0.10 to 0.20 g/210 L, duplicate analyses should agree within the range of 0.02 g/210 L. For standards or controls with concentration in excess of 0.20 g/210 L, agreement within 10% of the putative values is considered acceptable. Records of all blank analyses, control analyses, and subject breath analyses with the times and dates and location thereof should be a part of each final completed case report. Details of analysis of controls, blank analyses, and analysis of the sample taken from a subject differ according to the instruments employed and the corresponding directions for use of each should be rigorously followed. Presently, there is no valid procedure known for preservation of Breathalyzer reagent ampules and their contents after initial use (Dubowski, 1986). This issue is still infrequently raised in some jurisdictions as a result of appellate court decisions arising from the notorious Hitch case (*People v Hitch*, 1974).

Collection of a breath specimen or its content of alcohol with subsequent analysis at a different place and time is known as "remote sampling" and several procedures have been described. These include adsorption on anhydrous magnesium perchlorate, first used in the original Portable Intoximeter (Jetter et al, 1941) and later in the DPC Intoximeter (Forrester, 1964); on anhydrous calcium chloride with the Breathalyzer Remote Sampling Unit (Dubowski, 1970); indium tube encapsulation of breath for subsequent analysis by the *GC*-Intoximeter (Penton and Forrester, 1969); collection of breath in a glass tube (Hine et al, 1968), or in an evacuated metal container (Principe, 1974); and several other devices and procedures. A number of early remote sampling devices no longer in general use were described by Harger et al (1956). Adsorbed alcohol is usually recovered by aqueous elution or by distillation with subsequent analysis of the eluate following dilution with distilled water to a known volume.

REFERENCES

American Medical Association. Report of the Committee to Study Problems of Motor Vehicle Accidents. *JAMA* 108:2137, 1937; 112:2164–2166, 1939.

American Medical Association Committee on Medicolegal Problems. *Chemical Tests for Intoxication*, American Medical Association, Chicago, 1959. [See especially Friedemann, T.E., and Dubowski, K.M. Chemical testing procedures for the determination of ethyl alcohol, pp. 20–44; Appendix B, Procedures for analysis of breath for ethyl alcohol, pp. 45–56.]

American Medical Association. *Alcohol and the Impaired Driver. A Manual on the Medicolegal Aspects of Chemical Tests for Intoxication with Supplement on Breath Alcohol Tests*, American Medical Association, Chicago, 1970, 1972. Reprinted by National Safety Council, Chicago, 1976 [see especially pp. 94–100].

Anstie, E.F. Final experiments on elimination of alcohol from the body. *Practitioner* 13:15–28, 1874.

Borkenstein, R., Buck, R., Dubowski, K.M., et al. *Statement, Ad Hoc Committee on the Blood/Breath Alcohol Relationship*, Indiana University Law School, Indianapolis, Jan 1972.

Bouchardat, M.M., and Sandras, De la digestion des boissons alcooliques et de leur rôle dans la nutrition physique. *Ann. Chem. Physique. Ser.* 21:448–457, 1847.

Dubowski, K.M. Necessary scientific safeguards in breath alcohol analysis. *J. Forensic Sci.* 5:422–433, 1960.

Dubowski, K.M. Measurement of ethyl alcohol in breath. In *Laboratory Diagnosis of Diseases Caused by Toxic Agents* (F.W. Sunderman, Jr., ed.), Warren H. Green, St. Louis, 1970, pp. 316–342.

Dubowski, K.M. *Selected References on Chemical Tests for Alcoholic Influence*, 10th ed. University of Oklahoma, Oklahoma City, 1973.

Dubowski, K.M. Breath analysis as a technique in clinical chemistry. *Clin. Chem.* 20: 966–972, 1974.

Dubowski, K.M. Studies in breath-alcohol analysis: Biological factors. *Z. Rechtsmed.* 76:96–117, 1975.

Dubowski, K.M. Letter to the editor, National Safety Council Committee on Alcohol and Drugs. *Am. J. Forensic Med. Pathol.* 7:266, 1986.

Dubowski, K.M., and Essary, N.A. Alcohol analysis of stored whole-breath samples by automated gas chromatography. *J. Anal. Toxicol.* 6:217–221, 1982.

Ellin, R.I., Farrand, R.L., Oberst, F.W., et al. *Collection, Detection, Identification and Quantitation of Human Effluents*, Edgewood Arsenal Technical Report EB-TR-73007, EATR 4779, Dept. of the Army, Edgewood Arsenal, Aberdeen Proving Ground, Md, Oct 1973.

Ellin, R.I., Farrand, R.L., Oberst, F.W., et al. An apparatus for the detection and quantitation of volatile human effluents. *J. Chromatogr.* 100:137–152, 1974.

Federal Register 38 (Nov. 5): 30459–30463, 1973 [Erratum: Section 5.4.4., line 7, should read: "BAC's are within the range of 0.4–0.10 per. . . ."].

Federal Register 39 (Nov. 21): 41399, 1974.

Federal Register 44 (July 7): 3261, 1979.

Federal Register 45 (Sept. 11): 60103, 1980.

Federal Register 51 (April 9): 12257, 1986.

Forrester, G.C. *Chemical Tests for Alcohol in Traffic Law Enforcement.* Charles C Thomas, Springfield, Ill, 1960.

Forrester, G.C. *Manual for the DPC Intoximeter.* Intoximeters-Midwestern, St. Louis, 1964.

Haines, A., Metz, G., Delawari, J., et al. Breath-methane in patients with cancer of the large bowel. *Lancet* 2:481–483, 1977.

Harger, R.N., Forney, R.B., and Baker, R.S. Estimation of the level of blood alcohol from analysis of breath. II. Use of re-breathed air. *Q. J. Stud. Alcohol* 17:1–18, 1956.

Harger, R.N., Forney, R.B., and Barnes, H.B. Estimation of the level of blood alcohol from analysis of breath. *J. Lab. Clin. Med.* 36: 306, 1950.

Hine, C.H., Aitchison, J.P., and Parker, K.D. *The Accutube: A New Method for Determination of Alcohol in Breath.* Hine Laboratories, San Francisco, 1968.

Jetter, W.W., Moore, M., and Forrester, G.C. Studies in alcohol. IV. A new method for determination of breath-alcohol. *Am. J. Clin. Pathol.* 5:75–89, 1941.

Lauterburg, B.H., Newcomer, A.D., and Hofmann, A.F. Clinical value of the bile acid breath test. Evaluation of the Mayo Clinic experience. *Mayo Clin. Proc.* 53:227–239, 1978.

McCarroll, J.R., and Haddon, W., Jr. A controlled study of fatal automobile accidents in New York City. *J. Chron. Dis.* 15:811–826, 1962.

Manolis, A. The diagnostic potential of breath analysis. *Clin. Chem.* 29:5–15, 1983.

Mason, M.F. A note upon barometric pressure and breath-alcohol analysis. *J. Forensic Sci.* 19:325–326, 1974.

Mason, M.F., and Dubowski, K.M. Alcohol, traffic, and chemical testing in the United States: A resume and some remaining problems. *Clin. Chem.* 20: 126–140, 1974.

Mason, M.F., and Dubowski, K.M. Breath-alcohol analysis: Uses, methods and some forensic problems — Review and opinion. *J. Forensic Sci.* 21:9–41, 1976.

National Committee on Uniform Traffic Laws and Ordinances. Aug. 15–17, Washington, DC 1979.

National Committee on Uniform Traffic Laws and Ordinances. Uniform Vehicle Code and Model Traffic Ordinance, rev. ed. 1980; Section 11–902.1(a), *Michie Company*, Charlottesville, Va. [This publication may be obtained from the National Committee on Uniform Traffic Laws and Ordinances, 525

School St., S.W. Washington, DC 20024.]

National Highway Safety Bureau. *Highway Safety Program Manual*. Vol. 8, *Alcohol in Relation to Highway Safety*. U.S. Dept. of Transportation publication, 1968.

National Safety Council Committee on Tests for Intoxication, *Report: Chemical Test for Intoxication*. National Safety Council, Chicago, 1938.

National Safety Council Committee on Alcohol and Drugs. *A Model Program for the Control of Alcohol for Traffic Safety*. National Safety Council, Chicago, 1967.

National Safety Council Committee on Alcohol and Drugs. *Recommendations of the Ad Hoc Committee on Testing and Training*. National Safety Council, Chicago, 1968. [see appendix A for 66 relevant references to CO_2 in breath.]

National Safety Council Committee on Alcohol and Drugs. *Recommendations of the Ad Hoc Committee on Quantitative Breath Alcohol Instrumentation*. National Safety Council, Chicago, 1971.

National Safety Council *Ad Hoc* Committee of Committee on Alcohol and Drugs. *Comments on Standards for Devices to Measure Breath Alcohol*. National Safety Council, Chicago, 1974.

National Safety Council. *Minutes of the Executive Board of the Committee on Alcohol and Drugs*. National Safety Council, Chicago, Feb. 1975.

National Safety Council. *Recommendations of the Committee on Alcohol and Drugs, 1936–1977, p. 15*, National Safety Council, Chicago, 1979. [The Uniform Vehicle Code was amended to meet this recommendation in 1962.]

Pauling, L., Robinson, A.B., Teraneshi, R., et al. Quantitative analysis of urine vapor and breath by gas-liquid partition chromatography. *Proc. Natl. Acad. Sci. U.S.A.* 68:2374–2376, 1971.

Penton, J.R., and Forrester, M.R. A gas chromatographic breath analysis system with provisions for storage and delayed analysis of samples. In Proceedings of the Fifth International Conference on Alcohol and Traffic Safety. Schulz Verlag, Freiburg, West Germany, 1969, pp II-79–86.

People v Hitch, 527 P2d 372 (Cal. Sup. Ct., 1974).

Perman, J.A., Barr, R.G., and Watkins, J.B. Sucrose malabsorption in children: Non-invasive diagnosis by interval breath hydrogen determination. *J. Pediatr.* 93:17–22, 1978.

Principe, A.H. The Vacu-Sampler — A new device for the encapsulation of breath and other gaseous samples. *J. Police Sci. Admin.* 2:404–413, 1974.

Schneider, J.F., Schoeller, D.A., Nemchausky, B., et al. Validation of $^{13}CO_2$ breath analysis as a measurement of demethylation of stable isotope-labeled aminopyrine in man. *Clin. Chim. Acta.* 84:152–162, 1978.

Schoeller, D.A., Schneider, J.F., Solomons, N.J., et al. Clinical diagnosis with the stable isotope ^{13}C in CO_2 breath tests; Methodology and fundamental considerations. *J. Lab. Clin. Med.* 90:412–421, 1977.

Smith, W.C., Hardin, D.M., Biasotti, A.A., et al. Breathalyzer experiences under operational conditions recommended by the California Association of Criminalists. *J. Forensic Sci. Soc.* 9:58–64, 1969.

Subbotin, V. Ueber die physiologische Bedeutung des Alkohols für den thierischen Organismus. *Z. Biol.* 7, 361–369, 1891.

7

Methods for Breath Analysis

George E. Browne
Alvin Weathermon
Richard Baxter

In order to cover the subject of breath alcohol testing adequately, it is necessary not only to discuss the analytical methods and instruments employed, but also to provide a summary of the physiologic and pharmacologic aspects of breath alcohol testing. To accomplish this task, this chapter is divided into sections, including each of these topics.

The use of breath as a specimen to determine alcohol* concentration in living subjects was initially developed and is currently used primarily in traffic law enforcement to determine the presence and concentration of alcohol in automobile drivers. There are other applications for this technology. Breath alcohol testing may be and sometimes is used in conjunction with diagnostic procedures, employee screening, and in the investigation of accidents of vehicles other than automobiles.

Since 1980 there has been a growing public awareness in the United States concerning the death and injuries caused by the drinking automobile driver. This has prompted most states to enact more comprehensive legislation with stricter sanctions in order to combat this national tragedy. Citizen action groups, such as MADD (Mothers Against Drunk Drivers) and others have been very successful in demanding that more public resources and funds be made available to detect, apprehend, and convict the intoxicated automobile driver.

Some of the public funds made available to combat the drinking

*Unless otherwise specified, the term "alcohol" will refer to ethanol. For convenience, the terms will often be used interchangeably.

driver problem have been used by law enforcement officials to purchase breath alcohol testing devices. The expanded market has resulted in a proliferation of new breath alcohol testing instruments and allied equipment. It would not be practical to list and discuss in a single chapter all of the devices and various models that have been developed. New models or variations of existing models are being developed at such a rate that any attempt to produce a comprehensive review of each would be out of date by the time it was published. However, it is possible to classify breath test instruments by type. Currently, there are three distinct types of instruments.

1. *The passive sensor:* This device only detects the presence of ethanol. It is a hand-held unit that is designed to be used by law enforcement officers in a road block situation. In operation, the officer would hold the unit (usually built into the head of a flashlight) in close proximity to the driver's mouth. The driver is not required to blow into the device; thus the term "passive sensor." A suction fan draws the expired breath of the driver across sensors; an indicator light on the unit will be illuminated if alcohol is present. If alcohol is present the officer would have probable cause to do further investigation. If no alcohol is present, the driver would be released.
2. *The screening device:* There are numerous brands, types, and models of screening devices that use various technologies to detect and approximate the concentration of alcohol in a subject's breath. These are hand-held units that are designed to be used by the officer at the scene of the arrest of a suspected intoxicated driver. The driver is required to blow into the device which will analyze the breath and give an approximate concentration of the alcohol present. If sufficient alcohol concentration is present, the driver would be arrested and transported to a facility where an evidential test would be administered. Some screening devices have a "pass-fail" indicator, usually preset at 0.10 g ethanol/210 L of breath. Below this concentration a driver would "pass the test"; above this concentration, he would "fail." Other devices have a "pass-warn-fail" range. The pass range would be a breath alcohol concentration between 0.00 and 0.05 g/210 L. The warn range would be set between 0.05 and 0.10 g/210 L of breath. Other devices have a digital read-out which gives the approximate breath alcohol concentration. The screening devices are not designed or intended to be used for evidentiary purposes, but rather are used at the

roadside as another tool for the officer to determine if there is probable cause to make an arrest. In some jurisdictions, statutes prohibit their use. It should be noted that even though the screening devices do not have all of the safeguards required for evidential instruments and are intended only to give an approximate alcohol concentration, some units do, in fact, correlate very well with the more accurate and sophisticated evidential instruments.

3. *Evidential breath test instruments:* These are analytical instruments which, if used properly, will give extremely accurate results. The results of analyses conducted on these instruments are admissible in court trials; thus the term "evidential" instrument. Later in this chapter there will be a more detailed explanation of several types of evidential instruments that were being used in traffic law enforcement in the United States according to a 1984 survey. These evidential instruments utilize very basic analytical chemistry methods to determine the presence and concentration of alcohol in the breath. The trend in the newer instruments is to make them more compatible with computers and thus have the capability to not only analyze the alcohol concentration, but also provide statistical data about the testing operation. Laws differ from one jurisdiction to another and consequently there are different testing requirements. To comply with these requirements, some instruments have the capability to conduct duplicate and/or replicate analyses of breath sample. Others have the capability to collect and store samples for later analysis. There are numerous options available in modern evidential breath test instruments.

PHYSIOLOGIC AND PHARMACOLOGIC ASPECTS

There are certain physiologic aspects of the human body and pharmacologic aspects of ethanol that have a great bearing on the use of breath as a specimen for alcohol analysis. That alcohol is infinitely soluble in water is the premise on which all breath testing is based. Under properly controlled conditions, which includes suitable methods and equipment, proper training and continuing expert supervision of competent operators, and adequate control by professionals of equipment, reagents, and procedures, most breath testing equipment mentioned in this chapter will produce highly accurate results (Dubowski, 1960).

Breath and Blood Ratio

Historically, breath analyses have been reported in terms of blood alcohol by converting breath alcohol concentration by mathematical calculation. This calculation, necessary because most DWI laws are based on blood alcohol results, is based on the fundamental principal that the distribution of alcohol between circulating pulmonary blood and alveolar air occurs by simple diffusion and obeys Henry's law (Harger, 1931). Thus, at a given temperature, a constant ratio exists between the concentration of alcohol in the blood and the concentration of alcohol in the alveolar air. At 34°C (the average temperature of exhaled air) this ratio is approximately 2100:1, that is, 2100 mL of alveolar air (saturated with water and at 34°C) contains the same quantity of alcohol as 1 mL of circulating pulmonary arterial blood (American Medical Association, 1972; National Safety Council, 1953).

The word "approximately" in the above statement is responsible for a 30-year continuing courtroom battle over the accuracy of this ratio. A more current review of scientific data tends to confirm that the ratio is probably closer to 2300:1, but that the continued use of the 2100:1 ratio is warranted for law enforcement purposes (National Safety Council, 1979). Breath testing instruments, then, calibrated at 2100:1 would tend to report breath alcohol concentrations approximately 8.7% lower than a simultaneous blood sample. Any actual discrepancy would therefore give a proportionately lower result and without prejudice to the defendant. The "blood" in most comparisons is a venous specimen and thus, except after absorption and distribution has been completed, does not reflect precisely the concentration of alcohol being presented to the brain and the CNS, whereas the alcohol in alveolar air is in equilibrium with that of arterial blood plasma which is the concentration to which the brain *is* exposed (Mason and Dubowski, 1976).

Residual Alcohol

An alveolar breath specimen that is to be analyzed for ethanol can be contaminated by residual alcohol, that is, extraneous alcohol in the mouth either from alcoholic beverage, vomitus containing alcohol from regurgitation of stomach contents, or by eructation of gas containing a significant amount of alcohol.

The effects of residual alcohol may be nullified by careful and constant observation of the subject for the 15 minutes prior to the test (Harger et al, 1950a). This period of observation would ensure that neither eructation nor regurgitation has occurred nor has anything entered the subject's mouth prior to sampling. Alternatively, the mouth may be flushed with water followed by a six-minute delay to allow the residual water to equilibrate with alcohol in saliva and mucous membrane secretions (Dubowski, 1975). Otherwise, immediate sampling could give a falsely low result.

Variance in Body Temperature

Another physiologic factor that applies to breath testing is body temperature. The breath-blood alcohol ratio mentioned earlier depends on temperature and a change in body temperature may cause a change in this ratio and consequently in the validity of breath test analysis expressed in terms of blood alcohol concentration. Using the partition ratio data from Harger et al (1950b), an increase of 1°C of body temperature would theoretically increase the calculated blood alcohol concentration from a breath analysis by 6.5% over and above the actual blood alcohol concentration.

The distribution of alcohol between blood and breath, however, is a complex phenomenon involving not only the equilibrium diffusion process at the alveolar interface, but also sequential distribution of alcohol between the various components of respiratory tract air and exchanges of the water-soluble alcohol in the several breath components with the walls of respiratory dead space (Forster, 1964). These processes attenuate the theoretical variations attributable to temperature quite effectively. Thus, while breath alcohol concentration in various segments of a prolonged expiration does increase somewhat during expiration, the increase is not generally correlated with the observed increase in breath temperature (American Medical Association, 1972; Edwards et al, 1963).

Variance in Carbon Dioxide Content

Some of the older methods of breath alcohol analysis, such as the Portable Intoximeter, employ mixed expired breath. Methods dependent on mixed expired breath estimate the amount of alveolar air involved by measuring the carbon dioxide concentration, assuming that alveolar air contains 5.50% vol/vol CO_2, while atmospheric air contains 0.03% vol/vol of CO_2. However, alveolar CO_2 varies about 13% from men to women and can vary substantially among individuals (Dubowski, 1963b). This, as well as factors mentioned below, have led to breath alcohol devices dependent on alcohol-carbon dioxide ratios being supplanted by those employing deep lung air.

Other Physiologic Considerations

Factors that are more likely to cause variation in the blood-breath alcohol ratio are differential rates of equilibrium at different points in the repiratory tract, the length of time available for equilibration to take place (including the respiratory rate), and individual differences in breathing habits (Greenberg, 1960; Logge, 1965; Wright, 1966). Standard sampling will eliminate most of these potential sources of variation. It is recommended therefore that continuous exhalation be made against moderate pressure and that the initial two third of the sample be discarded (i.e., to obtain deep lung air) (American Medical Association, 1972).

OVERVIEW OF BREATH TEST INSTRUMENTATION

The instruments discussed herein were selected from the study by the National Highway Traffic Safety Administration (1984). The choice of instrumentation in any one jurisdiction is usually mandated by state statutes. The instruments currently being used can be classified under the following three methods of analysis: (1) oxidation-reduction, (2) infrared absorption, and (3) gas chromatography.

Oxidation-Reduction

Methods of analysis based upon oxidation-reduction are characterized by a chemical reaction between two substances wherein the oxidation number of both substances undergoes a change. Universally the substance whose oxidation number increases undergoes *oxidation*, while the chemical it reacts with decreases in oxidation number and is said to have undergone *reduction*; thus the term *oxidation-reduction reaction* (Quagliano, 1964).

Four instruments that operate on the oxidation-reduction method of analysis are currently being used for evidentiary testing (National Highway Traffic Safety Administration, 1984). These are: (1) Breathalyzer 900, (2) Breathalyzer 900A, (3) Breathalyzer 1000, (Chaney, 1975); and (4) the Photoelectric Intoximeter.

Breathalyzer 900, 900A, 1000 The analytical method of these instruments consists of three principal phases: (1) collecting the sample; (2) passing the sample through a potassium dichromate–sulfuric acid solution; (3) measuring the amount of potassium dichromate required to oxidize the alcohol.

In the 900 and 900A models the first phase involves having the subject blow with force into a heated plastic tube. The breath raises a piston in a metal cylinder. When the piston reaches the top of its stroke, it is held in this position by a small magnet aligned with two fixed pole pieces. Two holes just below the piston permit the breath to escape so that when blowing is stopped, the cylinder is full of the last breath.

When blowing stops, the piston drops from its supporting iron plate sufficiently to seal the holes.

A special valve is incorporated in the top of the sample chamber. It is designed to make leaks virtually impossible. The valve and magnet operate on the same shaft, rotated by the control knob on the panel. When the valve is in the TAKE position, the breath passes from the retractable sample tube to the sample chamber. The magnet is aligned with the fixed pole pieces and the piston is supported. When the valve is turned to ANALYZE the magnet is disaligned with the fixed pole pieces and the piston, by its own weight, forces the measured amount of air through 3 mL of 0.025% potassium dichromate in a 50% sulfuric acid solution.

The sample chamber delivers 52.5 mL of alveolar air to the solution. The sample chamber actually contains 56.5 mL. This is necessary because the breath is raised from mouth temperature (34°C) to 47°C to 53°C. The 52.5 mL of breath will occupy a larger volume at this higher temperature. Also, the delivery tube from the sample chamber to the test solution is full of room air before the test and full of breath after the test. This volume must be added to the cylinder volume. This adds up to 56.5 mL. The breath bubbles through the test solution in about 30 seconds. After 1.5 minutes, the reaction is complete.

Before the test is started, the test ampule of solution is balanced photometrically against a standard ampule. The reading light is moved back and forth between the two ampules until the nullmeter centers. This indicates that each of the two photocells is receiving the same amount of light. The position of the light is noted by setting the blood alcohol pointer to the baseline of the scale. After analysis, the reading light is again turned on. If part of the potassium dichromate has been consumed by alcohol, more light will reach the right-hand cell and the nullmeter will no longer be centered.

The light is moved until the balance is again established as indicated by the centering of the nullmeter. The distance the light was moved is directly proportional to the amount of potassium dichromate used, and this is directly related to the amount of alcohol in the breath. The scale is calibrated in percent blood alcohol.

Since 52.5 mL is 1/40 of 2100 mL (the amount of alveolar breath equal to 1.0 mL of blood), the alcohol figure must be multiplied by 40 to obtain milligrams of alcohol per milliliter of blood. This figure must be divided by ten to convert it to percent blood alcohol. These are the figures on the scale.

With this arrangement, line voltage affects each ampule and photocell the same, so changes in this voltage make no difference. For the same reason, changes in intensity of the reading light make no difference. The actual output of the photocells makes no difference since they are balanced before each test. The strength of the test solution is unimportant since only the dichromate used in the test is measured. Thus the instrument does not depend on constant conditions. The only factor that must be maintained is the accurate volume of the test solution. A special gauge is provided to check this volume in each ampule.

Breathalyzer 900A The Breathalyzer Model 900A employs the same principles as the Breathalyzer Model 900. The photometric and collection systems are identical. There are, however, two distinct differences in these systems. The first is the addition of a time delay circuit that does not allow the operator to activate the photometric system during the 90-second waiting period. The second is a modification of the photometric system that replaces the conventional galvanometer with a circuit amplifier and a jeweled panel meter (see Figures 7-1 and 7-2). The only change to the outer configuration is the addition of a light that indicates the end of the 90-second time delay. The operational procedure is identical with both systems except for the operator monitoring the read light.

The *timer circuit* is a resistor-capacitor delayed circuit in conjunction with a field effect transistor amplifier. When the power is applied by activation of the power switch, or by filling and emptying the sample chamber, the timer circuit is activated for a period of 90 seconds. The photometer light is connected in series through the lamp switch to a timing circuit. Utilizing a relay, the timer circuit does not allow power to illuminate the photometer lamp during the 90-second delay. At the conclusion of the delay, the relay is again energized and the photometer light can be illuminated.

Breathalyzer 1000 In this instrument the photometric system's function is to determine the change in light transmittance, which is directly related to the amount of alcohol in the sample, and convert it to a series of electrical impulses which are calculated to provide a reading. This is accomplished by using a balanced photometric system consisting of a pair of matched photocells, two blue filters, and a 50-cd lamp. On each side of the lamp is an ampule, a blue filter, and a photocell. The photocells are connected to a servodriver system. When both cells receive equal illumination, their output current cancels to give a zero input to the servodriver system.

Initially, the lamp is positioned by the servodriver and motor to yield equal output from the photocells. After allowing a sufficient reaction time, the servodriver repositions the lamp to reestablish equal cell output. The distance the lamp must be moved to reestablish balance is directly proportional to the amount of alcohol in the sample. The lamp is driven by a precision threaded shaft wheel. Each full turn of the counter pickup applies 16 impulses to the countercircuits of the control board. The ratio between the lamp carriage travel and the number of counts generated by the pickup is determined by the diameter of

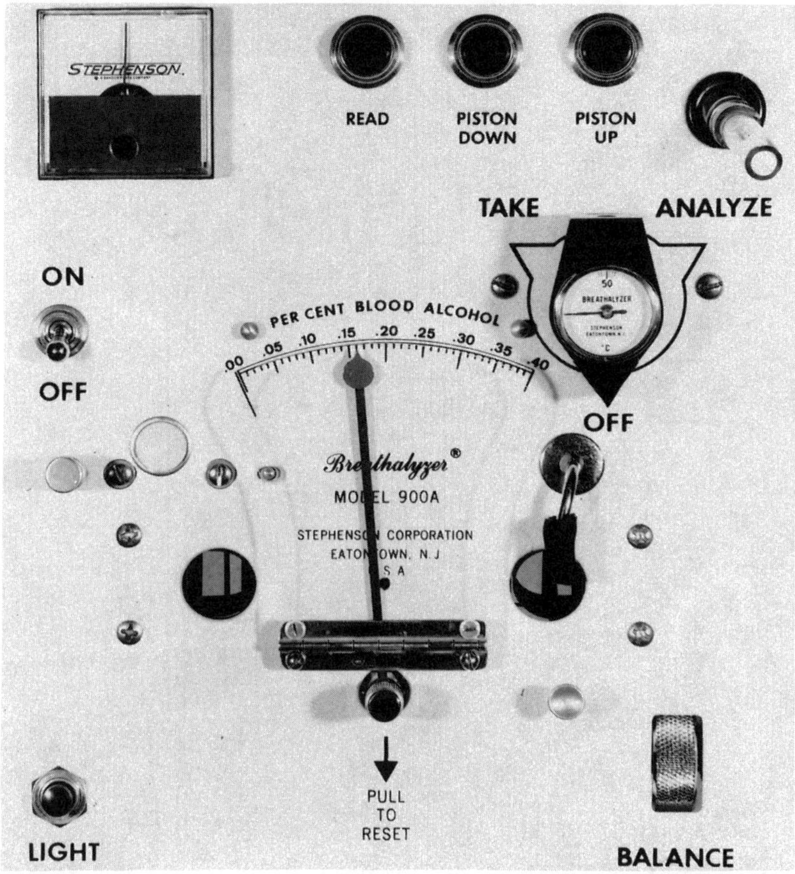

Figure 7-1 Breathalyzer Model 900. The sample chamber is designed to collect and deliver 52.5 mL of alveolar air into an ampule containing potassium dichromate as an oxidizing agent (Borkenstein, 1968).

the calibration wheel. Proper calibration is attained by selection of a calibration wheel with suitable diameter selected at final test.

Photoelectric Intoximeter The Photoelectric Intoximeter collects two samples of alveolar air. One is analyzed immediately in the device, and the other passes through a tube of anhydrous magnesium perchlorate, which absorbs the alcohol for later analysis. The two breath sampling cylinders are similar to the sampling cylinder of the Breathalyzer models 900 and 900A, and 1000. One cylinder contains a volume of 105 mL and the other has a volume of 210 mL, which are, respectively, 5% and 10% of 2100 mL. As the subject blows into the mouthpiece, the first portion of the breath is discarded into a plastic bag with a volume of 500 mL. The route valve is then turned to fill first the 210-mL cylinder, and then the 105-mL cylinder. On further turning of the valve the essen-

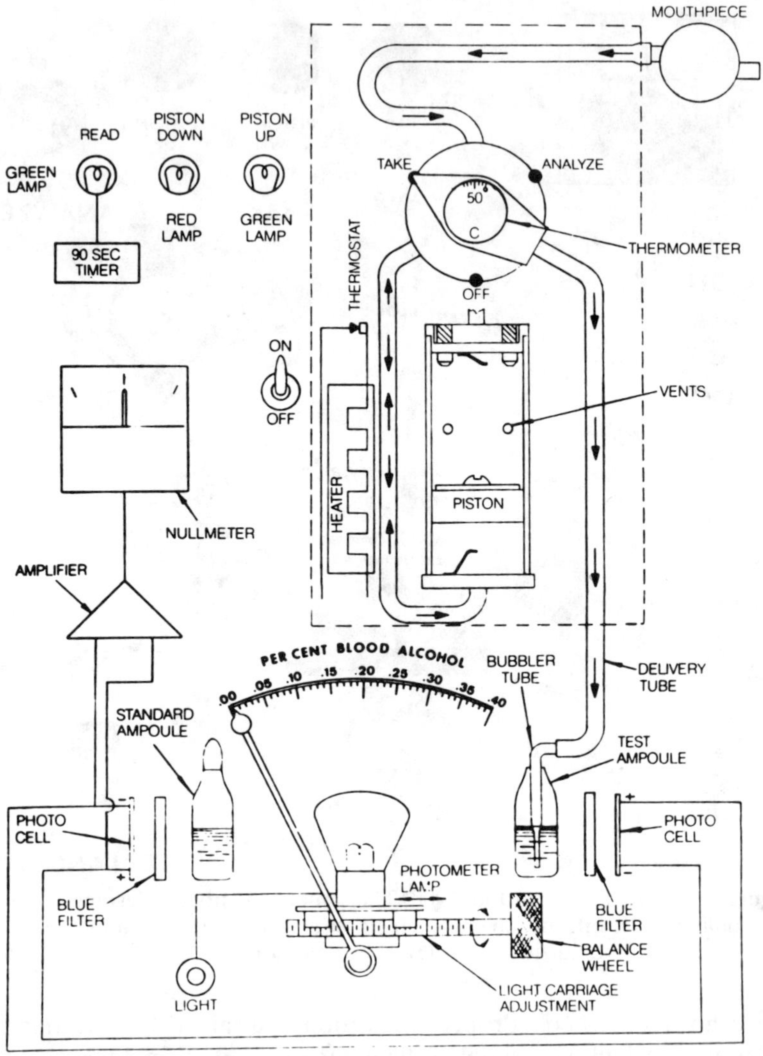

Figure 7-2 Diagrammatic illustration of the operation of the Breathalyzer Model 900. The ampules are balanced against each other before and after sampling by adjusting the "reading" light back and forth between the two until the nullmeter centers. The Model 900A has a time delay circuit to prevent activation of the photometric system during the 90-second waiting period, and replaces the galvonometer with a circuit amplifier (Chaney, 1975).

tially alveolar sample in the 105-mL cylinder is bubbled through the reaction ampule. This ampule contains 4 mL of a solution of 18N sulfuric acid and 0.021% potassium dichromate with a small amount of catalyst.

After a short reaction time the decrease in the yellow-colored potassium dichromate in the ampule is read via the photometer, which is a Klett colorimeter set at 420 mμ. The larger 210-mL sample is passed through the magnesium perchlorate tube to be absorbed for later analysis.

Infrared Absorption

Infrared absorption relies on a different physical mechanism than do other radiation analyses. The absorption of infrared radiation depends on increasing the energy of vibration or rotation associated with a covalent bond, provided that such an increase results in a change in the dipole moment of the molecule. This means that nearly all molecules containing covalent bonds will show some degree of selective absorption in the infrared region (Ewing, 1969).

Breathalyzer 2000 The Breathalyzer Model 2000 (Smith and Wesson, Springfield, Mass) is designed to quantitatively measure blood alcohol concentration by analyzing a breath sample. The incoming sample flows in series through a primary chamber, a secondary chamber, and then exits the instrument. The design of the collection chamber is essentially free flow. Within each chamber the sample passes through a collimated infrared beam approximately 12 in long. The beam originates from a light source external to the sealed sample area of the chamber, and terminates at a filter-detector assembly at the opposite end of the beam, also external to the sample area of the chamber. The primary chamber volume is 52.5 mL at 50°C.

Ethanol molecules absorb light energy in the 2- to 5-μ range in the infrared spectrum. The filter in each chamber allows only certain light wavelengths to reach the detector, screening out all other wavelengths of light present in the collimated beam. The primary chamber employs a band pass filter of a wavelength optimized for ethanol molecules. The secondary chamber employs a band pass filter of a wavelengh chosen for detection of acetone, or materials of equivalent infrared absorption in the breath, in addition to the detection of ethanol.

If only ethanol is present in a given sample, the primary and secondary chamber will quantitatively compare the ethanol concentration of the sample. Only the primary chamber will report the quantitative measurement for purposes of the test. If, however, acetone or materials of equivalent infrared absorption are present in a given test sample, the combined absorption seen by the detector in the secondary chamber will be greater than the absorption seen by the detector in the primary chamber. If the difference in energy absorption between the two chambers represents an apparent alcohol concentration that would cause a reading to be equal to or greater than 0.01% BAC (third place truncated), the instrument will revert to an INTERFERENCE mode, preventing completion of the test.

Additionally, each chamber is partitioned throughout its entire length. Concave reflectors, located externally to the breath sample area, serve to split the light source into two collimated beams. One beam passes through the breath sample side of the chamber, while the other passes through a sealed internal reference standard of nitrogen vapor. If variations in light source intensity occur during a test, the change in signal from the reference side of the chamber will be detected. The instrument will instantaneously adjust the signal from the sample side. This ensures that changes in the energy level seen by the detector and reported in the test results are due solely to energy absorption by the ethanol molecules present in the sample.

Intoximeter 3000 The Intoximeter Model 3000 (Intoximeters, Inc, St Louis) employs the well-established principles of nondispersive infrared (NDIR) molecular absorption. Each organic compound in the breath absorbs infrared energy in a combination of absorption bands at frequencies unique to the compound. The positions of these absorption bands do not change. However, the strength of a given absorption band will vary in direct relation to the change in the number of molecules within a fixed path.

The analyzers use a narrow band pass interference filter to isolate an absorption band at 3.39 μ, which is one of the strong absorption bands for alcohol. A heated element sends infrared energy through a two-chambered gas sample cell of fixed path length. With no absorbing gas in the sample half of the cell, the energy of the sample beam is ratioed against the energy passing through the reference half of the cell. The ratio is used to set the automatic gain control (AGC) and establishes the zero set point. The presence of alcohol in the sample cell will attenuate some of the sample beam energy. The amount of energy attenuated is proportional to the number of alcohol molecules in the sample cell.

The source is formed by embedding a Nichrome helix in a ceramic core. This assembly is then resistance-heated to 800°C. A single source is used to simplify the optics and electronics and to insure stability. It is used so that any change in source character will have no net effect on the system. Extensive source check-out and burn-in yields high reliability in operation. The source energy is modulated at 180 Hz in the sample and reference beams by a slotted chopper wheel.

The sample cell is of a unique two-chamber design. The lower portion is the sample chamber and is ported close to each end to allow rapid sample transfer. The upper portion is the reference chamber. The energy transmitted through the sample chamber is compared to the energy transmitted through the reference chamber. This establishes the zero and automatically corrects for any changes in the cell sensitivity. No reflective optics or surfaces are used inside the sample cell. Consequently, particulates or other coatings will not affect the cell sensitivity.

Polished sapphire flats are used as cell end windows. Diamond is the only other infrared window material that is harder or more chemically inert than sapphire. The unique two-chamber design minimizes optics and does not require critical alignment, which permits rapid cell interchange. The sample cell is heated to prevent water condensation. The temperature is typically set to 45°C.

A specially selected narrow band pass interference filter transmits infrared energy where the sample gas absorbs, while blocking all energy where interfering gases absorb. The filter is mounted on the detector for maximum stability.

The transmission characteristics of the filter do not change with time, ensuring long-term stability. Careful filter selection provides a read-out free from interferences. A solid-state photoconductive detector was chosen for its sensitivity and fast response. The detector is extremely rugged and is insensitive to mechanical shock and vibration.

Intoxilyzer omicron The Intoxilyzer (National Safety Council, 1976) (Omicron Systems Corp) operates on the principle of infrared spectrophotometry. The unit was designed to determine the alcohol content of the breath using no chemicals but utilizing the absorption of infrared energy by the alcohol vapor following the Lambert-Beer law of absorption.

A sample of breath is obtained for analysis by the subject who exhales or blows essentially alveolar air into the sample chamber through a tube fitted with a saliva-trap mouthpiece. Infrared energy from a highly stabilized source is modulated, then collimated by fused silica lenses, and directed through a specially designed sample chamber. At the exit end of the sample cell, a second set of fused silica optics focuses the energy onto the surface of an infrared photodetector. The unit is optically centered at a wavelength at which ethyl alcohol has shown substantial energy absorption.

As the amount of alcohol vapor increases in the cell the amount of infrared energy reaching the detector falls in a predictable exponential manner. The sample cell is heated to remove moisture condensation from the optics. The signal detected is electronically monitored at the source modulation frequency and then is processed through a high-gain, high-sensitivity, low-noise circuit and converted from an AC to a DC signal. This DC analog signal, which represents the exponential relationship between the energy transmitted through the cells and the concentration of alcohol in the cell, is linearized by a signal processing unit, then passed through an analog-to-digital converter and displayed on a three-digit display directly in alcohol concentration expressed as grams of alcohol per 210 liters of breath. A parallel connection operates a digital printer device which produces a hard-copy read-out.

Intoxilyzer CMI There are four models: (1) Intoxilyzer 4011, (2) Intoxilyzer 4011A, (3) Intoxilyzer 4011AS-A, and the (4) Intoxilyzer 5000 (Weathermon et al, 1984).

These instruments, offered by CMI (Colorado Mountain Industries, Mintern, Colo), are essentially similar to the Omicron Intoxilyzer. They are both infrared spectrophotometers, and the only differences between them revolve around the choice of selected filters and packaging. Whereas the Omicron Intoxilyzer uses a selected filter of 3.39 μ to evaluate alcohol concentration, the first units from CMI utilized a filter of 3.48 μ. Later versions utilized a dual filter system wherein alcohol was quantitated at 3.48 μ and a 3.39-μ filter was used to qualitate for acetone.

The latest instrument offered by CMI is the Intoxilyzer 5000 which again is an infrared until but is microprocessor-operated giving the user many more options adjunct to infrared spectroscopy (Figure 7-3).

BAC Verifier The BAC Verifier (Verax Systems, Inc, New York City) was conceived in the early 1970s and subsequently developed in West Germany. A diagrammatic illustration of the operating principles of the instrument is shown in Figure 7-4. Some of the features of the Verifier are:

- Beam path of infrared energy is 1.1 m (44 in.)
- Small sample chamber (52.5 mL)
- Built-in radio frequency interference detector
- Piston and cylinder arrangement that captures fixed amount of sample that can be stored for later analysis
- Quartz plate constant to internally check the electronics
- Differentiation of alcohol from substance with similar infrared-absorption characteristics
- Microprocessor technology: self-calibrating, self-zeros, and, upon request, print-out of a complete internal systems diagnostic check

Gas Chromatography

Gas chromatography is the most extensively employed of all instrumental *separation* methods. It provides a quick and easy way of

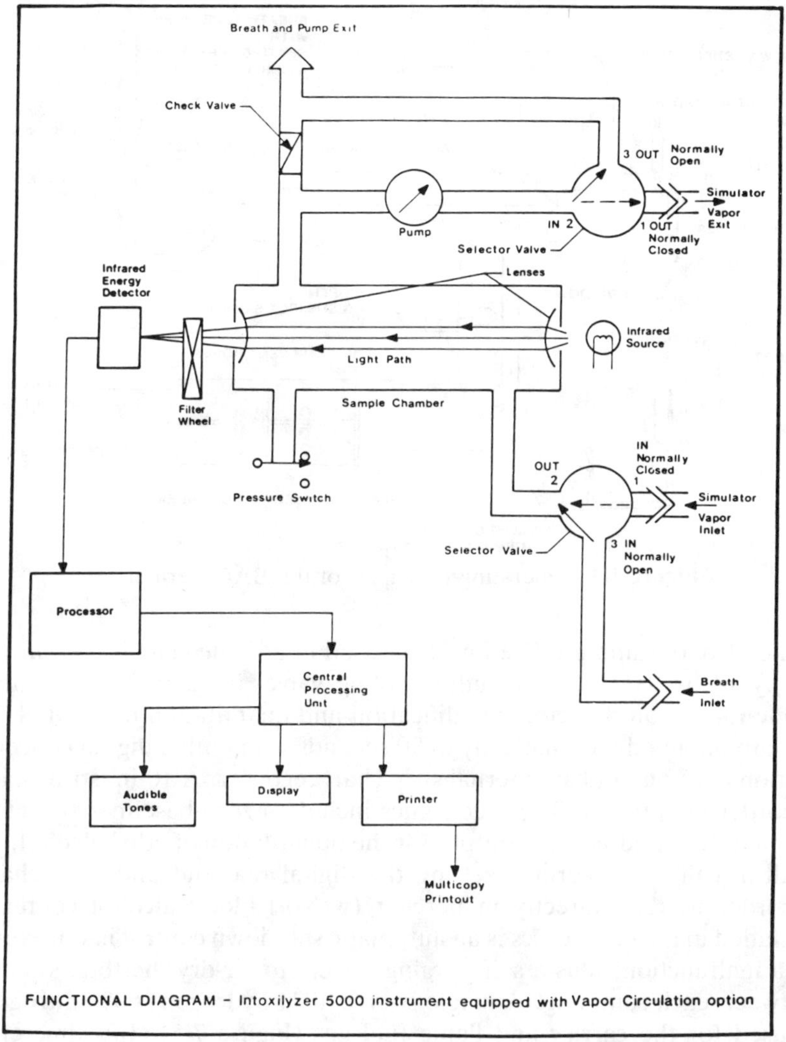

Figure 7-3 Intoxilyzer 5000. Infrared detection of alcohol with microprocessor operation.

determining the number of components in a mixture (Ewing, 1969). According to Ewing, its greatest usefulness may be in qualitative or semiquantitative work. The gas chromatograph can be an essential tool for those concerned with the characterization of covalent compounds of moderate molecular weight.

GAS Chromatographic Intoximeter The Gas Chromatographic Intoximeter (GCI) (Intoximeters, Inc) is a specially designed gas chromatograph which analyzes direct or field-collected breath, blood, and

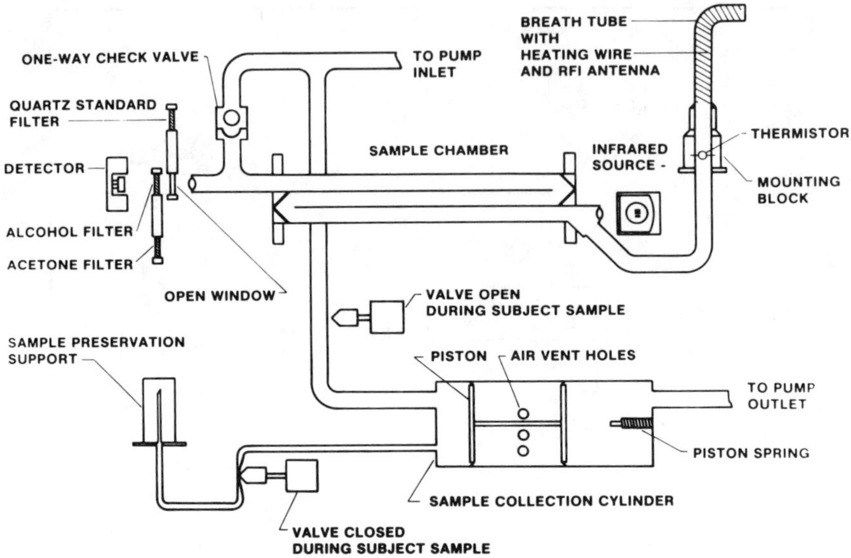

Figure 7-4 Operating principles of the BAC Verifier.

urine alcohol samples. The unit is housed in a single chassis measuring 18 by 14 by 9 in., with a multisampling valve, injector, column, and flame ionization detector. Qualification and quantitation of ethyl alcohol are obtained automatically in 90 seconds with both a digital concentration read-out and an internal strip chart recorder. A 10-in. strip chart recorder is optional. The electronics include a zero-baseline corrector and a differential-integral output for the quantitation of ethyl alcohol. A built-in calibrator permits setting the digital read-out and strip chart recorder to read directly in percent (wt/vol) blood alcohol content. Included in the electronics is an automatic shutdown control in the event of a malfunction, plus a self-purging system to air-dry the total system between each sampling. A single source 40% hydrogen–60% nitrogen is used for the carrier and flame fuel gas (Figure 7-5) (Intoximeters, Inc.).

The unit analyzes a 0.25 mL (fixed volume) sample of deep lung air in both the direct breath and the field-collected sample mode. The direct breath sample is collected in a sample loop after the tidal (upper lung) air is vented into a fixed colume waste bag (1200 mL). To analyze the sample of alveolar air, the operator activates the ANALYSIS button. The sample is carried through the column (separated) and detector (identified and quantitated), and the result is amplified (electrometer) and displayed on the recorder and digital readout as percent (wt/vol) blood alcohol content. Similarly, the field breath sample, collected in an indium tube 0.200 in. in diameter and 4 in. long with a specially designed

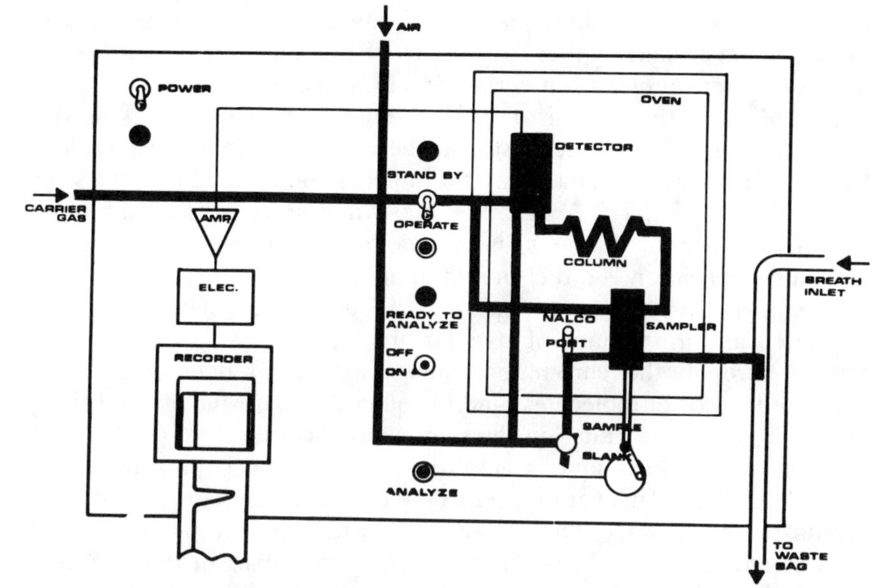

Figure 7-5 The Gas Chromatographic Intoximeter. The specially designed gas chromatograph analyzes direct or field-collected breath or body fluid samples.

Figures 7-2, 7-3, 7-4, and 7-5 were provided by courtesy of Patrick M. Harding, Chemist, Toxicology Section, State Laboratory of Hygiene, University of Wisconsin, Madison, Wiscn.

crimping device, is analyzed with the GCI. A crimped indium tube provides three hermetically sealed capsules of breath (0.25 mL). The capsules are analyzed by placing one capsule in the multisampling valve injector of the GCI and activating the ANALYSIS button. An impinger needle punctures the capsule, and the sample is swept into the column of the unit as above.

Standardization is conducted by a NALCO breath alcohol standard of known concentration. The NALCO standard contains a mixture of alcohol vapor and a dry inert gas. The contents of the NALCO are maintained in a single gas phase in the absence of water. The ratio of alcohol vapor to inert carrier gas is fixed and is totally independent of any temperature requirement. A regulator attached to the NALCO tank releases a fixed volume of gaseous mixture to simulate an ideal breath specimen containing a known percent (wt/vol) alcohol standard to standardize the unit.

ALCO-ANALYZER The oven of the Alco-Analyzer (Harger, 1974) contains two columns, one for direct analysis of liquid samples, and the other for breath or headspace air. Instead of a flame ionization detector, the 0.1-mL exit chambers from the columns each contain a thermistor probe, and the reading of the concentration of alcohol vapor in its fraction is made by thermal conductivity, using a Whetstone bridge in the manner employed in certain combustible gas meters. With the Alco-Analyzer, the thermistor in the unused chamber serves as the reference point for the thermistor in the active chamber. The conductivity differential between the two thermistors operates the pen of a strip recorder, AID No. 240. While the Alco-Analyzer may be used for the analysis of ethanol in blood, urine, saliva, headspace, or breath, its most common application is direct breath analysis.

As a breath instrument it operates in four phases: (1) collection of a measured uniform volume of alveolar breath, (2) passing of the breath sample through the chromatographic column, (3) detection of the separated bands of molecules, and (4) quantitation of the ethanol from the peak height recording on the strip chart recorder.

The specific technique is as follows: The selector knob is turned to BREATH, the oven lever raised to TAKE, and the zero on the recorder is adjusted if necessary. The subject blows with force through the plastic tube connected to the breath input on the oven. Part of the breath is passed through a collection loop, trapping the last 10.5 mL of breath. Moving the oven lever to ANALYZE allows the helium carrier gas to push the sample through a 0.125 in. by 4 ft column containing Porapak 80 to 100 mesh. The column terminates in a detector bridge circuit. The thermistor current change is proportional to the quantity of ethanol passing over it. The current change unbalances the bridge and is read as a voltage peak on the strip chart recorder or as a direct milligram percent of blood alcohol on the digital read-out.

The only expendable items are: (1) a plastic mouthpiece and (2) several inches of chart paper. Each analysis requires approximately three minutes. Analyses may be run continuously every three minutes. The electronics are designed for continuous operation; thus there is no warm-up requirement after the initial operating temperature is obtained.

REFERENCES

American Medical Association. *Alcohol and the Impaired Driver. A Manual on the Medicolegal Aspects of Chemical Tests for Intoxication with Supplement on Breath Alcohol Test.*, 1970, 1972. Reprinted by National Safety Council, Chicago, 1976, [see especially pp. 94–100].

Borkenstein, R.F. *Breathalyzer Model 900 Instruction Manual*. pp. 18–19, 1968, Stephenson, Red Bank, N.J.

Bouchardat, M.M. and Sandras, De la digestion des boissons alcoholiques et de leur rôle dans la nutrition physique. *Ann. Chem. Physique* Ser. 21:448–457, 1847.

Chaney, M.G. *Breathalyzer Maintenance*. Smith and Wesson. Springfield, Ma. 1975, pp. 7–12, 15–17, 31, 74, 79, 83–84.

Dubowski, K.M. Necessary scientific safeguards in breath-alcohol analysis. *J. Forensic Sci.* 5:422–433, 1960.

Dubowski, K.M. *Selected References on Chemical Tests for Intoxication*. University of Oklahoma, Oklahoma City, 1963a.

Dubowski, K.M. In *Alcohol Determination — Some Physiological and Metabolic Considerations*. (B.H. Fox, ed.) Public Health Service publication No. 1043, Government Printing Office, 1963b, pp. 91–115.

Dubowski, K.M. Studies in breath-alcohol analysis: Biological factors. *Z. Rechtsmed.* 76:93–117, 1975.

Edwards, A.W.T., Velasquez, T., and Farhi, L.E. Determination of alveolar capillary temperature. *J. Appl. Physiol.* 18:107, 1963.

Ewing, G.W. *Instrumental Methods of Chemical Analysis*. McGraw Hill, New York, 1969. pp. 119, 450.

Forster, R.E. Breathing tests for alcohol. *JAMA* 190:85, 1964.

Forrester, M.R. Advances in infrared technology for breath alcohol testing with particular reference to the Intoximeter Model 3000, in *Alcohol, Drugs and Traffic Safety*. (L. Goldberg, ed.) Almquist & Wiksell International, Stockholm, 1981, pp. 677–685.

Greenberg, L.A. Physiological factors affecting breath samples. *J. Forensic Sci.* 5:411, 1960.

Harger, R.N. Presented at the Meeting of the American Chemical Society, Indianapolis, Science, *Science News* 73: No. 1892, 1931.

Harger, R.N. *Recently Published Analytical Methods for Determining Alcohol in Body Materials — Alcohol Counter-Measures Literature Review*. U.S. Dept. of Transportation publication No. (HS)371-3-786. Final report, Oct. 1974, pp. 13–21.

Harger, R.N., Forney, R.B., and Barnes, H.B. Estimation of the level of blood alcohol from analysis of breath. *J. Lab. Clin. Med.* 36:306, 1950a.

Harger, R.N., Raney, B.B., Bridwell, E.G., et al. Partition ratio of alcohol between air and water, urine and blood. *J. Biol. Chem.* 183:197, 1950b.

Logge, D. The influence of breath temperature on assessments of blood alcohol level by breath analysis. *Q. J. Stud. Alcohol* 26:371, 1965.

Mason, M.F., and Dubowski, K.M. Alcohol, traffic and chemical testing in the United States. A resume and some remaining problems. *Clin. Chem.* 20: 9–41, 1974.

Mason, M.F., and Dubowski, K.M. Breath alcohol analysis: Uses, methods, and some forensic problems — Review and opinion. *J. Forensic Sci.* 21:9–41, 1976.

National Highway Traffic Safety Administration. *State Breath Alcohol Test Program*. U.S. Dept. of Transportation *Directory of Key Contacts*. Spring 1984.

National Safety Council. Committee on Tests for Intoxication. *Chemical Tests for Intoxication*, National Safety Council, Chicago, 1953.

National Safety Council Committee on Alcohol and Drugs. *A Model Program for the Control of Alcohol for Traffic Safety*, National Safety Council, 1967.

National Safety Council Committee on Alcohol and Drugs. *Recommendations of the Ad Hoc Committee on Testing and Training*. National Safety Council, Chicago, 1968. [see appendix A.]

National Safety Council Committee on Alcohol and Drugs. *Recommendations of the Ad Hoc Committee on Quantitative Breath Alcohol Instrumentation*, National Safety Council, Chicago, 1971.

National Safety Council: *Alcohol and the Impaired Driver*, National Safety Council, Chicago, 1976, pp. 240–262.

National Safety Council *Recommendations of the Committee on Alcohol and Drugs*, National Safety Council, Chicago, 1977, p. 83.

National Safety Council. *Recommendations of the Committee on Alcohol and Drugs, 1936–1977*, National Safety Council, 1979, pp. 15, 45.

Quagliano, J.V. *Chemistry*. Prentice-Hall, N. J., 1964.

Sabbotin, V. Ueber die physiologische Bedeutung des Alkohol für den thierischen Organismus. *Z. Biol.* 7: 361, 1891.

Weathermon, A.W. et al. *Texas Breath Alcohol Testing Program, Operators Manual*. Austin, TX 1984, pp. 4.1–4.7, 1984.

Wright, B.M. Influence of breath temperature on blood alcohol determination by breath analysis. *Q. J. Stud. Alcohol* 27:112, 1966.

8

Methods for Fluid Analysis — Colorimetric and Instrumental

Richard F. Shaw

Methods for the measurement of alcohol in fluids of biological nature such as blood, cerebral spinal fluid, urine, bile, vitreous humor, and infrequently saliva appeared in the scientific literature as early as 1860 (Jain and Cravey, 1972a; Smith, 1965). Bechamp (1865) is credited with the first method using potassium dichromate and sulfuric acid for the quantitative determination of ethyl alcohol. Since then, numerous analytical approaches have been suggested leading to literally hundreds of published or modifications of published methodologies. Generally, the methods have been classified as chemical, biochemical, and instrumental. Comprehensive reviews on the subject have been reported by Jain and Cravey (1972a; 1972b), Cravey and Jain (1974); the American Medical Association Committee on Medicolegal Problems (1973); Dubowski (1977); and Caplan (1982). A number of these methods require separation and isolation of alcohol from the biological matrix by procedures involving diffusion, aeration, distillation, or headspace production, while others require protein precipitation, or direct mixing of biological fluids with a diluent just prior to measurement of alcohol.

CHEMICAL METHODS

Alcohol, due to its volatility, is conveniently separated from biological samples by various techniques and, after separation, can be quantitatively measured by means of reaction with oxidizing agents such as dichromate, permangenate, or osmic acid. In the reaction with potassium dichromate and alcohol in strong sulfuric acid solution, the yellow-orange dichromate ion is reduced to the blue-green chromic ion while alcohol is oxidized to acetaldehyde, acetic acid, or carbon dioxide and water, depending on the condition of the reaction.

One of the earliest methods involving diffusion was that of Widmark (1922) utilizing a specially constructed spoon for suspending the biological sample over a known quantity of potassium dichromate solution in a stoppered flask. The flask was heated allowing for the simultaneous distillation and oxidation reactions to be completed. The cooled dichromate was then titrated with standard sodium thiosulfate using potassium iodide and starch as an indicator. Since 1922, a number of very suitable dichromate methods for determining ethyl alcohol in body fluids have been described (Harger, 1935; Cavett, 1938; Kozelka and Hine, 1941; Shupe and Dubowski, 1952; Sunshine and Nenad, 1953; Bradford, 1958; Kirk et al, 1958) involving distillation or desiccation coupled with conventional distillation apparatus, modified Erlenmeyer reaction flasks, or Conway diffusion cells.

One of the most reliable diffusion methods is that reported by Smith (1951). He used a 50 mL glass-stoppered Erlenmeyer flask with an attached glass cup, similar to that of the Widmark flask. The glass stem is fused to the center of the cup and a strip of filter paper is rolled around the stem and fitted into the cup. A known amount of blood or urine is added to the cup which is suspended over the dichromate solution of known concentration. The flask and its contents are heated in an oven for an hour or allowed to remain overnight at room temperature. The liquid specimen diffuses onto the filter paper and a highly exposed surface area provides for rapid evaporation. Any vaporized alcohol combines with the dichromate solution. Any residual dichromate is then determined either colorimetrically or by titration. Blystone and Collins (1984) described a procedure to measure the dichromate concentration directly at 444 nm with a microcomputer-controlled spectrophotometer. The spectrophotometer interfaced with an HP-85 desktop computer provided additional capability to average and store data.

BIOCHEMICAL METHODS

Alcohol dehydrogenase (ADH), an enzyme, is used in the measurement of alcohol in biological specimens. In the reaction, alcohol is oxidized to acetaldehyde by ADH in the presence of a coenzyme, nicotinamide adenine dinucleotide (NAD), which is further reduced to NADH. This reduced form can be measured spectrophotometrically at 340 nm. In a secondary reaction the NADH can be coupled to a diaphorase-chromagen system producing a red-colored formazan colloidal suspension that may be read spectrophotometrically at 500 nm. This procedure can be automated with microprocessor control and print-out providing rapid turn-around time. The enzyme does not react with methyl alcohol or acetone and only reacts to a lesser degree with isopropyl alcohol and butyl alcohol. Bonnichsen and Theorell (1951) described the first use of ADH for the analysis of ethyl alcohol.

Redetzki and Dees (1976) compared results obtained with four commercially available kits for enzymatic determination of ethyl alcohol in blood. Each of the kits yielded reliable results with acceptable reproducibility. Blood samples containing ethyl alcohol (0.045 g/dL) plus varying concentrations of methyl alcohol (0.05 g/dL; 0.15 g/dL) and isopropyl alcohol (0.05 g/dL; 0.15 g/dL) were analyzed to evaluate the specificity of the assays. As suspected, high concentrations of methyl alcohol increased apparent ethyl alcohol levels only insignificantly and isopropyl alcohol in low concentrations interfered in all kits.

Vasiliades et al, (1978) reported a case of ethyl alcohol and isopropyl alcohol ingestion that resulted in coma. Erroneous analytical results were obtained using the enzyme method because of the nonselectivity of ADH. In this case ethyl alcohol was overestimated and the significance of isopropyl alcohol was underestimated. Jung and Ferard (1978) described an automated enzymatic method for ethyl alcohol determination with a centrifugal analyzer by measuring the rate of the reaction catalyzed by ADH and coupled to aldehyde dehydrogenase. This new method has several advantages over an automated ADH method utilizing semicarbazide. Results show an improved linearity and sensitivity, in addition to the method being more rapid due to a shorter equilibrium time. A rapid electrochemical measurement of ethyl alcohol in blood was proposed by Cheng and Christian (1978). In their method, ethyl alcohol is oxidized by NAD^+ in the presence of alcohol dehydrogenase, and the NADH produced is aerobically oxidized by horseradish peroxidase. The rate of depletion of buffer-carried oxygen, which is directly proportional to the alcohol in the sample, is amperometrically monitored with a membrane oxygen-sensing electrode. Only 5 μL of blood is required, with no deproteinization, incubation, or dilution needed. Results, obtained in less than one minute, correlate well with those obtained by gas chromatographic and spectrophotometric methods.

Poklis and Mackell (1982) evaluated a new ADH enzymatic assay (ADH-glycine, Sigma Chemical Co) for ethyl alcohol in blood. The assay differs from Sigma's previous assay (ADH-pyrophosphate) in that glycine replaced pyrophosphate as the buffer and hydrazine replaced semicarbazide as the trapping agent. The standard curve for the assay was linear over blood alcohol concentrations of 0.05 to 0.50 g/dL. The major advantage of the ADH-glycine assay over the ADH-pyrophosphate assay is the shorter reaction time, ten minutes versus 30 minutes.

Whitehouse and Paul (1979) reported an enzymatic method that has been adapted to the Abbott Bichromatic Analyzer-100. Fully automatic, the method can accommodate up to 192 assays per hour. It requires only 2.5 μL of plasma and therefore is applicable to analysis for ethyl alcohol in blood by finger stick. Takel et al, (1985) described an enzymatic method for detecting ethyl alcohol in blood by use of membrane-bound microbial ADH (no EC number assigned). This enzyme catalyzes the reaction irreversibly and the rate of oxidation can be monitored by spectrophotometry of the reduction of the indicator dye. No pyridine nucleotides such as NAD^+ or $NADP^+$ were used. The specific activity of membrane-bound ADH is 300-fold greater than cytosol NAD–linked ADH (EC 1.1.1.1.) and its optimum pH is 4.0 as compared with pH 8.0 for cytosol ADH. Given these characteristics, the enzyme can be used to detect trace amounts of ethyl alcohol and the enzyme reaction can be performed in an acidic reaction mixture that includes the trichloroacetic acid used to deproteinize specimens of blood, plasma, or serum.

In the forensic laboratory, biochemical methods are not usually used for determining blood alcohol due to their lack of total specificity. Isopropyl alcohol and butyl alcohol interfere in the reaction. For forensic purposes, enzyme methods must be confirmed by an alternate technique (Garriott, 1983).

In 1984, Abbott Laboratories introduced a radioactive energy attenuation (REA) assay for the determination of ethyl alcohol on the TDx analyzer, a microprocessor-controlled automated fluorometer used for fluorescence polarization immunoassay for many therapeutically monitored drugs. In the REA method for ethyl alcohol, the enzyme-catalytic reactions of ADH and diaphorase result in the formation of a reduced iodonitrotetrazolium (INT), a red color chromogen which has an absorbance peak of 492 nm. Because the chromogen's absorbance overlaps the excitation and emission spectrum of fluorescein (a fluorescent indicator added to the reaction) the fluorescence intensity decreases logarithmically with increasing concentration of reduced INT. The concentration of ethyl alcohol is therefore proportional to the degree of inner filter effect on the fluorophore. In addition, no cross-reaction toward methyl alcohol, isopropyl alcohol, or acetone at concentrations that might be expected in toxic situations occurred (Cary et al, 1984).

Recently, Abbott Laboratories reformulated the ethyl alcohol assay by replacing the iodonitrotetrazolium violet dye (INT) with a thiazolyl blue dye (MTT). The reason for this reformulation was to eliminate a probe wash step required after every run in the original method. In the reaction, the reduced MTT now yields a purple color with an absorbance at 565 nm. The new formulation significantly reduces the bias found by the analysis of postmortem blood with the original REA reagent system. Abbott Laboratories recommends a sensitivity limit for ethyl alcohol in postmortem blood by the REA method of 0.015 g/100 mL. Determination of ethyl alcohol in serum, fresh whole blood, fresh or postmortem urine, and vitreous humor by REA demonstrated no bias whatever (Cary, 1986).

Caplan and Levine (1986) performed a similar study to evaluate the two Abbott TDx REA ethyl alcohol assays, INT and MTT, and compared them to a reference method using headspace gas chromatography. Serum, plasma, urine, and whole blood were analyzed by the three methods. While statistical evaluation by least square regression analysis revealed good correlation, it was found that postmortem whole blood specimens, at high and low ethyl alcohol concentrations, showed a greater variability than did the other specimen types. For the other specimens, the discrepancies occurred only at the lower concentrations of ethyl alcohol. Of the two methods, the authors felt that although both TDx ethyl alcohol assays are acceptable methods, the MTT method performed somewhat better at lower ethyl alcohol concentrations for analyzing serum, urine, and fresh blood. It was recommended that a larger study is needed to determine a proper cutoff for reporting ethyl alcohol concentration in postmortem blood.

GAS CHROMATOGRAPHIC METHODS

The most commonly used method for the forensic analysis of ethyl alcohol is gas chromatography. For the measurement of ethyl alcohol in biological fluids, several gas chromatographic methods, such as solvent extraction, protein precipitation, distillation, direct injection, or headspace techniques have been used (Jain and Cravey, 1972b; Gudzinowicz and Gudzinowicz, 1977). Earlier methods involving the separation of ethyl alcohol from biological specimens usually utilized solvent extraction, protein precipitation, and distillation. Recent methods involve direct injection and headspace techniques.

Extraction Techniques

One of the earliest methods was that of Cadman and Johns (1958) in which they reported a procedure using a Beckman GC-2 gas chromatograph equipped with a thermal conductivity detector (TCD) and a column containing 28 g of a mixture consisting of Flexol 8N8, diisodecyl phthalate, and polyethylene glycol 600 in a ratio of 15:10:3 by weight on 100 g of 42/60 mesh firebrick. The extraction technique consisted of pipetting 1 mL blood and 1 mL of *n*-propyl acetate into a 3 mL screw-capped vial containing 1 g of anhydrous potassium carbonate. The sample vial was mixed and shaken one minute on a mechanical mixer. The sample was centrifuged and a 35-μL aliquot of the *n*-propyl acetate was injected into the gas chromatograph. For purposes of quantitation, ethyl alcohol standards were prepared by adding measured amounts of ethyl alcohol to blood and the blood subsequently extracted and chromatographed under the same conditions as that of the unknown samples.

Lyon and Bard (1964) subsequently published a report using the same gas chromatograph as Cadman and Johns but utilized a column containing 15 g of the mixed liquid stationary phases (Flexol 8N8, diisodecyl phthalate, and polyethylene glycol in a ratio of 15:10:3) on 100 g of 30/60 mesh chromosorb. Extraction consisted of mixing the blood with calcium sulfate–sodium bisulfite mixture, then adding *n*-butanol. The tube was shaken and centrifuged. The *n*-butanol was removed and added to a tube containing anhydrous potassium carbonate, allowed to stand for five minutes, and an aliquot of the *n*-butanol injected into the gas chromatograph. Davis (1966) modified the method of Cadman and Johns using flame ionization detection and Steinberg et al, (1965) also modified the method using a column of 15% Hallcomid M-18 on 60/80 mesh, HMDS-treated Chromosorb W to effect separation of alcohols.

Distillation Techniques

The method of Fox (1958) involved the separation of ethyl alcohol from biological specimens based on adding measured amounts of blood, urine, or tissue homogenate into a distilling flask containing 25 mL of water, 3 mL of 50% sodium tungstate solution, and 5 mL of 1.0N sulfuric acid. The specimen was distilled and the distillate collected with a known amount of *n*-butanol added to the receiver flask. An aliquot of the distillate was then injected into a Perkin-Elmer Model 154B gas chromatograph equipped with a thermistor thermal conductivity detector. Two copper columns were employed: one a 30/60 mesh C-22 firebrick, glycerol, and tricresyl phosphate (50:30:20) and the second firebrick, glycerol and tricresyl phosphate (60:18:11). Temperatures for column 1 and column 2 were 106°C and 84°C, respectively. The use of two columns allowed the separation of ethyl alcohol from methyl alcohol or formaldehyde when these mixtures were encountered. McCord and Gladsden (1964) used a similar method of distillation as that of Fox with protein precipitation, addition of a water-immiscible solvent, and subsequent distillation. It differs from the method of Fox in that the distillate was chromatographed without regard to its water content.

Direct Injection Techniques

There are numerous direct injection techniques for the determination of ethyl alcohol in biological specimens by gas chromatography.

These techniques may vary according to the preparation of the sample for testing and may consist of (1) direct injection of the sample, (2) protein precipitation and subsequent injection, or (3) dilution of the sample prior to injection. Probably the easiest and fastest is the injection of a diluted sample with an appropriate internal standard into a gas chromatograph equipped with a flame ionization detector. A number of suitable methods have been described (Maricq and Molle, 1959; Chundela and Janak, 1960; Wesselman, 1960; Machata, 1962; Parker et al, 1962; Bonnichsen and Linturi, 1962; Hessel and Modglin, 1964; Mather and Assimos, 1965; Curry et al, 1966; Finkle, 1971; Jain, 1971; Solon et al, 1972; Blume et al, 1973), all involving direct injection techniques.

Solon et al (1972) and Baird (1973) described methods involving automated gas chromatographic analysis of ethyl alcohol in blood or urine. Solon used a Hewlett-Packard gas chromatograph, automatic liquid sampler, electronic integrator, and data processor with special software. Samples and calibrators are mixed in vials with *n*-propyl alcohol added as the internal standard. Vials are placed in position in the automatic liquid sampler which is controlled by a subroutine in the data processor software which advances the samples to each of its 36 positions automatically. Vials in position 1 and 2 are filled with heparin, rinse solution. Position 3 is filled with a calibrator and the remaining positions are filled with unknown samples. The processor advances the sampler to position 1 and then to position 3, where the standard is sampled and injected. The retention time and response factors relative to *n*-propyl alcohol are stored for later reference. The sampler then moves to position 1 to rinse the syringe and then to position 4, unknown samples. The sample is injected and the data analyzed. The overall relative standard deviation was shown to be +1.00% and linearity was excellent in the range 0.015 to 0.26 g/dL.

Baird described a modification of the method of Solon. Data reduction was ascertained by interfacing the Hewlett-Packard gas chromatograph and automatic liquid sampler with an Auto Lab System IV computing integrator. Other modifications included the use of a greater sample–internal standard dilution ratio (1:8), computing results on a wt/vol basis, and different operating conditions.

Manno and Manno (1978) described an ultramicro method utilizing direct sample injection for the simultaneous identification and quantification of ethyl alcohol in blood and urine. Aliquots of whole blood or urine and an internal standard, 1-propyl alcohol, are mixed together in equal parts. One μL of the mixture is then injected into a gas chromatograph equipped with a flame ionization detector. The glass column, 3 mm i.d. by 2 m long, is packed with 0.2% Carbowax 1500 on 80/100 Carbopak C. The column is filled with a precolumn glass insert filled with a loosely packed silanized glass wool plug that acts as a trap for the nonvolatile protein material of the blood or urine samples. The optimal operating conditions for the gas chromatograph are: column temperature 120°C; injected temperature 100°C; carrier gas flow 20 mL/min; hydrogen and air pressure set at optimal conditions for a hydrogen flame. When it is necessary to collect blood specimens in extremely small volumes, blood from a finger puncture can be collected in plain capillary tubes. One-half microliter of serum, plasma, or whole blood can be drawn into a 1.0 μL syringe from the capillary tube followed by 0.5 μL of internal standard. Contents of the syringe are then injected into the gas chromatograph. The peak area of the alcohol peak and the internal standard peak are measured and compared with known amounts of ethyl alcohol and internal standard and the concentration of ethyl alcohol present is calculated.

Headspace Techniques

Headspace techniques are based on Henry's law of physics, which states that the ratio of a dissolved substance in aqueous solution is dependent on temperature, pressure, and concentration in the aqueous medium. It follows, then, that volatile substances may be measured by analyzing the vapor which is in equilibrium with a liquid specimen such as blood. Typically, the blood sample is placed into a vial with appropriate internal standard and sealed with a septum and allowed to stand, usually at 37°C, until equilibrium is reached. A sample of the headspace is removed from the vial by syringe and injected into a gas chromatograph.

Wallace and Dahl (1966) described a method in which sodium chloride was added to the samples in amounts greater than those required for saturation, to minimize the variations in the gas-liquid partition ratio of ethyl alcohol ordinarily caused by differences in dissolved solvents. According to the authors, the addition of the salt markedly increases the vapor pressure of ethyl alcohol in the biological samples and permits quantitative analysis of the vapor phase for ethyl alcohol without the preparation of complex standards. In the method, after addition of sodium chloride to a flask containing blood, the flask is capped with a rubber stopper and the contents equilibrated for five minutes. A 1-mL vapor sample is then injected into a column packed with 1.5 g Flexol 8N8, 1.5 g diisodecyl phthalate, and 1.5 g polyethylene glycol 600 per 100 g 100/120 mesh Chromosorb P. With the method described, 1 SD (N=30) of a day-to-day quality control sample containing 0.098 g/dL ethyl alcohol concentration was 1.3.

Reed and Cravey (1971) in a search for a simple, rapid, specific, quantitative procedure for the analysis of ethyl alcohol from blood, investigated the advantages of headspace techniques that had been documented by Goldbaum et al (1964); Duritz and Truitt (1964); Wallace and Dahl (1966); Bassette and Glendening (1968); and Glendening and Harvey (1969). The authors selected 1,4-dioxane as an internal standard (Biasotti and Bradford, 1969) and to reduce the variation in the vapor phase–liquid partition ratios of blood and other aqueous fluids, sodium chloride was used (Wallace and Dahl, 1966). Compared with a widely used distillation-oxidation method (Kozelka and Hine, 1941), this headspace technique provided comparable accuracy with the advantage of speed, simplicity, and specificity. The unknown blood sample is measured accurately by means of 1 mL tc pipette to a small beaker containing 1 mL of 1% aqueous 1,4-dioxane and the pipette is washed in and out several times while swirling the beaker. An aliquot of the mixture is added to a vial containing sodium chloride. The stopper bottle is equilibrated for eight minutes and 1.5 mL of vapor phase is injected in a 0.25 in. by 8 ft stainless steel column packed with 40/60 firebrick impregnated with 28% by weight, the following mixtures: diisodecyl phthalate, Flexol 8N8, and Carbowax 600 in a ratio of 10:15:3 (Cadman and Johns, 1958).

Karnitis and Porter (1971) described a method which consists of equilibrating blood with *n*-propyl alcohol as the internal standard and then injecting the vapors into a 0.125 in. by 6 ft stainless steel column packed with Poropak S. Concentrations were linear over the range 0.00 to 0.35 g/dL blood ethyl alcohol. Correlation of blood ethyl alcohol concentration results were excellent when compared with a distillation method (Shupe and Dubowski, 1952). Dubowski (1976) described a new method for quantitating ethyl alcohol in equilibrated headspace gas of biological liquids by means of a solid state metal-oxide semiconductor (MOS) detector. After equilibration of the sodium chloride–saturated specimen at 40°C in a closed vessel, a Taguchi MOS sensor is momentarily exposed to the headspace vapor. The resulting DC voltage change from baseline conditions accurately reflects the alcohol concentration of the liquid specimen, and can be read in direct alcohol-concentration units.

Jones (1977) described a method for the determination of blood alcohol concentration by headspace analysis using an electrochemical detector. A determination can be made within two minutes and only 0.1 mL of blood is required for analysis. The detector response was linearly related to ethyl alcohol concentration up to 0.30 g/dL. The accuracy of the method based on comparison with an enzymatic technique (Buijten, 1975) was high, the mean recovery being 102.2% of the attributed concentration.

An Alcometer Evidential device was used and is based on an electrochemical ("fuel cell") principle for ethyl alcohol oxidation. The unit consists of a sampling head thermostated at 60°C between tests, containing the electrochemical detector and the aspirating sampling valve. A

SET button serves to activate the sampling valve and discharge the fuel cell and a READ button releases the sampling valve (causing aspiration of a 0.6-mL test sample) and activates the fuel cell. The detector signal is displayed on a digital voltmeter in DC voltage, which may be calibrated to blood alcohol units.

For headspace analysis, the sampling head of the Alcometer is fitted with a special nozzle connection to hold a Luer-fitting hypodermic needle in place of the mouthpiece normally used for breath alcohol. A blood sample of 0.1 mL is transferred into a 10-mL serum bottle and made airtight with a rubber septum. Samples are equilibrated in a water bath at 25°C for 15 minutes. The vapor phase above each blood sample is adjusted to atmospheric pressure prior to headspace sampling. The sampling head with the hypodermic needle attached is allowed to pierce the rubber septum of the serum bottle containing the sample and the SET button is pressed to activate the sampling mechanism. Immediately afterward the READ button is pressed to aspirate the headspace vapor sample for analysis. The final reading on the digital voltmeter is recorded and is proportional to the alcohol concentration in the headspace vapor. The SET button is pressed to discharge the detector in preparation for a new test. The ease of the operation and rapid analysis time make the method ideal for mass screening for ethyl alcohol in forensic laboratories.

Today, the most widely accepted headspace sampling method is based on one that was developed by Machata (1972) using a Perkin-Elmer Multifract F-40 system. This system consisted essentially of a gas chromatograph equipped with a flame ionization detector and a special electropneumatic valve dosing system in addition to a conventional injection port for manual sampling; a precision thermostated turntable water bath; and control unit, recorder and/or printing integrator. The principles of the system are three basic steps of headspace sampling: (1) equilibration, (2) pressurization, and (3) transfer of an aliquot of the headspace onto the column. After equilibrium is established in the vial, a needle connected to the carrier gas inlet is introduced through a rubber cap into the headspace of the vial. If the pressure in the vial is smaller than the carrier gas inlet pressure, part of the carrier gas flow will enter the vial and pressurize it until it reaches the inlet pressure. At this point the carrier gas supply is momentarily cut off for a specified time. This action causes the gas to flow from the vial into the column, barely injecting an aliquot of the headspace. Coefficients of variation below 3% have been reported. Detailed descriptions of the Multifract F-40, F-42, and F-45 are found in manuals published by the Perkin-Elmer Company, and more recently a detailed procedure was reported by Dubowski (1977).

In addition to the Multifract F-40, F-42, and F-45, the newest automatic headspace sampler is the Perkin-Elmer Model HS-100 mounted on a Sigma gas chromatograph. It combines the simplicity of CRT interaction with the versatility of the microprocessor-control, dual-channel gas chromatograph. The microprocessor control ensures precise thermostating and timing and also allows automatic unattended injection and analysis of up to 100 samples (Hurt and Welton, 1983). Christmore et al (1984) described solutions for two problems encountered in an automated headspace gas chromatograph method (Anthony et al, 1980). The first is the catalytic oxidation of ethyl alcohol by oxyhemoglobin, a process that is limited only by the amount of oxygen present in the sealed vial. This reaction was prevented by the addition of sodium dithionite. The second problem dealt with the lack of a suitable salting-out agent and led to the selection of ammonium sulfate which improved recovery of ethyl alchol as well as enhanced the precision of the method.

Penton (1985) modified an autosampler technique previously used for liquid injection into a gas chromatograph to function as an automatic headspace sampler by replacing the syringe with a 100-μL gas-tight syringe and shortening the needle that normally enters the vial for sampling. In addition, instead of the 1.0 to 1.5 mL of liquid sample, the vials contained 200 μL of liquid. The vapor above the liquid was injected into the gas chromatograph. Since the autosampler was not thermostated, the effect of temperature change was examined by placing the gas chromatograph and autosampler in an environmental chamber and analyzing a sample at various temperatures. The author states that the results were in general agreement with those reported by others (Hauck and Terfloth, 1969; Machata, 1975), that in headspace determination of blood ethyl alcohol the internal standard corrects for temperature fluctuations.

REFERENCES

Anthony, R.M., Sutheimer, C.A., and Sunshine, I. Acetaldehyde, methanol, and ethanol by headspace gas chromatography. *J. Anal. Toxicol.* 4:43–45, 1980.

Baird, W.W. Paper presented to Pacific Coast Conference on Chemistry and Spectroscopy, San Diego, Nov. 1973.

Bassette, R., and Glendening, B.L. Analysis of blood alcohol by direct headspace sampling and gas chromatography. *Microchem. J.* 13:374, 1968.

Bechamp, M.A. Sur la fermentation de l'urine normale et sur les organismes divers qui sont capables de la provoquer. *C. R. Acad. Sci.* 61:374, 1865.

Biasotti, A.A., and Bradford, L.W. Quantitative determination of ethanol by gas liquid chromatography after collection from the vapor phase on anhydrous magnesium perchlorate. *J. Forensic Sci. Soc.* 9:65–74, 1969.

Blume, P., Berchild, K.M., and Cawley, L.P. A gas chromatographic analysis of ethanol with identifying confirmation. *Anal. Biochem.* 54:429–433, 1973.

Blystone, P.G., and Collins, H.L. Determination of blood alcohol levels using a direct readout spectrophotometer. Presented at the Semi-Annual meeting of the California Association of Criminalists. Monterey, Calif., May 1984.

Bonnichsen, R., and Linturi, M. Gas chromatography determination of some volatile compounds in urine. *Acta. Chem. Scand.* 16:1289, 1962.

Bonnichsen, R., and Theorell, H. An enzymatic method for the microdetermination of ethanol. *Scand. J. Clin. Lab. Invest.* 3:58, 1951.

Bradford, L.W. Concepts and standards of performance in the technique of alcohol analysis of physiological specimens. Reprinted from the Proceedings of the Symposium on Alcohol and Road Traffic, Indiana University, Indianapolis, 1958, pp. 61–79.

Buijten, J.C. An automatic ultramicro distillation technique for determination of ethanol in blood and urine. *Blutalkohol* 12–393–398, 1975.

Cadman, W.J., and Johns, T. Gas chromatographic determination of ethanol and other volatiles from blood. Read to Ninth Annual Pittsburgh Conference on Analytical Chemistry and Applied Spectroscopy, March 1958.

Caplan, Y.H. The determination of alcohol in blood and breath. In *The Forensic Science Handbook* (R. Saferstein, ed.), Prentice-Hall, Englewood Cliffs, N. J., 1982, pp. 592–652.

Caplan, Y.H., and Levine, B. The analysis of ethanol in serum, blood, and urine: a comparison of the TDx REA ethanol assay with gas chromatography. *J. Anal. Toxicol.* 120:49–52, 1986.

Cary, P.L. Reformulated REA ethanol assay evaluated. *J. Anal. Toxicol.* 10: 38–39, 1986.

Cary, P.L., Whitter, P.D., and Johnson, C.A. Abbott radioactive energy attenuation method for quantifying ethanol evaluated and compared with gas-liquid chromatography and the DuPont *aca. Clin. Chem.* 30:1867–1870, 1984.

Cavett, J.W. The determination of alcohol in blood and other body fluids. *J. Lab. Clin. Med.* 23:543, 1938.

Cheng, F.S., and Christian, G.D. Enzymatic determination of blood ethanol, with amperometric measurement of rate of oxygen depletion. *Clin. Chem.* 24:621–626, 1978.

Christmore, D.S., Kelly, R.C., and Doshier, L.A. Improved headspace analysis. *J. Forensic Sci.* 29:1038–1044, 1984.

Chundela, B., and Janak, J. Quantitative determination of ethanol besides other volatile substances in blood and other body fluids by gas chromatography. *J. Forensic Med.* 7:153–161, 1960.

Committee on Medicolegal Problems American Medical Association. *Alcohol and the impaired Driver*. American Medical Association, Chicago, 1973.

Cravey, R.H., and Jain, N.C. Current status of blood alcohol methods. *J. Chromatogr. Sci.* 12:209–213, 1974.

Curry, A.S., Walker, G.W., and Simpson, G.S., Determination of ethanol in blood by gas chromatography. *Analyst* 91:742, 1966.

Davis, R.A. The determination of ethanol in blood or tissue by gas chromatography. *J. Forensic Sci.* 11:205–213, 1966.

Dubowski, K.M. Method for alcohol determination in biological liquids by sensing with a solid-state detector. *Clin. Chem.* 22:863–867, 1976.

Dubowski, K.M. *Manual for Analysis of Ethanol in Biological Liquids.* U.S. Dept. of Transportation report No. DOT-TSC-NHTSA-76-4, 1977.

Duritz, G. and Truitt, E.B. A rapid method for the simultaneous determination of acetaldehyde and ethanol in blood using gas chromatography. *Q. J. Stud. Alcohol* 25:498–510, 1964.

Finkle, B.S. Ethanol-type C procedure. In *Manual of Analytical Toxicology* (I. Sunshine, ed.), CRC Press, Cleveland, 1971, pp. 147–149.

Fox, J.E. Fast chromatographic analysis of alcohols and certain other volatiles in biological material for forensic purposes. *Proc. Soc. Exp. Biol. Med.* 97: 236, 1958.

Garriott, J.C. Forensic aspects of ethyl alcohol. *Clin. Lab. Med.* 3:385–396, 1983.

Glendening, B.L., and Harvey, R.A. A simple method using headspace gas for determination of blood alcohol by gas chromatography. *J. Forensic Sci.* 14: 136–145, 1969.

Goldbaum, L.R., Domanski, T.J., and Schloegel, E.L. Analysis of biological specimens for volatile compounds by gas chromatography. *J. Forensic Sci.* 9:63–71, 1964.

Gudzinowicz, B.J., and Gudzinowicz, M. *Analysis of Drugs and Metabolites by Gas Chromatography–Mass Spectrometry*. Marcel Dekker, New York, 1977, pp. 85–189.

Harger, R.N. A simple micromethod for the determination of alcohol in biological material. *J. Lab. Clin. Med.* 20:746, 1935.

Hauck, G., and Terfloth, H.P. Investigations on automatic blood alcohol determination according to the headspace method. *Chromatographia* 2:309–315, 1969.

Hessel, D.W., and Modglin, F.R. The quantitative determination of ethanol and other volatile substances in blood by gas-liquid partition chromatography. *J. Forensic Sci.* 9:255–264, 1964.

Hurt, S.G., and Welton, B. New microprocessor-controlled gas chromatographs. *Am Lab* 15:89–916, 1983.

Jain, N.C. Direct blood injection method for gas chromatography determination of alcohols and other volatile compounds. *Clin. Chem.* 17:82–85, 1971.

Jain, N.C., and Cravey, R.H. Analysis of alcohol. I. A review of chemical and infrared methods. *J. Chromatogr. Sci.* 10:257–262, 1972a.

Jain, N.C., and Cravey, R.H. Analysis of alcohol. II. A review of gas chromatographic methods. *J. Chromatogr. Sci.* 10:263–267, 1972b.

Jones, A.W. A rapid method for blood alcohol determination by headspace analysis using electrochemical detector. *J. Forensic Sci.* 22:283–291, 1977.

Jung, G., and Ferard, G. Enzyme-coupled measurement of ethanol in whole blood and plasma with a centrifugal analyzer. *Clin. Chem.* 24:873–876, 1978.

Karnitis, L., and Porter, L.J. A gas chromatographic method for ethanol in vapors of biological fluids. *J. Forensic Sci.* 16:318–322, 1971.

Kirk, P.L., Garbor, A., and Parker, K.P. Determination of blood alcohol. Improvements in chemical and enzymatic procedures. *Anal. Chem.* 30:1418, 1958.

Kozelka, F.L., and Hine, C.H. Method for the determination of ethyl alcohol for medicolegal purposes. *Ind. Engin. Chem. (Anal. Ed.)* 13:905, 1941.

Lyons, H., and Bard, J. Gas chromatographic determination of lower alcohols in biological samples. *Clin. Chem.* 10:429–432, 1964.

Machata, G. Die Routineuntersuchung der Blutalkoholkonzentration mit der Gas-Chromatographie. *Mikrochim. Acta.* 4:691, 1962.

Machata, G. Determination of alcohol in blood by gas chromatography headspace analysis. *Perkin Elmer Clin. Chem. Newsl.* 4:29–32, 1972.

Machata, G. The advantages of automated blood alcohol determination by headspace analysis. *Z. Rechtsmed.* 75:229–234, 1975.

McCord, W.M., and Gladsden, R.M. The identification and determination of alcohols in blood by gas chromatography. *J. Gas Chromatogr.* 2:38–39, 1964.

Manno, B.R., and Manno, J.E. A simple approach to gas chromatographic microanalysis of alcohol in blood and urine by a direct-injection technique. *J. Anal. Toxicol.* 2:257–2611, 1978.

Maricq, L., and Molle, L. Investigations on the determination of blood alcohol levels by gas chromatography. *Bull. Acad. Med. Belg.* (Ser. 6) 24:199–232, 1959.

Mather, A., and Assimos, A. Evaluation of gas-liquid chromatography in assays for blood volatiles. *Clin. Chem.* 11:1023–1035, 1965.

Parker, K.D., Fontan, C.R., Yee, L.L. et al. Gas chromatographic determination of ethyl alcohol in blood for medicolegal purposes. *Anal. Chem.* 34:1234–1236, 1962.

Penton, Z. Headspace measurement of ethanol in blood by gas chromatography with a modified autosampler. *Clin. Chem.* 31:439–441, 1985.

Poklis, A., and Mackell, M.A. Evaluation of a modified alcohol dehydrogenase assay for the determination of ethanol in blood. *Clin. Chem.* 28:2125–2127, 1982.

Redetzki, H.M. and Dees, W.L. Comparison of four kits for enzymatic determination of ethanol in blood. *Clin. Chem.* 22:83–86, 1976.

Reed, D. and Cravey, R.H. A quantitative gas chromatographic method for alcohol determination. *J. Forensic Sci. Soc.* 11:263, 1971.

Shupe, L.M., and Dubowski, K.M. Ethyl alcohol in blood and urine. A simple photometric method for its forensic determination. *Am. J. Clin. Pathol.* 901, 1952.

Smith, H.W. The specificity of the desiccation method for determining alcohol in biological fluids. *J. Lab. Clin. Med.* 38:762–766, 1951.

Smith, H.W. Methods for determining alcohol. In *Methods for Forensic Science* (A.S. Curry, ed.), Interscience, New York, 1965, vol. 4, pp. 1–97.

Solon, J., Watkins, J., and Mikkelsen, L. Automated analysis of alcohols in blood. *J. Forensic Sci.* 17:447–452, 1972.

Steinberg, M., Nash, J.B., and Walker, J.Q. Quantitation of alcohols using gas chromatography and a 15% hallcomid column. *J. Forensic Sci.* 10:201, 1965.

Sunshine, I., and Nenad, R. A modification of Winnick's method for the rapid determination of ethyl alcohol in biological fluids. *Anal. Chem.* 25:653, 1953.

Takel, H., Nakashima, K., Adachi, O., et al. Enzymatic determination of serum ethanol with membrane-bound dehydrogenase. *Clin. Chem.* 31:1985–1987, 1985.

Vasiliades, J., Pollock, J., and Robinson, C.A. Pitfalls of the alcohol dehydrogenase procedure for the emergency assay of alcohol: a case study of isopropanol overdosage. *Clin. Chem.* 24:383–385, 1978.

Wallace, J.E., and Dahl, E.V. Rapid vapor phase method for determining ethanol in blood and urine by gas chromatography. *Am. J. Clin. Pathol.* 46:152–154, 1966.

Wesselman, H.J. Quantitative determination of ethanol in pharmaceutical products by gas chromatography. *J. Am. Pharmacol. Assoc.*, 49:320, 1960.

Whitehouse, L.W., and Paul, C.J. Micro-scale enzymic determination of ethanol in plasma with a discrete analyzer, the ABA-100. *Clin. Chem.* 25:1399–1401, 1979.

Widmark, E.M.P. A micromethod for the estimation of alcohol in blood. *Biochem. Z.* 131:473, 1922.

9

Collection and Storage of Specimens for Alcohol Analysis

David R. Harper
Janet E.L. Corry

Ethanol levels in clinical specimens are sometimes challenged in court because it is alleged that the ethanol might be an artifact and not represent the level originally present in the subject. Conversely, loss of ethanol between taking a sample and its analysis could result in the acquittal of a person guilty of an offense, or misinterpretation of the factors influencing a crime. Whilst an acquittal is unlikely to trouble the defense lawyer, the analyst and those involved in law enforcement should be concerned about the validity and accuracy of the ethanol levels used for legal purposes. In addition to accurate analysis and interpretation, a storage system which is capable of maintaining the initial level of ethanol is necessary because forensic cases can take many months before all legal procedures have been exhausted, and the ability to repeat analyses in often useful.

This chapter is concerned with the optimal methods for collection and storage of forensic clinical specimens intended for ethanol analysis, with particular reference to microbial activity. Physical and chemical mechanisms that can result in the loss or gain of ethanol are also considered. Unless stated otherwise, all details refer primarily to practices in the United Kingdom.

RECOMMENDED METHODS OF COLLECTION AND STORAGE

The two fluids most commonly analyzed for ethanol are blood and urine; these will receive prime consideration here. Specimen containers should be glass bottles with metal screw caps and rubber liners, or glass vials sealed with rubber bungs and metal caps. Normally, 28-mL screw-cap bottles are used for urine samples from live subjects and for blood and urine specimens taken postmortem. However, if there is only a small volume of sample, a 7-mL screw-cap bottle can be used to reduce the air space (see Chemical Mechanisms of Ethanol Loss below). Blood from live subjects is often put into 5-mL glass vials. All bottles should be chemically clean, and those intended for unpreserved specimens should preferably be sterile. In the United States, blood is most commonly collected and stored in sterile Vacutainers; these have rubber stoppers with a silicone lubricant.

Preservation of Specimens

It is standard procedure to preserve all blood and urine specimens taken from live subjects suspected of drunken driving offenses. Until a few years ago, urine samples were submitted in 170-mL bottles containing tablets of phenylmercuric nitrate (50 mg) plus sodium fluoride (100 mg). The concentration of preservatives varied depending on the volume of urine in the bottle and the degree to which the tablet dissolved; the remains of the tablet in the bottom of the jar acted as a useful check that preservative was indeed present. Recently, concern about the toxicity of organic mercury salts prompted a change to the use of 300 to 400 mg of sodium fluoride in 28-mL bottles. Glass beads are dispensed into the bottles with the preservative and serve as a visual check that the sodium fluoride is present after the urine has been added. Microbiological examination of case-sample urine during the change-over period showed that there was little difference between the above methods of preservation (Table 9-1).

For blood samples, standard 5-mL glass vials containing sodium fluoride and an anticoagulant (potassium oxalate) are usually used. When dissolved in 2 mL of blood, concentrations of approximately 15 mg/mL and 4 mg/mL, respectively, are obtained. These concentrations tend to be somewhat lower in the United States; about 2.5 mg of sodium fluoride and 2 mg of potassium oxalate are added per milliliter of blood. Solutions of the additives are evaporated to dryness in the vials before use, and two 3 mm diameter glass beads are present to facilitate mixing. Sodium nitrite (0.13–2.5 mg/mL) has been used, in addition to the other two salts, by provincial laboratories in England and Wales to inhibit the oxidation of ethanol described by Smalldon and Brown (1973). However, this compound tends to produce a brown precipitate which makes analysis difficult and has no detectable antimicrobial effect in blood (Corry, unpublished observations, 1977).

Samples taken postmortem should ideally be divided into two

Table 9-1
Microbiological Survey Carried Out in January and February 1977 on Urine Samples Preserved With (a) Sodium Fluoride or (b) Sodium Fluoride Plus Phenylmercuric Nitrate

	Number of Contaminated Samples			
Number of Colony-Forming Units Detected Per mL	Preservative (a)		Preservative (b)	
<10	103	(66)*	84	(72)
10–100	22	(14)	12	(10)
100–1000	21	(13)	12	(10)
>1000	10	(6)	8	(7)
Total	156	(99)	116	(99)

*Numbers in parentheses indicate percentages.

portions, one with preservative and the other without; these can be submitted in similar vessels to those used for samples from live subjects.

Specimens from Live Subjects Suspected of Drunken Driving Offenses

In May 1983, evidential breath testing was introduced into the United Kingdom for ethanol determinations connected with drunken driving offenses. This has largely replaced certain of the procedures described below.

Blood is usually taken from the anterior cubital vein in the forearm by a qualified medical doctor. Police stations are supplied with kits comprising: two vials containing preservative and anticoagulant; a sterile disposable syringe with needle; and a sterile swab impregnated with a suitable disinfectant to clean the skin before the blood sample is taken. Although it is quite obvious to the forensic scientist that the use of a disinfectant containing ethanol and/or propanol (see Measurement of Ethanol below) could distort the blood alcohol level of the sample, it can be overlooked by the doctor. There have been occasions in this laboratory when extremely high blood ethanol levels have been observed, and subsequent inquiries have revealed that the skin was disinfected with ethanol.

The blood sample is distributed between the two vials, and the contents thoroughly mixed to ensure that the preservative is well dispersed and clotting prevented. Appropriate labels and forms are completed and the bottles are sealed in plastic Securitainers (Johnson and Jorgensen, London, UK). One is given to the defendant for an independent analysis and the other is sent, as rapidly as possible, to be analyzed at the forensic science laboratory. Police officers are instructed to refrigerate samples before dispatch, and samples are stored at 4°C when they reach the laboratory.

A similar system operates for the collection of urine samples. Clean, nonsterile plastic cartons are supplied, into which the suspect urinates; a fresh carton should be used for each suspect. The urine is then divided between two sample bottles and treated as described above. Analysis of blood and urine is normally done within one to three days. Analytical results are not reported if more than 2 weeks have elapsed since the samples were taken.

Specimens Taken Postmortem

Collection of samples from corpses should be done as soon as possible after death to minimize the possibility of microbial contamination. Urine samples should be taken through the intact bladder wall using a sterile syringe. Blood from the heart is not ideal because it may contain high levels of glucose which, if microbes are present, can rapidly give rise to ethanol. The most suitable source of blood is a vein, particularly the femoral vein, since the spread of microbes postmortem takes place largely from the intestine via the arteries (Fallani, 1961; Corry, 1978). Leg veins contain large numbers of valves which resist blood movement from the intestine. However, the veins of the head and neck contain fewer valves and are therefore second choice for postmortem blood samples. Blood from the thoracic or abdominal cavity ought only to be sampled if it is impossible to find any elsewhere; it is likely to contain large numbers of microbes. If possible, blood should be taken using a sterile syringe; a needle, which could puncture surrounding tissue, is unnecessary.

MECHANISMS OF ETHANOL LOSS

Physical Loss from Containers

The volatile nature of ethanol creates problems during the storage of samples for alcohol analysis. Brown et al (1973) reported the loss of ethanol from blood specimens by diffusion from inadequately sealed containers; 553 containers were examined, of which 31 exhibited closure failure.

Because samples may be subjected to different conditions, for example, type of container, storage time and temperature, it is impossible to estimate the physical losses of ethanol. If samples are required to be stored for extended periods, containers should be carefully sealed and the temperature should be as low as possible. Brown et al (1973) demonstrated that the rate of ethanol loss was almost zero at a storage temperature of −20°C.

Chemical Mechanisms of Ethanol Loss

In sealed containers the ethanol levels of blood samples can be lowered by an erythrocyte-associated, temperature-dependent oxidation (Smalldon and Brown, 1973). An oxyhemoglobin intermediate and methemoglobin have been implicated in the oxidation of ethanol to acetic acid via acetaldehyde. The extent of alcohol loss is also affected by the amount of air held within the specimen container (Scapelhorn, 1970). Smalldon and Brown (1973) suggested that oxyhemoglobin could be formed from the oxygen in the air space of the container and subsequently utilized during ethanol oxidation. In practice, they observed losses of 20 to 40 mg/100 mL from samples with air spaces, following storage for extended periods; losses did not appear to be directly related to the initial ethanol concentrations. To reduce the oxygen availability, blood sample containers should therefore be as full as possible.

Although the ethanol content of urine samples also decreases during storage, changes in concentration are considerably smaller than those associated with blood samples (Hayden et al, 1977). Absence of the erythrocyte oxidation mechanism probably accounts for this, and the loss is probably due to a physical mechanism.

Microbial Mechanisms of Ethanol Loss

A wide variety of microbes are capable of utilizing ethanol as a source of carbon and energy. However, they are unlikely to have any great effect on ethanol levels unless they are present in relatively high numbers.

Blood taken from a healthy person should be sterile, and if it is refrigerated and contains a preservative, the likelihood of ethanol loss due to microbes is negligible. Adequately preserved urine from healthy persons will contain low numbers of microbes which likewise should not reduce the ethanol level.

The rapid loss of ethanol from unpreserved samples containing high numbers of microbes has frequently been observed in this laboratory. It is particularly marked when a large air space is present in the specimen container; conditions may favor the aerobic metabolism of bacteria. In full containers, ethanol loss due to microbial activity appears to be more rare. However, there are mechanisms by which ethanol can be utilized anaerobically (eg, for the synthesis of fatty acids by *Clostridium* spp; Wood, 1961) and these should be considered.

MECHANISMS OF ETHANOL GAIN

Extraneous Contamination

As described above, the use of ethanol to swab the skin before blood is taken from a live subject can give rise to high ethanol levels in either of the duplicate samples that are provided for analysis. Comparison of the two blood samples will usually yield quite different ethanol levels because the contamination is not evenly distributed.

Instances have been encountered in which blood taken postmortem from a neck vein appears to have been contaminated by ethanol from gastric fluid refluxed into the esophagus. There are also reports concerning the possibility of postmortem leakage or diffusion of alcohol from the stomach into fluid in the abdominal or thoracic cavities, or even into blood in neighboring organs such as the heart (Bowden and McCallum, 1949; Gifford and Turkel, 1956). However, Hansman (1967) is critical of certain aspects of the research on which conclusions regarding alcohol diffusion from the stomach were based.

Chemical and Biochemical Mechanisms

Bogusz et al (1970; 1972) have suggested that ethanol can be produced from lactate in putrefying blood. Since blood often contains relatively high levels of lactate — 240 to 350 mg/100 mL (Franks et al, 1974; Corry, 1978) — this could be a common occurrence. However, it is not clear whether this can occur in the absence of high numbers of microbes; ethanol production in blood without microbes has not been observed in this laboratory.

Microbiological Mechanisms

Microbiological mechanisms were comprehensively reviewed by Corry in 1978 (Corry, 1978). There is no doubt that microbes are capable of producing significant quantities of ethanol in body fluids such as blood and urine, particularly in samples taken postmortem; up to 400 mg/100 mL (Corry, 1978; see Case Histories below). Concentrations of suitable substrates for microbial fermentation (glucose, glycerol, fatty acids, ribose, etc) tend to be much higher postmortem. Ethanol production can occur both in the corpse and after the samples have been taken. It should be understood, however, that ethanol is not invariably produced in putrefying tissues; production depends on the number and nature of the organisms present and the type and quantity of substrates. The predominant microflora that exist during the early stages of putrefaction of a corpse is primarily determined by the intestinal microflora during life. Temperature is also important and exogenous contamination may exert an influence. Evidence suggests that there is a progressive change in the microflora of corpses during decomposition. There is evidence too, of a succession of organisms — facultative anaerobes such as members of the Enterobacteriaceae, streptococci, certain lactobacilli, and staphylococci being succeeded by obligate anaerobes such as *Clostridium* spp, other lactobacilli, and *Bacteroides* spp.

Glucose is the substrate most likely to vary in concentration in tissues either postmortem or in living subjects. Severe shock immediately prior to death — not uncommon when death is caused by an accident or a criminal act — or death by asphyxia, can cause the glycogen reserved in the liver to be mobilized, converted to glucose and distributed throughout the blood system (Hamilton-Paterson and Johnson, 1940; Hill, 1941; Plueckhahn, 1967; Corry, 1978). In addition, glycogen normally present in the muscles and liver is spontaneously hydrolyzed to glucose after death. Hydrolysis of fat produces glycerol, and hydrolysis of nucleic acids yields ribose.

The Effect of Embalming

During the embalming process as practiced in the United Kingdom, blood is drained from the vascular system of the dead body and replaced with fluids which may include formaldehyde, phenol, methanol, glycerol, and ethanol. Thus, it is clear that determination of the "blood" alcohol level following this type of embalming would be meaningless. On occasion, the analysis of vitreous humor or urine might prove useful but only if the ethanol concentration is found to be zero, or if it can be established that there was no ethanol in the embalming fluid (see also chapter 5).

PRESERVATIVES

Fluoride

The use of sodium fluoride to preserve blood in forensic science seems to have occurred more by chance than by design, and was probably due to its use within hospitals as a preservative for blood samples taken for glucose analysis. Fluoride is an inhibitor of enolase, a key enzyme in the Embden-Meyerhof-Parnas glycolytic pathway, and hence it is used to prevent the fermentation of glucose to lactate, which normally occurs in blood when the supply of oxygen ceases. As an inhibitor of microbial ethanol production or utilization, fluoride may well be much less effective. Fortuitously, fluoride at the high level employed above (1%–2% wt/vol) has an antimicrobial effect, although this tends to be growth-inhibitory rather than lethal.

In spite of its deficiencies, fluoride is an adequate preservative for blood taken from live subjects since large numbers of microorganisms are only rarely encountered. The previous use of contaminated instruments to sample this type of specimen may become evident upon subsequent microbial examination, because organisms that are introduced in this way can often survive for extended periods even though their ability to multiply might be impaired. It has been noticed that an automatic sampler (Perkin-Elmer Ltd, Beaconsfield, UK), which removes blood from glass storage vials by passing a nonsterile needle through their septa, does not cause significant microbial contamination when preservative is present in the sample. This appears to be partly due to a mechanical cleansing action; considerable contamination has been observed when vials are opened and sampled directly with a nonsterile needle. In both of these instances a diluent containing sodium bisulphite was used to flush out the needle between consecutive samples (Corry and Gunewardene, unpublished observations, 1979).

The ability of certain microbes to survive in the presence of sodium fluoride can be of assistance when examining preserved samples taken postmortem. Although many of the organisms originally present will probably not be detected, isolates from these samples can give an indication of the numbers and effects prior to preservation.

Preserved urine samples from live subjects are sometimes found to contain greater than 10^5 colony-forming units (CFU) of microbes per milliliter. Large numbers of one or two pathogens could indicate that the suspect had a bladder infection. Mixed cultures of more than two organisms are more likely to indicate either that the urine was contaminated by the microflora in and around the external meatus of the urethra, or that a contaminated vessel was used, or that the fluid in the vessel is not urine. Attempts at deception have been made by suspects spitting into urine samples. These attempts were detected because the samples were found to contain a preponderance of facultative and obligate anaerobes in combination with an unusual foaming quality, lack of yellow pigment, absence of creatinine, and presence of amylase.

A major disadvantage of using sodium fluoride as a preservative is that certain fungi are capable of multiplying and affecting ethanol levels even when it is present in quite high concentrations (Table 9-2). This effect was known and even exploited in the brewing industry at the end of the last century (Arthus and Huber, 1892; Effront and Duclax, 1894) when fluoride was added to inhibit unwanted bacteria whilst allowing the yeast to grow; no reference was made to likely effects on the consumer! Another drawback with regard to samples submitted for forensic examination is that fluoride tends to be most effective in acid

Table 9-2
Effect of Sodium Fluoride on Ethanol Production*

Yeast	Ethanol Produced (mg per 100 mL of growth medium)				
		% (w/v) Sodium Fluoride			
	No Sodium Fluoride	pH 7.4		pH 6.0	
		1.2	0.6	1.2	0.6
A: unidentified (from unpreserved postmortem urine)	249	1.5	163	1.5	1.6
C: *Saccharomyces cerevisiae* (wine strain)	258	ND	1.4	1.1	1.6
F: *Candida albicans* (clinical strain)	215	1.1	153	1.3	209
G: unidentified (from corpse flesh)	185	ND	82.8	1.0	1.3
I: unidentified (from unpreserved postmortem blood)	202	1.0	148	1.1	223
J: unidentified (from urine containing 0.3% w/v sodium fluoride)	166	1.0	25	ND	20

*The six strains of yeast were incubated at 25°C for 21 days in heart infusion broth (Difco Laboratories, Surrey, UK) containing 0.5% (w/v) glucose.
ND = none detected.

solution; however, blood usually has a pH of 7.4, and the pH of urine can vary from 6 to 8. Occasionally, large numbers of yeasts have been isolated from preserved samples taken either from live subjects or postmortem. The samples had usually been stored for several weeks before being analyzed, and there is evidence to suggest that the yeasts had multiplied and not merely survived. Levels of fluoride in the above samples were generally rather low, but strains have been found growing in urine containing 1% (wt/vol) sodium fluoride. The multiplication of one strain, isolated from urine containing 0.7% (wt/vol) sodium fluoride, has been observed experimentally after incubation for several months in heart infusion broth containing 1.6% (wt/vol) sodium fluoride.

It is apparent that when yeasts are able to multiply they usually affect ethanol levels. Table 9-2 shows the effect of sodium fluoride on ethanol production by several strains of yeast. Table 9-3 shows the effect of fluoride on ethanol utilization. Two out of eight strains tested were able to utilize ethanol at pH 7.4 in the presence of 1.2% (wt/vol)

Table 9-3
Effect of Sodium Fluoride on Ethanol Utilization*

Yeast	Ethanol Utilized				
		% (w/v) Sodium Fluoride			
	No Sodium Fluoride	pH 7.4		pH 6.0	
		1.2	0.6	1.2	0.6
A†	+	−	+	−	+
B: unidentified (from postmortem urine containing 0.7% w/v sodium fluoride)	+	+	+	−	+
C†	+	−	−	−	−
E: unidentified (from urine containing 0.4% w/v sodium fluoride)	+	−	±	−	−
F†	+	−	+	−	±
G†	+	−	+	−	+
I†	+	−	+	−	+
J†	+	+	+	−	+

*The strains of yeast were incubated at 25°C for 21 days in heart infusion broth containing 100 mg of ethanol per 100 mL of growth medium.
†See Table 9-2 for details of yeast strain.
+ = ethanol level reduced substantially; ± = ethanol level reduced slightly; − = ethanol level unaffected.

sodium fluoride; both strains were isolated from urine that contained fluoride.

Alternative Preservatives

An extensive survey of alternative preservatives to fluoride was undertaken in this laboratory. Most were rejected because:

a. they were likely to interfere with toxicological assays for drugs other than ethanol
b. they were active only at low pH
c. they were not stable

A study with urine was carried out to compare the effect of various combinations of *p*-aminobenzoic acid esters (parabens), quaternary ammonium compounds, sodium fluoride, phenylmercuric nitrate, and various antibiotics. Mixtures of fungi and gram-negative and gram-positive bacteria were added to portions of the urine, and their survival and effect on ethanol levels were monitored at different pH values in the presence or absence of glucose or ethanol (Corry and Loveder, 1976, unpublished report). The most satisfactory preservative was found to be a mixture of benzethonium chloride (0.5% wt/vol) and pimaricin (Upjohn Ltd, Crawley, UK; 100 μg/mL). A subsequent report from the Home Office Central Research Establishment, Aldermaston, UK, (Law and Moffat, 1980) indicated that benzethonium chloride, but not pimaricin, would interfere with enzyme immunoassays and radioimmunoassays for barbiturates. A combination of pimaricin with sodium fluoride was subsequently tested to determine whether it would solve the problem of yeast proliferation in urine samples and the accompanying changes in ethanol levels. Considerable improvement was found over the use of fluoride alone (Table 9-4; Corry, unpublished observations). Thus, it is recommended that this mixture be employed for the preservation of urine samples and postmortem blood samples; pimaricin is not required as an additional preservative for blood samples taken from live subjects.

MICROBIOLOGICAL PROCEDURES FOR EXAMINATION OF SAMPLES

The following paragraphs summarize the methods currently employed in the Metropolitan Police Laboratory. The test system aims to determine two factors: (1) the numbers of microbes present in samples; (2) the ability of the strains of microbes present to produce and/or utilize ethanol.

Determination of Numbers of Microbes

Figure 9-1 shows the relationship between the number of CFU of a species of bacterium and the ethanol level of the glucose-containing medium in which it is multiplying. It is apparent that ethanol is not detected until the number of bacteria exceeds about 10^8 CFU/mL. However, the ethanol level continues to rise after the number of CFU has reached a maximum and long after it has started to fall. Figure 9-2 shows a similar relationship for a species of yeast. In this example, ethanol is evident when the number of CFU reaches about 10^6/mL.

In practice, it is difficult to be certain that all organisms have been detected, particularly if a sample is old or if it contains a preservative. The strains of microbe present in a sample are usually examined further if more than 10^5 CFU of bacteria per milliliter or 10^3 CFU of yeasts per milliliter are detected. A microscopic examination, as well as a viable count, is carried out to detect nonviable organisms or cells that do not

Table 9-4
Comparison of 0.6% (w/v) Sodium Fluoride With and Without 100 μg of Pimaricin per mL, as a Preservative for Urine*

	Ethanol Produced (mg/100 mL)				Ethanol Utilized (mg/100 mL)				
	0.5% (w/v) Glucose				90 mg Ethanol/100 mL Urine				
	Sodium Fluoride + Pimaricin		*Sodium Fluoride Only*		*Sodium Fluoride + Pimaricin*		*Sodium Fluoride Only*		
Yeast[†]	Log_{10}CFU/mL	Ethanol Level	Log_{10}CFU/mL	Ethanol Level	Log_{10}CFU/mL	Ethanol Level	Log_{10}CFU/mL	Ethanol Level	
A	ND	13	6.41	270	ND	90	4.34	53	
B	NT	NT	NT	NT	3.34	90	6.3	63	(0)[‡]
E	NT	NT	NT	NT	ND	87	5.1	71	(83)
F	ND	13	4.94	257	ND	84	5.0	64	
G	ND	21	ND	12	ND	92	4.97	39	(87)
H	NT	NT	NT	NT	ND	90	4.88	37	(72)
I	ND	12	3.48	272	ND	87	5.53	64	
J	ND	12	5.18	8	ND	90	5.14	68	
L	ND	12	4.8	242	ND	86	5.24	64	
M	ND	12	4.69	5	ND	88	5.54	63	
N	ND	12	5.18	15	ND	88	5.85	76	
O	ND	12	4.7	5	ND	97	3.53	69	
Uninoculated control	ND	12	ND	12	ND	90	ND	89	

*Approximately 10^4 cfu of yeasts per mL were inoculated into the urine (pH 7.4); incubation was for 22 days at 25°C.
[†]See Tables 9-2 and 9-3 for details: L = clinical strain of *Candida albicans*; M = isolated from unpreserved post-mortem urine; N = isolated from preserved urine (0.82% w/v sodium fluoride); O = isolated from preserved blood (1.15% w/v sodium fluoride); NT = not tested; ND = none detected.
[‡]Figures in parentheses are from duplicate bottles — quoted only if grossly different.

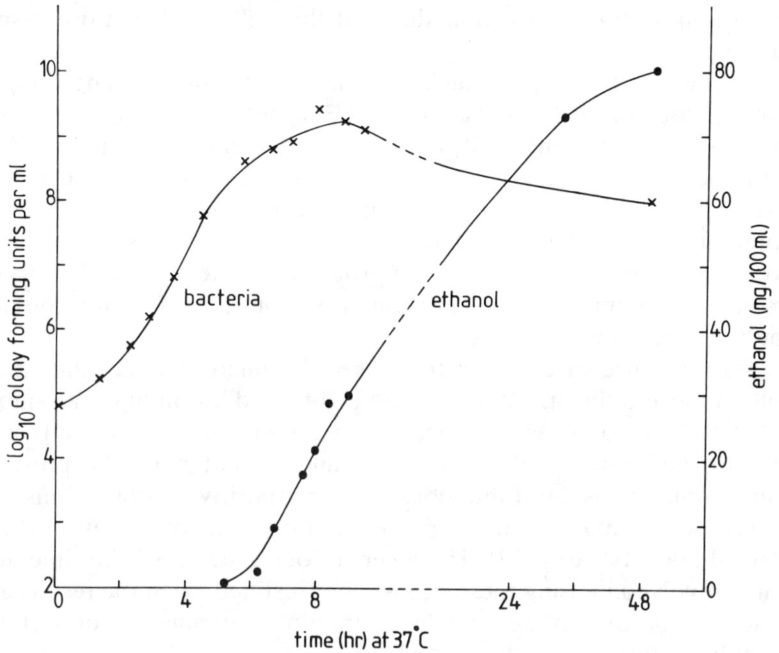

Figure 9-1 Relationship between ethanol level and numbers of the bacterium *Enterobacter aerogenes* (isolated from a putrefying corpse), during growth in heart infusion broth (Difco) containing 0.5% (w/v) glucose.

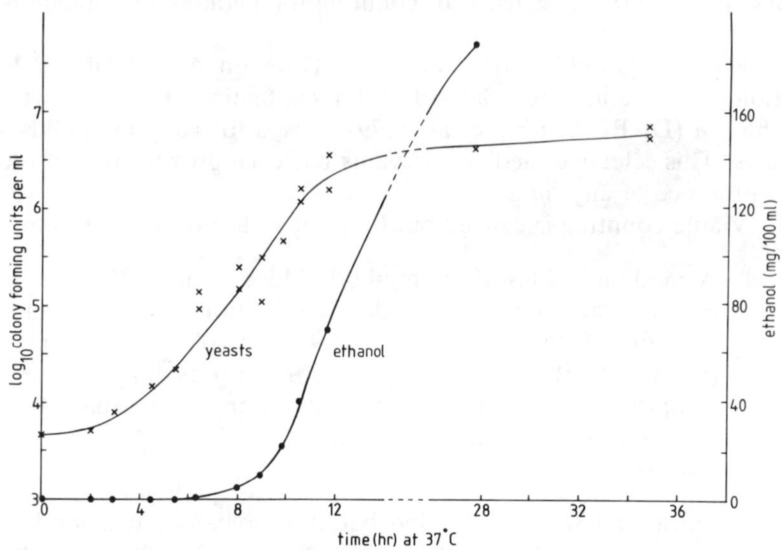

Figure 9-2 Relationship between ethanol level and numbers of the yeast *Candida albicans* (clinical isolate), during growth in heart infusion broth (Difco) containing 0.5% (w/v) glucose.

form colonies on the growth media. But this will not detect organisms that have died and then lysed.

Relatively clear liquids such as urine are examined using a high-power, phase-contrast microscope. A 1/30th-mL drop of sample, containing 10^6 organisms/mL, will give one to five organisms per microscopic field under a 22 by 22 mm coverslip at a magnification of 1000 times. More accurate microscopic counts can be carried out by using a hemocytometer (Cruickshank, 1965), or by adding to the samples a suspension of yeast cells, or latex particles of appropriate diameter (Prof B. Jarvis, personal communication, 1977) standardized using a Coulter counter (Coulter Electronics Ltd, Luton, UK).

The presence of erythrocytes makes the microscopic examination of blood more difficult. Therefore, an eightfold dilution of each sample in sterile distilled water is prepared to disperse the blood cells and facilitate the counting of any microorganisms that might be present. Gram staining is useful if microbes are gram-positive. Other stains can be used which make gram-negative organisms visible (Davis, 1976; Kronvall and Myhre, 1977). However, in our experience the time and trouble involved in using these stains is not justified when the results are considered, because blood samples containing high numbers of bacteria may still be missed.

Viable counting *Media:* Heart infusion agar (Difco Laboratories, East Molesey, Surrey, UK) with 5% (vol/vol) defibrinated horse blood (HIBA) is used for counting total colony-forming units of microbes.

Rose bengal chloramphenicol agar (London Analytical and Bacteriological Media Ltd, Salford, UK) containing 0.0002% (wt/vol) dichloran (DRBCA; King et al, 1979) is used for counting molds and yeasts. This selective medium prevents bacterial growth from masking the presence of any fungi.

Viable counting is carried out by using either of the following:

1. A modified Miles-Misra method (Miles et al, 1938) which involves the preparation of decimal dilutions in an aqueous solution of sodium chloride (0.9% wt/vol) and peptone (0.1% wt/vol), and surface plating on quarters of agar plates
2. A Spiral Plater (Spiral Systems Marketing, Bethesda, Md: supplied by Don Whitley Scientific Ltd, Shipley, Bradford, UK) which is a mechanized surface-plater

Duplicate HIBA plates are incubated aerobically and anaerobically for three days at 30°C and the DRBCA is incubated aerobically at 30°C for three days. Colonies growing on DRBCA are checked microscopically to confirm that they are fungal.

Media for Testing Ethanol Production and Utilization

Glucose and ethanol are sterilized by filtration. The appropriate aseptic additions are made to the basal medium to give final concentrations of 0.5% (wt/vol) and 100 mg/100 mL, respectively. The medium is distributed aseptically in 3-mL quantities in 7-mL bijou bottles (for the growth of aerobes), or in 28-mL quantities in 28-mL McCartney bottles (for the growth of anaerobes), with metal screw caps and rubber liners.

Yeasts, molds, aerobic, and facultatively anaerobic bacteria

a. Ethanol production. Heart infusion broth (HIB; Difco) containing 0.5% (wt/vol) glucose
b. Ethanol utilization. HIB (Difco) containing 100 mg of ethanol/100 mL

Anaerobic bacteria

a. Ethanol production. Reinforced clostridial medium (RCM; Oxoid Ltd, Basingstoke, Hampshire, UK; Hirsch and Grinsted, 1954) containing 0.5% (wt/vol) glucose. Some isolates will not grow in this but will grow in cooked meat medium (CMM; Southern Group Laboratory, London, UK) to which glucose can be added.
b. Ethanol utilization. RCM (made up from basic ingredients but without glucose) containing 100 mg of ethanol/100 mL.

Prior to inoculation all media for anaerobic bacteria are heated for ten minutes in a boiling water bath to remove residual oxygen.

Tests for Ethanol Production and Utilization

Representative strains of microbes are isolated from samples containing more than 10^5 CFU of bacteria per milliliter or more than 10^3 CFU of fungi per milliliter, and from samples where the microscopic count has indicated that levels of microbes are in excess of these figures.

Various microorganisms die in urine containing fluoride at rates that depend on the strain of microbe, the temperature of storage, and the concentration of fluoride (Table 9-5). Some bacteria survive well in blood preserved with sodium fluoride when stored at 5°C (Table 9-6). Even at levels of 5% (wt/vol) sodium fluoride, the survival rate was high for most of the strains tested. At 25°C survival was much poorer for some organisms but still good for others — for example, an unidentified bacillus isolated from a preserved, road traffic offense, blood sample.

It is impossible to be certain of the original numbers of microbes in preserved samples, and isolates are often examined for their effects on

Table 9-5
Numbers of Survivors After 7 Days Storage at 5°C or 25°C in Urine (pH 6.3) Containing Various Concentrations of Sodium Fluoride.

Organism	Temperature (°C)	Initial Number ($\log_{10}$CFU/mL) of Organisms	Numbers ($\log_{10}$CFU/mL) of Survivors at Various Concentrations of Sodium Fluoride (% w/v) 0.5	1	2	5
Escherichia coli	5	7.1	6.0	6.4	3.8	1.7
	25	7.1	6.6	4.5	ND	ND
Staphylococcus epidermidis	5	5.6	5.0	5.2	2.8	4.8
	25	5.6	ND	ND	3.3	2.7
Streptococcus faecalis	5	7.2	7.1	7.9	5.9	6.2
	25	7.2	6.6	7.1	7.2	ND
Unidentified yeast	5	5.4	5.1	3.2	2.1	1.4
	25	5.4	6.0	ND	ND	ND

ND = none detected.

Table 9-6
Numbers of Survivors After 7 days Storage at 5°C or 25°C in Postmortem Blood Containing Various Concentrations of Sodium Fluoride

Organism	Temperature (°C)	Initial Number ($\log_{10}$CFU/mL) of Organisms	Numbers ($\log_{10}$CFU/mL) of Survivors at Various Concentrations of Sodium Fluoride (% w/v) 0.2	1	2	5
Escherichia coli	5	5.3	5.5	5.6	5.4	5.6
	25	5.3	5.8	ND	ND	ND
Enterobacter aerogenes	5	5.7	4.9	6.6	5.7	4.5
	25	5.7	6.8	6.1	ND	ND
Proteus sp.	5	6.1	6.6	5.8	5.3	5.9
	25	6.1	6.8	6.7	3.3	3.7
Streptococcus faecalis	5	6.1	6.5	5.8	6.6	6.4
	25	6.1	5.3	5.0	4.7	4.2
Unidentified gram-negative bacillus from preserved blood	5	6.5	6.4	4.6	6.7	7.1
	25	6.5	5.8	6.3	6.6	7.2

ND = none detected.

ethanol levels when detected at less than 10^5 CFU of bacteria or 10^3 CFU of fungi per milliliter.

Isolates are inoculated into the test media (see above) and incubated at 30°C until growth is apparent. Sterile portions of media are also incubated, as described above, to act as controls for ethanol determination.

Samples from "fresh" corpses If corpses are stored at low temperatures (below 10°C), and samples are taken within 24 hours of death, with reasonable aseptic precautions, microbial counts should be low. One preserved and one unpreserved sample of both blood and urine are recommended for purposes of comparison. Unpreserved samples that are examined promptly, and preserved samples, usually contain small numbers of microbes.

Samples from older or putrefied corpses When a body has been left at a temperature exceeding about 20°C for more than 24 hours, it is wise to take more samples. Each specimen should be divided into two, one part being preserved and the other unpreserved. Blood should be collected from at least two different sites, and a urine sample should also be taken. The number of organisms in the preserved specimen may give an indication of the microbial quality at the time of sampling, whereas the organisms present in the unpreserved sample can be tested for their effects on ethanol levels. Any difference in ethanol level between the preserved and unpreserved samples demonstrates the most likely result of microbial metabolism. However, equal levels of ethanol in the two samples do not necessarily mean that there has been no microbial action.

On occasion, it can be useful for postmortem samples from putrefied corpses to be inoculated directly into prereduced CMM with added glucose or ethanol, particularly if there is difficulty in isolating the obligately anaerobic bacteria which are often present. This method yields mixed cultures and sometimes demonstrates ethanol production or utilization when pure cultures from the same sample show none.

Measurement of ethanol Gas chromatography is used for the determination of ethanol levels. Two Perkin-Elmer F45 gas chromatographs fitted with flame ionization detectors are used for duplicate analyses of the samples. One instrument is equipped with a column of 0.2% (wt/vol) polyethylene glycol 1500 on mesh 60–80 Carbopak C, the other with a column of 10% (wt/vol) polyethylene glycol 400 on mesh 100–120 Chromosorb W. Stainless steel tubing 1.22 m long and 2.1 mm i.d. is used for the preparation of the columns. Analysis time is extended from the usual three minutes to eight minutes, thus avoiding interference between samples caused by any microbial metabolites that have longer retention times. *N*-propyl alcohol is used as internal standard.

However, this compound is produced by some microbes (Corry, 1978) and hence could cause underestimation of the level of ethanol. Therefore forensic samples in which microbial effects are suspected should also be analyzed without the internal standard to show whether *n*-propyl alcohol is present. If it is, isolates should be checked for their ability to produce *n*-propyl alcohol.

EXAMINATION FOR METABOLIC PRODUCTS OTHER THAN ETHANOL

Microbial metabolites other than ethanol are often present in specimens containing high numbers of microbes. Acetic acid is common, as are higher molecular weight compounds such as propionic, butyric, valeric, and caproic acids. These can be quantified by gas chromatography (GC) using, for instance, the method of Jones and Kay (1976) or Larsson et al (1978). Lactic acid can also be determined by GC, but is often present even in sterile tissue postmortem, and in blood from live subjects. The presence of these metabolites is a useful indicator that the ethanol is of microbial origin (Harper, 1984). However, failure to detect them when high numbers of microbes are present does not necessarily rule out microbial ethanol production. This is because metabolic products vary, depending particularly on the type of organism and also on the conditions of growth. Gas chromatography has been used successfully in this laboratory to refute a claim that the presence of ethanol in a preserved urine sample was due to infection with *Escherichia coli* (Corry et al, unpublished observations, 1977). This organism produces large quantities of lactate and acetate when fermenting glucose, and lesser quantities of ethanol.

An alternative method of quantifying organic acids is isotachophoresis (van de Hoeven et al, 1978). The advantage of this technique is rapid estimation of the compounds from small samples without any prior treatment. It has been used recently to study the microbial metabolites associated with the production of ethanol in urine by *E coli* NCTC 10538 (Harper and Martin, 1983). Indications are, that unless glucose is available for growth, and organic acid metabolites are subsequently detected, any ethanol found in the urine would not have been produced by this organism.

INTERPRETATION OF THE RESULTS OF MICROBIOLOGICAL AND CHEMICAL TESTS

In this laboratory samples with reported ethanol levels just above the legal limit (81–94 mg/100 mL of blood; 108–125 mg/100 mL of urine), from persons suspected of drunken driving offenses, are checked for microbial contamination. Any sample that has unusual features is also examined, for example, if the container appears to have been tampered with, if the sample appears to have been tampered with, or if there is a delay between dispatch and receipt at the laboratory. In these cases the fluoride level is measured using an electrode with a single-crystal lanthanum fluoride membrane (Orion Research Inc, Cambridge, Mass).

Preserved blood samples from live subjects should never contain many bacteria or fungi provided that sterile or chemically clean equipment has been used during collection. If grossly contaminated samples are encountered they should be considered unsuitable for the analysis of ethanol.

In general, greater numbers of microbes are tolerated in preserved urine samples taken from live subjects because a certain amount of contamination during collection is unavoidable. However, the presence of microorganisms could be indicative of genitourinary tract infection, or more usually of failure to follow the recommended procedure at the police station. Inquiries should be made as to whether instructions concerning the use of fresh containers for each subject are being followed. Urine samples containing preservative are regarded as "normal" with regard to microbiological contamination if they contain less than 10^3 CFU/mL.

All samples taken postmortem and unpreserved samples taken from live subjects are checked for the presence of microbes. Reasonable conclusions can usually be drawn from the microbiological examinations of unpreserved samples if very few or no organisms are detected; the ethanol levels should have remained constant during storage. But care must be taken when interpreting the results obtained from the examinations of samples that have been stored for extended periods. Death and lysis of any microbes originally present could have occurred and they might not be detected either by microscopic or viable counts. The case histories in the following section demonstrate further how the results of microbiological examinations can be interpreted.

CASE HISTORIES

Case 1

The details provided in Table 9-7 refer to a murder case which was received in this laboratory during August 1978. The body had been left at ambient temperature and was not recovered until two days after death. The numbers of bacteria were high in all samples. The level of ethanol in the blood preserved with sodium fluoride was 89 mg/100 mL, whereas it was 128 mg/100 mL in the unpreserved sample. All samples contained high numbers of the anaerobe *Clostridium sordellii*, which

Table 9-7
Numbers of Bacteria and Concentrations of Ethanol (mg per 100 mL) in Samples Taken From a Corpse Found in August, 2 Days After Death

	Numbers of Bacteria (CFU/mL)		
Sample	Anaerobes	Aerobes	Ethanol Concentration
Blood			
(unpreserved)	6×10^6	5×10^5	128
(preserved)	2×10^6	3×10^3	89
Urine			
(unpreserved)	2×10^8	1×10^8	95

has been isolated on other occasions from corpses, and which is capable of producing about 150 mg of ethanol/100 mL of reinforced clostridial medium containing 0.5% (wt/vol) glucose.

The conclusions drawn from the microbiological data and the levels of ethanol were that the deceased definitely had not more than 89 mg of ethanol/100 mL of blood at the time of death, and that at least part of the 89 mg/100 mL found in the preserved blood sample could have been produced postmortem by bacteria.

The defense council, during the ensuing trial, argued that the deceased had been aggressive due to a level of blood ethanol higher than 89 mg/100 mL, which had been reduced postmortem by the bacteria. The microbiological data, including the evidence that none of the strains of bacteria isolated were able to reduce the ethanol level in the test system, refuted this.

Case 2

Table 9-8 shows levels of ethanol detected in three unpreserved samples from a corpse which was found about a week after death. The samples were stored at 10°C in a refrigerator and reanalyzed subsequently. Ethanol levels were raised in all samples after storage; in one blood sample from 50 to 320 mg of ethanol/100 mL. An increase in

Table 9-8
Concentrations of Ethanol (mg per 100 mL) in Samples of Unpreserved Blood and Urine Taken From a Corpse Found in January, About 1 Week After Death

		Ethanol Concentration After Storage of Samples for:		
Sample	Initial Ethanol Concentration	13 weeks	14 weeks	17 weeks
Blood	116	189	93	ND
Blood	50	315	313	320
Urine	11	56	25	2

ND = none detected.

the ethanol concentration of the urine is of particular interest since some workers assume that urine does not contain a suitable substrate for microbial ethanol production. All three specimens contained high numbers of bacteria, most of which were capable of producing ethanol. However, the increase of ethanol observed during storage appeared to be associated with the growth of a mold, *Mucor racemosus*, which produced over 200 mg of ethanol/100 mL of a glucose-containing test medium. The loss of ethanol observed in two samples was possibly due to the introduction of air during sampling; the third specimen had a much smaller air space in the bottle and did not lose ethanol.

The above data indicated that it was impossible to ascertain whether the deceased had been drinking prior to death. Nevertheless, even if alcohol were imbibed, the ethanol levels in the blood and urine at death would have been low.

Case 3

The information presented in Table 9-9 is from a "suspicious death" case received in this laboratory in the summer of 1982. The venous blood and urine were analyzed and found to contain 11 mg/100 mL and 8 mg/100 mL of ethanol and 10^4 CFU/mL and 2×10^7 CFU/mL of bacteria, respectively. Subsequently, samples were stored in a refrigerator for 3 weeks. During this time the ethanol level of the urine decreased to 4 mg/100 mL, and the quality of the venous blood deteriorated, thus preventing its reanalysis. A blood sample from the right atrium was examined; this had also been refrigerated for 3 weeks. It had an ethanol level of over 400 mg/100 mL, and contained large numbers of bacteria, many of which were capable of producing ethanol — up to 123 mg of ethanol/100 mL of a glucose-containing test medium.

These results suggest that bacteria had increased the concentration of ethanol in the blood from the heart.

VITREOUS HUMOR SAMPLES

Samples of vitreous humor are not routinely submitted to this laboratory for ethanol analysis. Only on those occasions when satisfactory blood or urine samples cannot be obtained is vitreous humor considered.

In the past, certain workers have advocated the use of vitreous humor for the estimation of ethanol (Leahy et al, 1968; Felby and Olsen, 1969; Coe and Sherman, 1970). Various reasons have been given, as follows: The sample is easy to obtain. It is anatomically well isolated, particularly from potential sources of microbes; the ethanol concentration is an accurate indicator of that in the rest of the body, and remains constant for substantial periods of time after death.

Recent research (Harper, in preparation) has provided an indication of the microbiological stability of vitreous humor (Table 9-10). Blood and vitreous humor samples were taken from each of ten cadavers and subsequently stored at 4°C until required for analysis. Sterile

Table 9-9
Concentration of Ethanol (mg per 100 mL) in Samples of Unpreserved Blood and Urine Taken From a Corpse Found in May, 3 days After Death

Sample	Initial Ethanol Concentration	Ethanol Concentration After Storage of Samples for 3 Weeks	Numbers of Bacteria (cfu/mL)
Blood (from iliac vein)	11	NT	10^4
Blood (from right atrium)	NT	401	2×10^8
Urine	8	4	2×10^7

NT = not tested.

Table 9-10
Comparison of the Numbers of Microorganisms Detected (log_{10}CFU/mL) in Postmortem Blood and Vitreous Humor Samples From Each of Ten Cadavers

Cadaver No.	Sample Type	Log_{10}cfu Bacteria/mL	Log_{10}cfu Fungi/mL
1	Blood	9.73	ND
	Vitreous humor	<2	ND
2	Blood	5.04	ND
	Vitreous humor	<2	ND
3	Blood	4.49	ND
	Vitreous humor	<2	ND
4	Blood	5.83	<2
	Vitreous humor	ND	ND
5	Blood	6.23	ND
	Vitreous humor	<2	ND
6	Blood	9.04	ND
	Vitreous humor	ND	ND
7	Blood	7.08	<2
	Vitreous humor	<2	ND
8	Blood	9.11	2.32
	Vitreous humor	<2	ND
9	Blood	4.62	<2
	Vitreous humor	2.44	ND
10	Blood	2.64	<2
	Vitreous humor	ND	ND

ND = none detected.

syringes, and when necessary sterile 21-gauge needles, were used for the removal of samples into sterile glass universal bottles (28 mL). Vitreous humor samples contained either small numbers of bacteria or no microbes at all, whereas many of the blood samples were grossly contaminated.

It should be noted that vitreous humor provides a good medium for the growth of certain microorganisms, and they can proliferate even if introduced at low levels. The samples must therefore be adequately preserved (eg, with sodium fluoride) and refrigerated to reduce the risk of changes in their ethanol contents during storage.

CONCLUSIONS

Routine checks for the effects of microorganisms on ethanol levels of samples submitted for forensic examination should be part of normal practice in all laboratories. Particular emphasis should be placed on samples taken from corpses more than a few hours after death, and to samples that have been stored at relatively high temperatures.

All samples should be taken aseptically, or in such a way that has been demonstrated not to cause contamination.

All samples should be stored at low temperatures in containers with sealed lids; the use of plastic bottles is not recommended since leakage may occur.

REFERENCES

Arthus, M., and Huber, A. Ferments solubles et ferments figurés. *Arch. Exp. Pathol. Pharmakol.* 24:651–663, 1892.

Bogusz, M., Guminska, M., and Markiewicz, J. Studies in the formation of endogenous ethanol in blood putrefying *in vitro*. *J. Forensic Med.* 17: 156–168, 1970.

Bogusz, M., Guminska, M., and Markiewicz, J. Studies on the formation of ethanol and of pyruvate as its precursor from some di-and tricarbonic compounds in putrefying blood *in vitro*. *Forensic Sci.* 1:229–237, 1972.

Bowden, K.M., and McCallum, N.E.W. Blood alcohol content: some apsects of its postmortem uses. *Med. J. Aust.* 2:76–80, 1949.

Brown, G.A., Neylan, D., Reynolds, W.J. et al. The stability of ethanol in stored blood. Part 1. Important variables and interpretation of results. *Anal. Chim. Acta* 66:271–283, 1973.

Coe, J.I., and Sherman, R.E. Comparative study of postmortem vitreous humor and blood alcohol. *J. Forensic Sci.* 15:185–190, 1970.

Corry, J.E.L. Possible sources of ethanol ante- and postmortem: its relationship to the biochemistry and microbiology of decomposition. *J. Appl. Bacteriol.* 44:1–56, 1978.

Cruickshank, R. *Medical Microbiology*. Livingstone, Edinburgh, UK, 1965.

Davis, J.C., A Gram stain for smears of blood cultures, body fluids and tissues. *Am. J. Med. Technol.* 13:417–423, 1976.

Effront, J., and Duclax, M. De l'influence des composés du fluor sur les levures de bières. *C.R. Acad. Sci.* 118:1420–1423, 1894.

Fallani, M. Contributo allo studio della circolazione ematica post-mortale. *Minerva Med.* (Torino) 81:108–115, 1961.

Felby, S., and Olsen, J. Comparative studies of postmortem ethyl alcohol in vitreous humor, blood and muscle. *J. Forensic Sci.* 14:93–101, 1969.

Franks, W.R., Kempton, A.R., Anderson, I.H., et al. Postmortem myocardial tissue lactate and potassium levels in fatal aircraft accidents. *Aerospace Med.* 45:980–986, 1974.

Gifford, H., and Turkel, H.W. Diffusion of alcohol through stomach wall after death. A cause of erroneous postmortem blood alcohol levels. *JAMA* 161: 866–868, 1956.

Hamilton-Paterson, J.L., and Johnson, E.W.M. Postmortem glycolysis. *J. Pathol. Bacteriol.* 50:473–482, 1940.

Hansman, F.S. Points of view. The validity of using heart's blood from the cadaver for alcohol assessment. *Med. J. Aust.* 2:130–131, 1967.

Harper, D.R. Demonstration of microbial action in specimens of wine analyzed for ethanol. Proceedings of the International Meeting of the International Association of Forensic Toxicologists. Brighton, U.K. Sept. 267–269, 1984.

Harper, D.R., and Martin, P.D. Isotachophoretic detection of microbial metabolites associated with ethanol production in urine. Proceedings of the Ninth International Conference on Alcohol, Drugs and Traffic Safety, San Juan, P.R., November 1983, pp. 609–621.

Hayden, P.M., Layden, M.T., and Hickey, M.D. The stability of alcohol content in samples of blood and urine. *Ir. J. Med. Sci.* 146:6–11, 1977.

Hill, E.V. Significance of dextrose and non-dextrose reducing substances in postmortem blood. *Arch. Pathol.* 32:452–473, 1941.

Hirsch, A., and Grinsted, E. Methods for the growth and enumeration of anaerobic spore-formers from cheese, with observations on the effect of nisin. *J. Dairy Res.* 21:101–110, 1954.

Jones, D.W., and Kay, J.J. Determination of volatile fatty acids $C_1 - C_6$ and lactic acid in silage juice. *J. Sci. Food Agric.* 27:1005–1014, 1976.

King, A.D., Hocking, A.D., and Pitt, J.I. Dichloran rose bengal medium for enumeration and isolation of moulds from foods. *Appl. Environ. Microbiol.* 37:959–964, 1979.

Kronvall, G., and Myhre, E. Differential staining of bacteria in clinical specimens using acridine orange buffered at low pH. *Acta. Path. Microbiol. Scand.* 85:249–254, 1977.

Larsson, L., Mardh, P., and Odham, G. Detection of alcohols and volatile fatty acids by head-space gas chromatography in identification of anaerobic bacteria. *J. Clin. Microbiol.* 7:23–27, 1978.

Law, B., and Moffat, A.C. *The Evaluation of an Homogeneous Enzyme Immunoassay (Emit) and Radioimmunoassay for Barbiturates.* Home Office Central Research Establishment, Aldermaston, U.K., Report No. 333, 1980 p. 20.

Leahy, M.S., Farber, E.R., and Meadows, T.R. Quantitation of ethyl alcohol in the postmortem vitreous humor. *J. Forensic Sci.* 13:498–502, 1968.

Miles, A.A., Misra, S.S., and Irwin, J.O. The estimation of the bactericidal power of the blood. *J. Hyg. Camb.* 38:732–749, 1938.

Plueckhahn, V.D. The significance of alcohol concentrations in autopsy blood samples. *Med. J. Aust.* 1:939–943, 1967.

Scaplehorn, A. *Storage of Blood Samples.* Home Office Central Research Establishment, Aldermaston, U.K. Report No. 35, 1970, p. 4.

Smalldon, K.W., and Brown, G.A. The stability of ethanol in stored blood Part II. The mechanism of ethanol oxidation. *Anal. Chim. Acta* 66:285–290, 1973.

van de Hoeven, J.S., Franken, H.C.M., Camp, P.J.M., et al. Analysis of bacterial fermentation products by isotachophoresis. *Appl. Environ. Microbiol.* 35:17–23, 1978.

Wood, W.A. Fermentation of carbohydrates and related compounds. In *The Bacteria* (I C Gunsalus and R Y Stanier, eds). Academic Press, New York, 1961, vol. 2, 59–149.

10

Quality Assurance

Patricia H. Field

A rigorous quality assurance program is necessary to ensure that analytical results for alcohol are accurate, reproducible, and acceptable in court. Quality assurance refers not only to the quantitative determinations of the procedure, but to all aspects of the laboratory that can affect the results, including personnel selection and training, method development, instrument maintenance, record-keeping, and sample handling and storage (Field, 1981).

LABORATORY

The laboratory should be clean, well-lighted and well-ventilated, with adequate space for the instruments, specimens, personnel, and paperwork. It should have a secure, refrigerated specimen storage area. An adequate electrical supply with a stable voltage is required. Temperature and humidity should be controlled within a range that will not affect analytical results. Finally, all employees should know and follow sound chemical and biological safety procedures.

PERSONNEL: SELECTION AND TRAINING

Personnel assigned to alcohol analysis should have a scientific education appropriate for the needs of the laboratory. Typically, candidates with at least a BS degree in chemistry, medical technology, or a related field are chosen. It is prudent to check candidates' backgrounds for evidence of serious driving offenses or felony convictions, since such a record can later affect the person's credibility in court, no matter how competent an analyst he or she is. The interview process should include an opportunity to evaluate the candidate's ability to answer questions clearly and concisely and to admit when he or she does not know the answer to a question, since these characteristics are vital when presenting testimony in court. It is good practice to initially assign new employees for several weeks or months to analyses that are not likely to result in subpoenas for testimony, since this gives the supervisor a chance to evaluate the employee's performance and demeanor, and gives the employee a chance to acquire valuable laboratory experience before his first court appearance.

On-the-job training should include a demonstration of the method of analysis and associated record-keeping, a thorough review of the principles of the analytical methods employed, and emphasis on the necessity of following methods exactly, without substitutions. This is vital if it later becomes necessary for the supervisor to reconstruct the employee's exact method of analysis when the employee is no longer available. This should be followed by a trial period during which the employee analyzes standards, controls, and multiple aliquots of samples previously analyzed by another employee known to be competent, in order to demonstrate and document his or her proficiency in quantitative terms of accuracy and precision. At the completion of this period, the supervisor will review the data before giving formal approval for the employee to begin analyzing actual subjects' samples and reporting results. The new analyst may be required to perform analyses in duplicate for some period beyond the initial training period, in order to demonstrate continuing competence.

Preparation for testimony in court should be a part of the analyst's training, and should begin well before the first subpoena is received. The analyst should be familiar with any laws or administrative code regulating both the analysis itself and licensure and certification of personnel and laboratories, and have some knowledge of the laws concerning the offenses for which the results of the analyses are relevant. He or she should be able to describe the method of analysis and all other areas of laboratory responsibility (sample collection kit, if any, notification of results, and record-keeping procedures) fluently and in simple language that is readily understandable to the lay person. Courtroom procedure should be described in detail, and the employee should be given the opportunity to participate in a mock trial covering both direct and cross-examination, and to accompany other analysts to court, if possible, prior to his or her first appearance. The lawyer issuing the summons for the employee's first testimony should be informed of this fact, and employee and lawyer should meet together prior to the trial to review the questions that will be asked. At this time, the employee should provide an up-to-date resume of his or her pertinent experience.

METHOD DOCUMENTATION

The method of analysis should be chosen for accuracy, reliability, and specificity, and should conform to any relevant statutory requirements.

Other chapters describe methods of analysis for alcohol. The laboratory's method book should describe in detail the method of analysis. It should be signed and dated by the supervisor, and reviewed regularly. Employees must understand that no changes may be made without the express consent of the supervisor. The method description should include operating parameters of the instrumentation, a list of reagents, standards and controls, information on their stability and frequency of replacement, a detailed stepwise description of the method itself, information on sources of error and trouble-shooting, and instructions on the steps to take if standard and control values do not fall within the expected range. It should include documentation of the source of the method and/or the steps taken by the laboratory to demonstrate its reliability (accuracy, precision, linearity, specificity, and detection limits).

INSTRUMENT DOCUMENTATION

An instrument maintenance log should also be part of the laboratory's documentation. It should describe routine preventive maintenance procedures for each instrument and have a place for the dates and initials of when and by whom such procedures were performed. These records may be prominently displayed at each instrument, or kept in a logbook near the instrument or at a central place in the laboratory. Instrument repair records (Figure 10-1) should also be readily accessible, and can be incorporated into instrument maintenance logbooks for convenience and completeness of documentation.

SAMPLE PRESERVATION AND CHAIN OF EVIDENCE

The laboratory has a responsibility for recommending appropriate procedures for collecting and preserving specimens and maintaining their integrity and evidentiary value while they are being conveyed to the laboratory. Many laboratories provide specimen collection kits with suitable containers, preservatives, labels and seals to facilitate this process. Sample collection and storage are discussed in detail in chapter 9.

A record should be kept of all persons who had access to the specimen from the time it was collected until it was analyzed. This is called the chain of custody or chain of evidence. At trial, each person who had access to the evidence (the sample) may be required to appear and testify about what he or she did with it. For this reason, it is advisable to strictly limit accessibility to legal alcohol samples. Court rulings have established that use of the US Postal Service does not break the chain of

INSTRUMENT MAINTENANCE RECORD

Page No. 4

Model No.(s) HEWLETT - PACKARD 5890 GC ; 3392A INTEGRATOR and 7672A AUTO SAMPLER

Serial No.(s): 2423A01907 2408A02670 2430A03339

Date	Initials	Description of Problem	Action taken / Comments
11/10/86	PH	Printhead element on 3392 A Integrator burned-out	replaced printhead assembly (PN 03390-60880)
5/12/86	PH	Sampler skipping numbers, especially in the 70's	adjusted pin alignement, cleaned pins with degreaser
6-13-86	TE	Skipping (Missing) Numbers	Disassembled and Cleaned Contacts
7-5-86	TE	Auto Sampler Carriage moving Slowly	Lubricated Guide Rails

Figure 10-1 Instrument maintenance record.

evidence, but mailroom employees may become involved in the chain—especially if certified or registered mail is used, since someone must sign for the package. It is advisable to have the alcohol analyst receive specimens directly from the mailroom. This is easier if the specimen is clearly labeled and packaged differently from other specimens which do not have legal implications.

Lockboxes designed for limiting the chain of custody are useful within institutions or courier systems that do not use the US Postal Service. They may have a key available (or combination known) only to the laboratory supervisor and the alcohol analyst, or a uniquely numbered tamperproof seal which is broken by the analyst just before the specimen is logged in and processed.

The employee who is about to analyze a specimen should make a record of whether it is securely sealed, how it is labeled, and whether the sample container (and, implicitly, the anticoagulant and preservative therein) is of the kind recommended by the laboratory, and should make note of any atypical observations, such as whether the sample is clotted, discolored, malodorous, leaking, or under pressure. The analyst should not break the seal until he or she is ready to analyze that particular sample, and should complete the entire sample preparation (except centrifugation) and label all the tubes and bottles containing that sample before proceeding to examining the next specimen.

QUALITY CONTROL OF ETHANOL ANALYSIS

Standards

Each time samples are analyzed for ethanol, a suitable selection of standards and controls should be run. Ethanol standards can be prepared from Gold Seal 100% ethanol. This reagent is hygroscopic (ie, it absorbs water after it is opened); therefore only freshly opened bottles should be used for preparing ethanol standards. A good quality of 95% ethanol, which is a more stable reagent, is equally suitable for preparing standards. When calculating the volume of ethanol required for a standard, it is essential to consider that the density of ethanol is less than 1.0 and varies with the temperature. Most standards are expressed as *weight* of ethanol per *volume* of sample. Certified ethanol standards at the 100, 150, and 200 mg/dL (0.10%, 0.15%, and 0.20% wt) levels are available from the College of American Pathologists, 7400 North Skokie Blvd, Skokie, IL 60077.

Laboratories using gas chromatographic techniques should employ an internal standard to improve the accuracy of quantitation. They may also wish to have available quantitative standards for alcohols other than ethanol which may be detected. It is a good idea to have a method of analysis for formaldehyde available in the laboratory, since if formaldehyde is detected in a postmortem sample, it is an indication that the specimen has been contaminated with embalming fluid. Gas chromatographic methods for alcohol analysis usually do not distinguish between methanol and formaldehyde.

Controls

Controls may be prepared by adding stock solutions of ethanol to preserved whole blood, serum, or urine, mixing thoroughly and freezing in small aliquots. The batch size should be sufficient that the mean and standard deviation can be obtained by analyzing ten to 20 different aliquots, with sufficient samples left over to analyze with several months' subsequent tests. Frozen samples of ethanol in biological materials should be stable for at least 6 months if the aliquots are tightly capped and the freezer maintains a constant temperature.

Standards and quality control materials should not be prepared by the same person on the same day, to avoid the possibility of an error in preparation compromising both. Purchasing either standards or quality control materials from a commercial source is one way to prevent this potential problem. New standards should not be introduced into the laboratory on the same day new quality control materials are analyzed.

New batches of quality control materials should be prepared sufficiently in advance that their target value can be established before supplies of the old quality control material are exhausted. It is preferable to introduce new quality control materials into the laboratory one at a time, rather than all at once.

Each run of alcohol analyses should be preceded by a series of standards covering the expected range of results, demonstrating the linearity, accuracy, and precision of the method. Quality control materials representing each type of biological matrix to be analyzed should be dispersed throughout the run, or grouped for analysis at the same time as unknown specimens of the same type. Throughout the run, every fifth sample for short runs (less than 30 specimens) or every tenth sample for long runs should be a standard or control. This assures that any deviations from the expected results are observed and corrected early in the process, and provides a high level of certainty about the accuracy of the analytical results throughout the run. A randomly selected portion of the unknowns (eg, every sample with a work sheet number ending in "5") should be analyzed in duplicate. Finally, if none of the samples is negative for alcohol, a blank should be run to demonstrate that the reagents, instrumentation, and laboratory environment are not a source of alcohol. It is good laboratory practice to run a blank just after the highest standard to fulfill this function and also to demonstrate the absence of carry-over of alcohol from one specimen to the next. Figure 10-2 is a work sheet from our laboratory showing the conditions of analysis, standards, quality controls, and target values, and the results on all samples, including duplicates.

The Use of Quality Control Results

Day-to-day variability in quality control results can be used to establish the precision of the method. Two thirds of the results can be expected to come within 1 standard deviation (SD) above or below the mean, 95% within 2 SD, and more than 99% within 3 SD. This information can be used to calculate the chances that a given result could have been greater or less than another, arbitrary, figure if analyzed repeatedly. This gives the laboratory worker a scientific means of addressing the question, "You say the result was 0.109% wt. What are the chances that it could have been 0.100% wt? 0.099? . . ." The comparability of a given analyst's own results on duplicate analyses within a given run is another powerful statistic for evaluating the certainty of a given result and the probability of that analyst reporting erroneous results.

The analyst's training and the written method description should include criteria for deciding when a series of analyses is acceptable, based on the results obtained on standards and quality control materials.

Alcohol Determination

HP 5790A GC with 7672A sampler and 3390A integrator instrument 3

temp	init.	final
inj.	150	150
oven	75	75
det.	150	150

Date Nov 8 1984 Page 1 of 1 Analyst TJE

#	Lab. #			#	Lab. #		
1	STD B	.151		19	A49105I	.090	
2	STD A	.076		20	A49106 I	.158	
3	STD C	.301		21	A49107 T	neg	
4	Con 92	.101		22	STD A	.076	
5	A49095I	.231	> .231	23	A49108T	.145	
6	A49095I	.231		24	A49109	neg	
7	A49096I	.153		25	A49110	neg	
8	A49097 I	.282		26	A49111T	.141	
9	A49098I	.116		27	A49112 I	.160	
10	STD B	.153		28	Con 94	.201	
11	A49099 I	.050		29	A49113 I	.171	
12	A49100I	.244		30	A49114 I	.319	> .320
13	A49101 I	.395	+ acetone + isopropanol	31	A49114 I	.322	
14	A49102 I	.272		32	A49101 I	.395	+ acetone + isopropanol
15	A49103 I	.085		33	STD C	.306	
16	Con 93	.059		34	ComB B	.149	+ acetone + isopropanol + methanol
17	A49104I	.160		35			
18	A49105I	.090	> .090	36			

STANDARDS		CONTROLS (MEAN VALUE)		
A	0.075	BLOOD	92	0.102
B	0.151	BLOOD	93	0.060
C	0.302	BLOOD	94	0.204
		URINE	95	0.295
		URINE	96	0.145

VALUES ARE % ETHANOL BY WEIGHT

Figure 10-2 Laboratory work sheet.

Typically, if any standard or quality control result is not within 2 SD of its target value, the analyst must take action or consult the supervisor before continuing. Suitable actions include analyzing another aliquot of the same control, and evaluating the results on the other standards and controls. The following criteria are adapted from Westgard et al (1981): If any result is more than 3 SD from its target value, reject the run or take corrective action. If two successive results are both 2 SD higher than the target value or both 2 SD lower than the target value, reject the run or take corrective action. If the range between the highest number of SD above the target value and the greatest number of SD below the target value is 4 SD or greater, reject the run because of excessive variability. If four consecutive standard or control results are all at least 1 SD above the target value or all at least 1 SD below the target value, reject the run or take corrective action. Finally, if ten consecutive results are all above the target value or all below the target value, reject the run or take corrective action.

These shifts and trends in control values can be readily observed by charting the mean, standard deviation limits, and actual results on graph paper. Suitable actions other than restandardizing include checking the records to see whether new standards or quality control materials were introduced at the same time the change was noted, checking the instrument maintenance records to see that all needed preventive maintenance has been performed, and checking the instrument itself along with all associated apparatus (ie, pipettes, diluters, and diluents) to see that everything is functioning properly. The final step in any series of diagnostics in response to a quality control result out of the expected limits should be to notify the supervisor and review any corrective action(s) with her before continuing with the analysis.

In our laboratory, a single record sheet shows each day's information on routine maintenance, changes of compressed gas cylinders, the results on each quality control material, retention times for ethanol and the internal standard, the number of injections on each chromatographic column, who was responsible for cleaning up the instrument and work area, and comments. This is a convenient single source for troubleshooting, and for the supervisor to keep an eye on the status of the instrumentation and results. Unfortunately, these record sheets, when filled out, contain too much information to reproduce legibly as an illustration for this chapter. People needing assistance in developing a similar form may wish to consult the author.

External Proficiency Testing

The National Highway Traffic Safety Administration (NHTSA, Transportation Systems Center, Kendall Square, Cambridge, Mass 02142) (Flores, 1977) and several states conduct external proficiency testing programs for alcohol, in which participating laboratories receive samples for ethanol analysis and, later, after they report their results, summaries which compare their performance with those of other participants and reference laboratories. Regular satisfactory participation in such programs is the best proof of the laboratory's competence, since the target values are unknown to the participants at the time they are conducting the analyses, and satisfactory results demonstrate the absence of certain problems which might go unnoticed within the laboratory, such as inaccurate standards. Toxicology proficiency testing programs from the College of American Pathologists, American Association for Clinical Chemistry (Washington, DC 20006), and the Centers for Disease Control (Atlanta, GA 30333) have included specimens for alcohol analysis occasionally, but not with sufficient frequency to rely on as a way of validating one's alcohol analysis program.

A new Blood Alcohol Survey Program, sponsored by the American Association for Clinical Chemistry and the College of American Pathologists (CAP) and available from the latter (address above), provides four shipments per year, each consisting of three whole blood specimens for alcohol analysis and an aliquot of CAP's aqueous ethanol standard. This program cost $212 for the 1986 calendar year. In addition to summaries of results, participants receive continuing education materials on alcohol analysis and related issues.

Wisconsin's alcohol proficiency testing program (Patricia Field, PhD, 465 Henry Mall, Madison, WI 53706) (Laessig et al, 1975) is particularly noteworthy, since laboratories receive at least two specimens each month, and whole blood, serum, and urine are represented in the samples. The program costs $100 per year. Programs which provide samples only infrequently are less useful, since poor performance by a participating laboratory could conceivably go unnoticed and uncorrected for months.

Alcohol analysis is one of the few toxicology tests that is not routinely confirmed using a different analytical technique. Because it is a simple and specific test, not subject to interferences, and because positive results are the rule rather than the exception, most toxicologists are confident of the validity of a single analysis for alcohol. Some laboratories follow the rule which governs analyses for most other drugs, and confirm all positive alcohol results using a different analytical technique. Examples of confirmation systems for alcohol analysis include gas chromatographic and enzymatic methods of analysis, and headspace and direct injection gas chromatographic techniques using two different chromatographic column packing materials. Another alternative is to screen for alcohol using a colorimetric technique, and confirm and quantitate using a more specific (eg, gas chromatographic) technique.

REPORTS

The supervisor should review and approve all records of analyses before results are reported out of the laboratory. This is the final check for the acceptability of standard and quality control values, the analytical data themselves (eg, sharp peaks, low blanks, and smooth baselines), consistency of the results with the case history, and the absence of mathematical and transcription errors. Statute or custom may dictate who will receive reports of the analysis. All reports should state the period the specimen will be retained in case further analyses are required.

RECORD-KEEPING

All records of the analysis and relevant quality control and proficiency testing records should be retained for as long as the results of the analysis may be required in court, which is several years for civil cases in many jurisdictions. Bulky records may be microfilmed or stored off-site, but it is essential that the filing system allow ready access to the records as needed. Laboratory and analysts' permits should be retained even though they may be renewed and replaced each year, since the year in question for a particular analysis is likely not to be the current year. The sample itself should be retained for a reasonable period of time to permit reanalysis by an independent laboratory. After the sample is no longer suitable for analysis, it is still useful to retain the container in order to demonstrate the label and seal.

REFERENCES

Field, P.H. Quality assurance and proficiency testing. In *Introduction to Forensic Toxicology* (R.H. Cravey and R.C. Baselt, eds.), Biomedical Publications, Davis, Calif., 1981.

Flores, A.L. The National Highway Traffic Safety Administration's Blood Alcohol Proficiency Test Program. *J. Anal. Toxicol.* 1:139–141, 1977.

Laessig, R.H., Becker, R.V., Basteyns, B.J., et al. Performance evaluation of Wisconsin laboratories performing implied consent alcohol determinations. *Health Lab. Sci.* 12:82–90, 1975.

Westgard, J.O., Barry, P.L., Hunt, M.R., et al. A multi-rule Shewhart chart for quality control in clinical chemistry. *Clin. Chem.*, 27:493–501, 1981.

11

State and Federal Regulations Concerning Driving While Intoxicated With Alcohol

Nancy Berk Pilchen

In recent years, public opinion in this country has altered significantly with regard to drunk driving. What once was viewed by many people as simply another traffic offense is now referred to as the "most frequently committed violent crime in America today." This change in public perception, due in large part to the efforts of grassroots victims' groups, has not escaped the attention of legislators at all levels across the country. And conversely, the state legislatures were one of the first targets on the agenda of the grassroots organizations in *their* quest for changes in the system.

The states have responded in a variety of ways. Over 40 state and local task forces were appointed in efforts to develop a comprehensive set of recommendations, many of which resulted in new approaches and tougher sanctions being employed. Since 1982, for example, 29 states have raised their minimum legal drinking age to 21 years old. Most of these same states had experimented with lowering the age in the early 1970s, many in response to pressure relative to the 18-year-old draft age. The result of these lower drinking ages was a significant rise in fatalities of 18- to 21-year-old drivers. A study done by Alexander C. Wagenaar at the University of Michigan Highway Safety Research Institute (1980) found that lowering the minimum legal drinking age from 21 to 18 years resulted in a 35% increase in alcohol-related crashes for 18- to 20-year old Michigan drivers. When the drinking age was raised in Michigan in 1978, the state experienced a 31% decline in fatalities in that same age group. Similar studies in other states have confirmed these findings.

Efforts were made to strengthen the ability to obtain DWI (driving while intoxicated) convictions as well. Twenty-eight states adopted a per se blood alcohol level definition of intoxication, ranging from 0.15 to 0.08 g/dL with the vast majority settling at 0.10 g/dL. By strictly linking the BAC (blood alcohol concentration) to the offense, the defense attorney is now curtailed in his or her ability to argue that, despite a high BAC, the defendent was in control of the vehicle. In those states with a per se law, the defense is virtually limited to arguing only that the chemical test was not conducted properly.

Studies that indicated license revocation, if swift and certain, to be an effective countermeasure prompted 44 states to take a new look at this sanction. Now, those states will administratively revoke a driver's license in the event of a refusal to submit to a BAC test, or if the BAC test was 0.10 g/dL or above. This sanction, which occurs after arrest but before conviction, is independent of any criminal penalties that may also be imposed after conviction. Twenty-eight states also instituted mandatory jail sentences, ranging from 24 hours to 30 days, for first or second offenders. In sum, not one state failed to enact some significant change to their pre-1981 laws dealing with the drinking driver.

Most recently, states are reviewing their youthful offender statutes, in some cases linking any alcohol-related offense, regardless of whether it occurred in a motor vehicle, to driver license restrictions and revocations. Victims' groups, which once focused much of their energy on tougher sanctions, are now moving beyond this and are examining initiatives designed to make the often-unwieldy judicial process more responsive to the victim. Requirements that victims be notified of court date changes affecting their cases are beginning to surface. Impact statements are making their way into more and more courtrooms as a presentencing requirement, and drunk-driving victims are being added to the list of persons eligible for restitution from victims compensation funds. Although not necessarily a legislative initiative, sobriety checkpoints are no longer being viewed as unwarranted intrusions but instead are considered valuable enforcement tools by a sympathetic public. Finally, overall emphasis is being placed on the development of self-sufficient programs that utilize mandatory assessments and are thus less dependent upon political winds that do not always blow favorably.

The drinking driver has not escaped the attention of federal lawmakers as well. Constitutionally, the responsibility for traffic enforcement lies with the states, yet federal input can serve a variety of purposes. Congressional support can be utilized to highlight the problem and provide a national forum on which the media can focus. Additionally, Congress may structure legislation that functions as either a carrot or a stick in prodding states to action without actually violating a state's sovereignty. On this issue, all three approaches have been employed.

In late 1981, Congress passed a resolution urging President Reagan to establish a National Commission Against Drunk Driving. With the signing of Executive Order 12358 on April 14, 1982, this became a reality. The charge of the new 1-year commission was to encourage state and local governments, as well as the private sector, to implement programs to reduce the carnage caused by the drunk driver. To highlight the need for such programs, the Commission undertook a series of national public hearings during the remainder of 1982 and listened to victims of drunk-driving crashes, enforcement officers, prosecutors, judges, and probation personnel. A wide range of experts from other fields including educators, legislators, health professionals, religious leaders, members of the media, and business executives also contributed their views on the problem and its possible solutions. An Interim Report was issued in December 1982 and a Final Report, based upon further review of the Interim Report, was issued in November 1983 (The Presidential Commission on Drunk Driving, 1982, 1984).

The Final Report of the Presidential Commission on Drunk Driving outlined a series of 37 recommendations encompassing public awareness and education, the private sector, alcohol beverage regulation, enforcement, prosecution, adjudication, licensing administration, and treatment. Among the legislative recommendations were:

The need for a 21-year-old minimum legal drinking age

Dram shop liability

Open container prohibitions

Creation of a dedicated funding source to include offender fines and fees (similar to the New York STOP-DWI program)

Effective tracking and reporting system for police, prosecutors, and the courts

Safety belt and child restraint laws

Implied consent laws encompassing the use of preliminary breath tests, police choice of chemical test, and mandatory testing of all fatally injured drivers or if there is probable cause that alcohol was involved in a fatal or serious personal injury crash

Prohibition against reducing DWI charges to nonalcohol offenses

Adoption of 0.10 g/dL per se and 0.08 g/dL presumptive as legal definitions of DWI

Mandatory 90-day license suspension and either 48 hours jail or 100 hours community service for first offenders; mandatory 1-year license suspension and 10 days jail for second offenders; 3-year license suspension and minimum 120 days jail for third offenders

Classifying the causing of death or serious injury while DWI as a felony

Elimination of pretrial diversion programs, instead requiring the charge to be rendered and education and treatment to be a condition of the sentence

Adoption of provisional licenses for young drivers which would be withdrawn for DWI conviction or implied consent refusals

Although the commission was merely an advisory panel, it did help to maintain the visibility of the issue in a national forum. Further, its Final Report proved useful for jurisdictions attempting to weigh the efficacy of various changes to the system.

While the Commission was developing its recommendations, Congress was considering other legislative alternatives, particularly ones employing the carrot-or-stick approach. In October 1982, legislation was enacted giving $125 million to the states over a 3-year period to combat drunk driving and upgrade the national driver register. The law made available incentive grants of up to 50% of a state's Section 402 funds that covered federal aid for state and local highway safety programs.

The 50% grant was administered under two provisions: The Basic Incentive Grant of 30% was available to states that adopted three legislative provisions: (1) 0.10 g/dL per se; (2) 90-day prompt license revocation upon probable cause for first offenders or upon refusal to submit to chemical testing, and a 1-year license suspension for second offenders or refusals; and (3) 48 consecutive hours in jail or ten days community service for subsequent offenders within a 5-year period. In addition, a state must provide increased enforcement and education programs. Later rule-making clarified "prompt revocation" to mean within 45 days of arrest for first offenders. If a state was unable to meet that timetable, but was revoking licenses within 90 days and could submit a plan detailing future compliance with the 45-day revocation, then the 45-day revocation would be waived for purposes of meeting the requirements for the Basic Incentive Grant only (30%). Prompt license revocation was also defined as at least 30 days hard suspension (no restricted license available) for first offenders and 1-year hard suspension for second offenders.

Once the Basic Incentive Grant requirements, including the 45-day revocation period, were met, a state was eligible for the Supplemental Incentive Grant. Twenty-one alternatives, including many of the Presidential Commission recommendations, were provided in the supplemental grant. To obtain the maximum 20% additional funding, a state would have to adopt any eight of the alternatives; they could qualify for 10% by adopting four of the alternatives.

Seventeen states took advantage of this carrot offered by Washington by tailoring their legislative initiatives toward compliance with the requirements for the additional federal funding. The majority of the participating states, however, qualified in the first 18 months of the program's existence; at the end of the 3-year appropriation period, there were still funds available although no new states appeared close to compliance.

Congress has also used sanctions to spur state activity. This time the effort was directed at raising the drinking age. Several bills were introduced which attempted to raise the age through the Constitution's Commerce Clause. Although Congress does not have express authority to regulate alcohol sales within a state's border, it may regulate "commerce between the states" through the use of the Commerce Clause. Thus Congress could regulate stores that received alcohol which had moved through interstate commerce, and thereby effectively regulate virtually all of the alcohol sold in this country. Although this approach would likely have passed judicial muster as it had been used by Congress in the 1960s to enact the civil rights legislation, the approach that ultimately prevailed was much more direct.

Under legislation enacted in 1984, states that failed to raise their drinking age to 21 years by October 1, 1986 faced a 5% cut in federal highway aid. If the age was not raised by October 1, 1987, the funds would be cut by 10%. For those states that failed to act in the first year, but did act by the second year, the 5% cut would be restored.

This statutory scheme has prodded some recalcitrant states such as Hawaii, where the loss of federal funds was specifically mentioned in the conference committee report of their successful 1986 drinking age legislation. Other states, however, have proved less easy to persuade. Iowa and Louisiana passed legislation in 1986, but specified that it would be valid unless the federal law was overturned or repealed. Since their laws have not yet taken effect, it is unclear what the ramifications of such legislative statements will be on enforcement efforts. South Dakota sued the federal government, claiming the law violated the Twenty-first Amendment, which provides for state regulation of alcohol transportation and importation and that the federal government lacks authority to withhold highway funds (*South Dakota v Dole*, 1986). The case was dismissed by the US District Court for the Western District of South Dakota, an action upheld by the US Court of Appeals for the Eighth

Circuit. The Court of Appeals held that the federal law did not alter South Dakota's right to maintain a lower drinking age. Since the state has no right to the funds absent congressional action, the fact that the federal government attaches strings to the dollars does not mean that the state *must* change its law. Since the state is thus not denied its power to regulate use and possession of alcoholic beverages within its border, the court concluded that the law does not violate the Twenty-first Amendment. Although the Court of Appeals appeared to apply settled principles in upholding the District Court's ruling, the US Supreme Court surprised many legal and policy observers by agreeing to review the case in the 1987 term. After hearing arguments in April 1987, the Court issued its opinion in June of the same year. In a 7-2 decision, the Court upheld the two lower court rulings and sanctioned Congress' use of its spending power to effect higher State minimum drinking age laws. The Court noted that Congress perceived a national problem and developed a legislative strategy reasonable related to solving that problem. The Court dealt very little with South Dakota's main argument that the 21st Amendment precluded federal intervention into State alcohol regulation, other than to note that Congress merely "offered relatively mild encouragement to the States to enact higher minimum drinking age laws". After three judicial reviews, the issue appears settled and by the end of 1987, all states with the exception of Wyoming raised their drinking ages.

Other states reviewed the possibility of a 15% cut over 2 years, and decided that the cut in funds did not merit raising the legal drinking age. There was discussion in some state legislative committees that it would be more productive to take the 15% cut rather than risk the loss of alcohol tax revenues over the long haul. As the federal legislation read, after 1988 there would be no further action by the federal government and funding would revert back to normal levels.

In April 1986, however, Congress amended the law to make the sanctions permanent. There is also a provision allowing a state to pass legislation yet implement it in stages until 1989, and not lose any of the federal dollars. This action appeared to turn at least one state around. Governor Anthony Earl of Wisconsin called the legislature back for a special session after it had officially adjourned in 1986, and passed Senate Bill I (SBI) raising the minimum legal drinking age in Wisconsin from 19 to 21 years.

Obviously, legislation is a critical part of the picture. But strong laws are only as good as the police community which must enforce them, the prosecutors who must try the cases, and the judges who must mete out the sanctions in accordance with the legislative intent. If the penalties are severe but there is no per se law, then convictions will be more difficult to obtain. If there are mandatory penalties for second offenders, but no reliable mechanism to identify the second offenders, then effective alcohol treatment programs will be next to useless. If there are long license revocation penalties, but also ample opportunity to delay their imposition, then this strongly negates the penalty's deterrent effect in the first place.

Eliminating the problem of drinking drivers has engendered a very complicated system where it is often difficult to separate the various components in order to determine the shortfalls. A problem in one area can rapidly bring down another part of the system, and so it may not matter, in the final analysis, how tough the actual statutes may be. For if laws are only a theoretical part of the overall system, then they will not have much impact on the result. Enacting legislation is not a panacea, but rather a first step in solving the complicated problem of the drinking driver. Thus it is critical that the laws be viewed in this context and with an understanding of their inherent limitations.

REFERENCES

Presidential Commission on Drunk Driving Final Report, Nov. 1983. Publication No. 0-4-428/368. Government Printing Office, 1984.

Presidential Commission on Drunk Driving Interim Report, Dec. 13, 1982. Government Printing Office.

South Dakota v Dole, 791 F.2d 628, 634 (8th Cir. 1986).

Wagenaar, A.C. *Traffic Safety Effects of the Raised Legal Drinking Age on Motor Vehicle Accidents in Michigan*, University of Michigan Highway Safety Research Institute, Ann Arbor, 1980.

ALABAMA

1985 Legislation: H6 — Raises drinking age from 19 to 21 yrs. Grandfather clause for persons 19 yrs. by 10/1/85. Effect. As long as fed'l law applying sanctions is in effect. Eff. 5/29/85.

1984 Legislation: None passed.

Per Se: .10 Drinking Age: 21 yrs. (new, see above). Dram Shop Law: Yes, §6-5-90. Open Container Prohibition: None. Section 408 Grant: Received $556,418 Alcohol/Traffic Safety Grant (Basic only. In order to qualify for Supplemental Incentive Grant, state must revoke lic. within 45 days of arrest, or within 90 days of arrest and submit plan to reduce it to 45 days.)

Refusals to Submit (admissible):
1st refusal: 30 days hard lic. revoc., 60 days restricted.
2nd refusal: 1 yr. lic. revoc. If acquitted of criminal DUI, revoc. may be reduced.

Driving under Revoc. License: Misdemeanor, $100–500, 180 days jail. Additional 6 mos. lic. revoc.

	Penalties	Jail/CommSvc	LicRevoc/Rehab/ Therapy	Other
1st Offense	$250–500,		30 days hard lic. revoc., 60 days restricted revoc. Rehab.	
2nd Offense w/in 5 yrs.	$500–2500,	Mand. 48 hrs.–1 yr. jail or 20 days comm. svc.	1 yr. lic. revoc.	
3rd Offense w/in 5 yrs.	$1000–5000,	Mand. 60 days–1 yr. jail,	3 yrs. lic. revoc.	
Homicide by m.v.	$500–2000,	1–5 yrs. jail.		

ALASKA

1985 Legislation: Nothing passed.

1984 Legislation: Nothing passed.

Per Se: .10 Drinking Age: 21 yrs. Dram Shop Law: Applies to businesses only (not private hosts) and only if the person served was already intoxicated. Open Container Prohibition: None. Section 408 Grant: Received $262,000 Alcohol/Traffic Safety Grant (Basic and Supplemental). PBTs: Allowed, refusal is admissible in court.

Refusals to Submit, or if .10 BAC: Same penalties as for criminal offenses (see below). Lic. revoc. are administratively imposed and all hard revocs. (no restricted lic. avail.). Lic. revocs. for DWI and refusal/.10 BAC admin. can run either consecutively or concurrently.

Driving under DWI Revoc. License:
1st Offense: Min. $500, mand. 30 days jail.
2nd Offense: Min. $1000, mand. 90 days jail.

	Penalties	Jail/CommSvc	LicRevoc/Rehab/ Therapy	Other
1st Offense	Min. $250,	Mand. 72 consecutive hrs. jail,	30 days hard. admin. lic. revoc., 60 days restricted admin. lic. revoc., rehab.	
2nd Offense w/in 10 yrs.	Min. $500,	Mand. 20 consecutive days jail,	1 yr. hard admin. lic. revoc., rehab.	Possible vehicle impoundment.
3rd Offense w/in 10 yrs.	Min. $1000,	Mand. 30 days jail,	10 yrs. hard admin. lic. revoc., rehab.	Possible vehicle impoundment.

Miscellaneous: *Cannot refuse BAC if death/physical injury* occured.

ARIZONA

1986 Legislation: HB2089 (Ch.39) — If DWI/underage, mand $250 or 80 hrs. comm. svce.

1985 Legislation: Nothing enacted.

1984 Legislation:

HB2307 (Ch.257) — Clarifies that if blood is taken from a "refuser" for any reason, police have right to a sample. Info on prior convictions/pending charges are admissible (at court's discretion) any time prior to start of trial. New punishment for DWI and driving without lic. Mand. 6 mos. jail before any parole/probation can be offered.

HB2027 (Ch.2) — Deletes provision for 1st offenders allowing probation and only fine instead of other penalties.

HB2149 (Ch.67) — Raised legal drinking age from 19 to 21 yrs. old. Provides 2 yr. lic. revoc. if underage DWI, or if 2nd offense of underage possession.

Per Se: .10 Drinking Age: 21 yrs. (1984) Dram Shop Law: No statute, and case law does not appear to support such 3rd party liability in absence of statute. Open Container Prohibition: Partial; illegal to drink while driving. Section 408 Grant: Received $701,413 Alcohol/Traffic Safety Grant (Basic and Supplemental).

Refusals to Submit: 1 yr. admin. lic. revoc., admissible as evidence.

Driving under Revoc. License: Class 1 misdemeanor, mand. 48 hrs. jail, double original lic. revoc.

	Penalties	Jail/CommSvc	LicRevoc/Rehab/ Therapy	Other
1st Offense	Class 1 mis-demeanor, mand. $250	Mand. 24 hrs. jail. 8–24 hrs. comm. svc.	Mand. 90 days lic. revoc., rehab.	*OR* probation, same penalties except no rehab. or comm. svc.
1st Offense if BAC less than .20 and no injury	Mand. $250.	8–24 hrs. comm. svc.	Rehab. 30 days hard lic. revoc, 60 days restricted.	*OR* probation, but same penalties (new).

	Penalties	Jail/CommSvc	LicRevoc/Rehab/ Therapy	Other
2nd Offense w/in 5 yrs.	Class 1 mis- demeanor, mand. $500	Mand. 60 days jail	Mand. 1 yr. hard lic. revoc., rehab.	*OR* probation but same penalties.
3rd Offense w/in 5 yrs	Class 5 felony	Mand. 6 mos. jail	Mand. 3 yrs. lic. revoc., rehab.	

Miscellaneous: Jurisdictions may establish *minimum security facilities for drunk driving* jail terms of less than 180 days.

ARKANSAS

1985 Legislation:
HB148 (PA108) — Must complete rehab before eligible for lic. reinstatement.
HB186 (PA113) — Increases lic. revoc. penalties.
SB516 (PA1034) — Estab. conditions for 1st offenders to obtain restricted licenses.

1984 Legislation: None; did not meet.

Per Se: .10 Drinking Age: 21 yrs. Dram Shop Law: None. Open Container Prohibition: None.

Refusals to Submit (not strictly administrative, lic. pulled, but temporary lic. issued until trial.):
1st refusal: 6 mos. lic. revoc.
2nd refusal w/in 3 yrs.: 1 yr. lic. revoc.

Driving under Revoc. License: 10 days jail, 90 days vehicle impoundment.

	Penalties	Jail/CommSvc	LicRevoc/Rehab/ Therapy	Other
1st Offense	Mis- demeanor, $150–1000.	24 hrs.–1 yr. jail or comm. svc.	Min. 90–120 day lic. revoc., pre- sentencing assessment. Rehab or probation (no expungement of record). Restricted lic. available	
2nd Offense w/in 3 yrs.	$400–3000,	7 days–3 yrs. jail.	Min. 1 yr–16 mth lic. revoc., pre- sentencing assessment. Rehab, no restricted lic.	
3rd Offense w/in 3 yrs.	$900–5000,	90 days–1 yr. jail.	Min. 2 yr–30 mth lic. revoc., pre- sentencing assessment. Rehab, no restricted lic.	

	Penalties	Jail/CommSvc	LicRevoc/Rehab/ Therapy	Other
4th Offense	Felony, $900–5000,	1–6 yrs. jail.	Min. 3 yr. lic. revoc., pre-sentencing assessment. Rehab, no restricted lic.	

CALIFORNIA

1985 Legislation:

AB144 (Ch1256) — If BAC .20+ or refusal, court can use for sentence enhancement or probation review.

AB331 (Ch735) — Enhances refusal penalties if subsequently convicted on the DWI charge. 48 hrs. jail-1st refusal, 96 hrs.-2nd, 10 days-3rd, 18 days-4th refusal.

AB740 (Ch1071) — 3 yr. lic. revoc. if previously convicted of vehicular manslaughter & BAC of .10+.

AB1414 (Ch1013) — Penalties for riding bicycles under the influence & estab. implied consent law.

AB2464 (Ch374) — Req. add'l counties to deposit $50 for each DWI conviction regardless of whether fine is imposed upon defendant.

SB127 (Ch 1455) — Alcohol/Drug Educ. to be incorp. into student driver ed. programs.

SB500 (Ch1330) — 2 yr. lic. revoc. for 2nd refusal.

SB735 (Ch337) — If DWI & emergency equipment/personnel needed, defendant liable for max. $500.

SB923 (Ch1475) — 48 hrs. jail or 10 days comm. svce. for 2nd offenders.

SB924 (Ch902) — Sentence enhancement if DWI felony & bodily injury occurs to 2 or more people. 1 additional year in state prison for each victim up to maximum of 3 yrs.

SB925 (Ch925) — Increases lic. suspension for 2nd offense w/no bodily injury from 1 yr. to 18 mths. Prohibits reissuing lic. for 3rd offense unless treatment is completed.

SB1278 (Ch244) — Tech. allows court to accept as evidence, a printout from DMV of defendent's driving record for purposes of determining if current offense is 1st or subsequent offense.

1984 Legislation:

SB1441 (Ch326) — Increases lic. revoc. to 3 yrs. for refusal after 2 prior offenses.

SB1411 (Ch658) — Provides for lic. revoc. for minors who commit any DWI offense (even where lic. revoc. is not part of existing penalties, such as open container violation).

SB1522 (Ch1142) — Relates to vehicle impoundment for 2nd and 3rd offenders.

AB3834 (Ch722) — DWI misd. does not have to occur in presence of police officer (as other misdm. do) Example: Intoxicated driver in car on road, but not driving can be DWI charged.

AB3509 (Ch3509) — Statutorily mandates no drinking and driving as one term of probation. DMV records to show driver on probation. Requires probation agreement to include mand. 2 days jail if BAC. .04 while on probation. Requires all plea bargained to "wet-reckless charge" to be considered as alcohol-offenses for purposes of DWI sentence enhance.

Per Se: .10 Drinking Age: 21 yrs. Dram Shop Law: Liability specifically forbidden by statute although it is illegal to sell to intoxicated person; BP§25602. Open Container Prohibition: Yes.

Refusals to Submit:

1st refusal: 6 mos. admin. lic. revoc, if convicted on DWI, add'l 48 hrs. jail.

2nd refusal: 2 yrs. lic. revoc., if convicted on DWI, add'l 96 hrs. jail.

3rd refusal: 3 yrs. lic. revoc., if convicted on DWI, add'l 10 days jail. (4th offense-18 days jail) If hearing requested, revoc. stayed pending outcome. Defendant has choice of tests. If choose breath, police can require blood/urine for drug detection.

Driving under DWI Revoc. License:

1st Offense: Max. $500, 10 days–6 mos. jail, or probation, 10 days jail.

2nd Offense: Max. $1000, 30 days–1 yr. jail, or probation, max. 30 days jail.

Youth Offender Legislation: If convicted of DWI, lic. revoked until 18th birthday, 1 yr. or period specified in statute, whichever is longest.

	Penalties	Jail/CommSvc	LicRevoc/Rehab/ Therapy	Other
1st Offense, no injury	$390–500,	96 hrs.–6 mos. jail,	6 mos. lic. revoc.	
If probation,	$390–500,	48 hrs.–6 mos. jail,	6 mos. lic. revoc.	
OR	$390–500,		90 days restricted lic.	
2nd Offense w/in 5 yrs., no injury	$375–1000,	90 days–1 yr. jail,	1 yr. lic. revoc.	
If probation	$390–1000,	10 days–1 yr. jail,	1 yr. lic. revoc.	
OR	$390–1000,	48 hrs.–1 yr. jail,	1 yr. hard lic. revoc., 2 yrs. restricted, 1 yr. rehab.	
3rd Offense w/in 5 yrs., no injury	$390–1000,	120 days–1 yr. jail,	3 yrs. lic. revoc.	
If probation	$390–1000,	120 days–1 yr. jail,	3 yrs. lic. revoc., 1 yr. rehab.	
4th Offense w/in 5 yrs., no injury	$390–1000,	180 days jail,	4 yrs. lic. revoc.	
If probation	Same.			
1st Offense, injury occured	$390–5000,	90 days–1 yr. jail,	1 yr. lic. revoc., rehab.	
If probation	$390–1000,	5 days–1 yr. jail,	1 yr. lic. revoc., rehab.	
2nd Offense w/in 5 yrs., injury occured	$390–5000,	120 days–1 yr. jail,	3 yrs. lic. revoc.	
If probation	$390–1000,	Min. 120 days jail,	3 yrs. lic. revoc.	
OR	$390–1000,	30 days–1 yr. jail,	1 yr. hard lic. revoc., 2 yrs. restricted lic. revoc., 1 yr. rehab.	

	Penalties	Jail/CommSvc	LicRevoc/Rehab/ Therapy	Other
3rd Offense w/in 5 yrs., injury occured.	$1015–5000,	2–4 yrs. jail,	5 yrs. lic. revoc.	
If probation	$390–5000,	Min. 1 yr. jail,	5 yrs. lic. revoc., 1 yr. rehab.	Restitution
Vehicular Mans- laughter while DWI & gross negligence		4–8 yrs. jail		
Vehicular Mans- laughter while DWI & not gross negligence		16 mos.–4 yrs. jail.		

*All penalties min. mand. unless noted.
Possible 1–30 day vehicle impoundments added to above penalties. Judge may order pre-sentence evaluation. Limits on plea bargains, info. must be recorded.

Miscellaneous: Probation Officer to notify victims of all sentencing proceedings and also give info. on victim's right to civil recovery and opportunity for compensation from Restitution Fund.

COLORADO

1985 Legislation:
HB1046 — Requires alcohol info. to be taught in K-12.
HB1124 — Allows info. relating to defendant's prior alcohol offense to be used at trial for driving under revoked license.
HB1258 — Illegal to give i.d. to underage person for underage person to buy alcohol. Also illegal to purchase alcohol for underage person.

1984 Legislation: HB1249 — Allows use of PBTs. Not admissible as evidence.

Per Se: .15 Drinking Age: 18 yrs. for 3.2 beer, 21 yrs. for everything else. Dram Shop Law: Only if previous written notification not to serve individual is given (13-21-103). Open Container Prohibition: None. PBTs: See HB1249.

Refusals to Submit: Mand. 1 yr. admin. lic. revoc., runs consect. with criminal disposition. .15 BAC: Mand. 1 yr. lic. revoc., if then convicted on crim. charges, lic. revoc. period run concurrently.

Driving under Revoc. License:
1st Offense: Misdemeanor, $500–1000, mand. 30 days–1 yr. jail.
2nd Offense: $500–3000, mand. 90 days–2 yrs. jail, 4 yr. lic. revoc.

	Penalties	Jail/CommSvc	LicRevoc/Rehab/ Therapy	Other
1st Offense DWI (.15)	$300–1000	Mand. 5 days–1 yr. jail or rehab. Mand 48–96 hrs. comm. svc.	No specific lic. revoc. period, court has option if public safety in danger.	
2nd Offense DWI w/in 5 yrs	$500–1500	Mand. 90 days–1 yr. jail or 7 days jail & rehab. Mand. 60–120 hrs. comm. svce.	Mand. lic. revoc. (generally until rehab completed).	
1st Offense DWI w/in 5 yrs. of 1st offense DWAI (below .15)	$450–1500	Man. 70 days–1 yr. jail. *OR* 7 days jail and rehab. Mand. 56–112 hrs. comm. svce.	Rehab.	
1st Offense DWAI (below. 15)	$100–500	Mand. 2–180 days jail or rehab and 24–48 hrs. comm. svc.	No specific lic. revoc. except mand. 1 yr. for provisional licenses	*OR* probation, no mand. sentence if complete rehab.
2nd Offense DWAI (below .15 BAC) w/in 5 yrs.	$300–1000	Mand. 45 days–1 yr. jail. *OR* 5 days jail and rehab. incl. 1 yr. abstinence from alcohol. Mand. 48–96 hrs. comm. svc.	No specific lic. revoc. period.	
1st Offense DWAI w/ in 5 yrs. of 1st offense DWI	$400–1200	Mand. 60 days–1 yr. jail. *OR* 6 days jail and rehab. Mand. 52–104 hrs. comm. svc.	Mand. lic. revoc.	
3rd Offense (any combination)	Habitual offender, $400–1200	Mand. 60 days–1 yr. jail. *OR* 6 days jail and rehab. Mand. 52–104 hrs. comm. svc.	Min. mand. 2 yr. lic. revoc.	
Vehicular Homicide	Class 4 felony		Mand. lic. revoc.	
Vehicular Assault	Class 5 felony		Mand. lic. revoc.	

Miscellaneous: Additional $50–60 assessment to fund Alcohol and Drug Driving Safety Program. Victims eligible for Crime Victim Compensation Program.

CONNECTICUT

1985 Legislation:

H5076 (PA264) — Raises drinking age from 20 to 21 yrs. Effective 10/1/85.

HB5158 (PA387) — Increases and. penalties, adds mand. jail for 1st offenders.

HB6275 (PA529) — Estab. Crim. Injuries Compensation Fund, $15 educ. fee used to fund.

H5429 (PA596) — Allows defendant the right to contact attorney before agreeing to BAC test.

H7433 (PA147) — Expands manslaughter with m.v. to include DWI.

1984 Legislation: Nothing passed.

Per Se: .10 per se, .07–.10 Driving While Ability is Impaired (infraction). Drinking Age: 21 yrs. (new 1985) Dram Shop Law: Maximum $20,000 per person injured, max. $50,000 per incident. Notice must be given to 3rd party within 60 days (Ch.545§30-102 [1935]). Open Container Prohibition: No law, except there is prohibition against drinking and driving.

Refusals to Submit:

1st refusal: 24 hr. lic. revoc. on spot + 6 mos. admin. lic. revoc.
2nd refusal: 24 hr. lic. revoc. on spot + 1 yr. admin. lic. revoc.
3rd refusal: 24 hr. lic. revoc. on spot + 3 yrs. admin. lic. revoc.

Driving under Revoc. License: $500–1000, mand. 5 days–1 yr. jail.

.10 BAC Administrative License Revocation: 24 hrs.

Youth Offender Legislation: If DWI & 18 yrs old, lic. revoc. until 18 yrs, or as set forth in penalty section, whichever longer.

	Penalties	Jail/CommSvc	LicRevoc/Rehab/ Therapy	Other
1st Offense	$500–1000,	Mand. 48 hrs–6 mths jail or 100 hrs. comm. service.	1 yr. lic. revoc., rehab.	*OR* pre-trial alcohol educ., $250, 8 rehab. sessions, lic. revoc. during rehab. Upon completion, charges are dismissed, but record of participation given to DMV.
2nd Offense	$500–2000,	Mand. 10 days–1 yr. jail	2 yrs. lic. revoc., rehab.	
3rd Offense	$1000–4000	Mand. 30 days–2 yrs. jail	3 yrs. lic. revoc., rehab.	
4th Offense	$2000–8000	Mand. 1–3 yrs. jail.	Permanent lic. revoc., rehab.	
Assault-2nd degree w/m.v.	Class D felony, $5000	Max. 5 yrs. jail.	1 yr. lic. revoc.	

	Penalties	Jail/CommSvc	LicRevoc/Rehab/ Therapy	Other
Manslaughter -2nd degree w/m.v.	Class C felony, $5000.	Max. 10 yrs. jail.	1 yr. lic. revoc.	

Miscellaneous: *Plea bargaining* to non-alcohol offense prohibited if BAC is .10+.

DELAWARE

1985 Legislation: Nothing passed this year. Bills pending, will carry over to 1986, incl. open container prohibitions, judicial appeals of administrative lic. revoc. & new penalties.

1984 Legislation: None.

Per Se: .10 Drinking Age: 21 yrs. Dram Shop Law: No specific statute, but illegal to sell to intoxicated person. Case law available to support liability of vender under this statute. Open Container Prohibition: None. Section 408 Grant: Received $262,000 Alcohol/ Traffic Safety Grant (Basic and Supplemental). PBTs: Allowed.

Refusals to Submit (administratively imposed, admissible as evidence):
1st refusal: 1 yr. hard. lic. revoc., rehab.
2nd refusal: 18 mos. hard lic. revoc., rehab.
3rd refusal: 24 mos. hard lic. revoc., rehab.

.10 BAC Administrative Penalties (separate from crim. disposition):
1st Offense: Mand. 3 mos. lic. revoc.
2nd Offense: Mand. 1 yr. lic. revoc.
3rd Offense: Mand. 18 mos. lic. revoc.

Driving under DWI Revoc. License:
1st Offense: Mand $200–500, 30 days–6 mos. jail. Min. 90 days vehicle impoundment.
2nd Offense: Mand. $500–1000, mand. 60 days–1 yr. jail. Min. 1 yr. vehicle impoundment.

	Penalties	Jail/CommSvc	LicRevoc/Rehab/ Therapy	Other
1st Offense	Mand. $200–1000	*&/OR* 60 days–6 mos. jail.	1 yr. lic. revoc., additional 6 mos. lic. revoc. or rehab.	
1st Offense if BAC less than .20 and no injury Pre-trial diversion program			Mand. 1 yr. lic. revoc., work restricted lic. avail. after 16 hrs. rehab and 90 days lic. revoc. have elapsed.	

	Penalties	Jail/CommSvc	LicRevoc/Rehab/ Therapy	Other
2nd Offense w/in 5 yrs.	Mand. $500–2000	Mand. 60 days–18 mos. jail.	Mand. 1 yr. lic. revoc., additional 6 mos. revoc. or rehab.	
3rd Offense w/in 5 yrs.	Mand. $500–2000	Mand. 60 days–18 mos. jail	Mand. 18 mos. lic. revoc., additional 6 mos. revoc. or rehab.	

FLORIDA

1986 Legislation: SB115 — Creates Alcohol/Drug Abuse Education program and Trust Fund funded until 7/89 by fines. Eff. 1/88, if less than 18 yrs. old, must complete course before obtaining drivers lic.

1985 Legislation:

SB1 (Ch285) — Raises drinking age from 19 to 21 yrs. Grandfather clause if born prior to 6/30/66. Effective 7/1/85.

SB106 (Ch326) — Establ. victim compensation/witness svce program. Funded by $20 surcharge.

SB964 (Ch337) — Add'l $25 fine imposed upon DWIs to go to Emergency Medical Svces Trust Fund.

1984 Legislation: HB360 (Ch84-359) — Allows out-of-state convictions to be used when determining prior offenses. Allows comm. svc. in lieu of fine if defendant financially unable. Youth offender leg.: if lic. used to misrepresent age, can revoke lic. for 1 yr. and order max. 40 hrs. comm. svc.

Per Se: .10 Drinking Age: 21 yrs. (New, 1985 see above) Dram Shop Law: No dram shop law, but it is illegal to furnish to habitual drunkard if written notice has been given by immediate family. Open Container Prohibition: None. PBTs: Used, refusal not admissible.

Refusals to Submit (admissible as evidence):
1st refusal: 6 mos. lic. revoc.
2nd refusal: 1 yr. lic. revoc.

Driving under Revoc. License:
1st Offense: 2nd degree misdemeanor, $500, 60 days jail.
2nd Offense: 1st degree misdemeanor, $1000, 1 yr. jail.

	Penalties	Jail/CommSvc	LicRevoc/Rehab/ Therapy	Other
1st Offense	$250–500.	Max. 6 mos. jail. Mand. 50 hrs. comm. svc.	180 days–1 yr. lic revoc. Rehab. Work-restricted lic. avail. upon completion of rehab.	Mand. 1 yr. probation.

	Penalties	Jail/CommSvc	LicRevoc/Rehab/ Therapy	Other
2nd Offense w/in 3 yrs.	$500–1000.	Mand. 10 days–9 mos. jail.	Min. 5 yrs. lic. revoc. (if 2nd offense w/in 5 yrs.), no work-restricted lic. avail. Rehab.	
3rd Offense w/in 5 yrs.	Habitual offender, $1000–2500.	Mand. 30 days–12 mos. jail.	Min. 10 yrs. hard lic. revoc. (if 3rd offense w/in 10 yrs.). Rehab.	
DWI/serious bodily injury/ property damage	3rd degree felony, $5000.	Max. 5–10 yrs. jail.		*OR* above penalties, whichever is tougher.
Vehicular homicide	3rd degree felony, max. $5000	Max. 5 yrs. jail.		

GEORGIA

1985 Legislation:

HB72 (PA562) — Raises drinking age to 21 yrs. over 2 yr. period. Eff. 9/30/85 — 20 yrs., 9/30/86 — 21 yrs.

HB90 (PA563) — Expands implied consent to anywhere in state, not just on roadways; if DWI while on restricted lic., automatic 5 yr. hard lic. suspension; other provisions.

HB558 (PA717) — Dept. of Revenue to be notified by County if alcoh. licensee charged with selling to minor.

HB142 (PA564) — Making it criminal offense for underage drinker to misrepresent age to obtain alcohol. Also adding penalty for 2nd offense of supplying minors with alcohol.

SB35 (PA366) — Tech. allows Comm. to enter reciprocal agreements to approve Driver improve. Courses.

SB30 (PA526) — Tech. relating to payment for police who attend admin. hearings on admin. lic. revoc.

1984 Legislation:

SB61 — Restricts court from changing sentence after judgement is rendered.

SB426 — Technical change

SR362 — Resolution establishing Problem Drinker and Highway Safety Study Committee.

HB1200 — DMV will suspend GA drivers' lic. for DWI conviction in another state.

Per Se: .12 Drinking Age: 21 yrs. (new, see above) Dram Shop Law: Limited to parents' right of action against person giving alcohol to minor children. Open Container Prohibition: None.

Refusals to Submit: 12 mos. hard admin. lic. revoc., admissible as evidence.

Driving under Revoc. License: $500, 2 days–6 mos. jail, additional 1 yr. lic. revoc.

Driving under Revoked License and Habitual Offender: $750, 1–5 yrs. jail.

Youth Offender Legis.: If under 18 yrs., must complete 6 hr. drug/alcohol course before obtaining lic.

	Penalties	Jail/CommSvc	LicRevoc/Rehab/ Therapy	Other
1st Offense	Mand. $300–$1000	10 days–1 yr. jail	Mand. 1 yr. lic. revoc. *OR* 120 days + ASAP + $25. Work-restricted lic. avail.	*OR* plead no contest, rehab, no lic. revoc.
2nd Offense w/in 5 yrs.	Mand. $600–$1000	Mand. 48 hrs.–1 yr. jail or 10 days comm. svc.	Mand. 3 yrs. lic. revoc. *OR* 120 days + ASAP + $25. Work-restricted lic. avail.	
3rd Offense	Habitual offender, mand. $1000	Mand. 10 days–1 yr. jail or 30 days comm. svc.	Indefinite lic. revoc.	
Homicide by m.v. while DWI	1st degree homicide	2–15 yrs. jail	Mand. 3 yr. hard lic. revoc.	
Habitual Offender DWI and homicide by m.v.	1st degree homicide	3–15 yrs. jail		

HAWAII

1986 Legislation:

HB26 — Increases drinking age from 18 to 21 yrs.

HB1726 — Expands open container prohib. to incl. scenic lookouts, alleys, bridges etc.

HB2170 — Prohibits civil liab. of qualif. people who withdraw blood for police.

HB2337 — Req. abusers to obtain treatment. Current law applies only if certified as having dependen.

SB2266 — Upgrades penalties for driving under influence of drugs.

1985 Legislation:

HB329 — Increased penalties for driving under revoc. lic.

SB125 — Techn. reiterates lic revoc. period is 30 days hard, 60 days restricted, not either/or.

SB644 — Allows open containers in limousines if barrier between driver/passengers.

SB843 — Add'l penalties for refusals.

1984 Legislation:

HB1629 — Sets up procedures for police to conduct roadblocks. All vehicles or vehicles in specific numbered sequence to be stopped. Uniformed police officers in sufficient quantity to assure speedy compliance. Minimum safety precautions must be met.

HB2103 — Establishments selling liquor must post DWI penalties.

HB2142 — Revisions to qualify for Sec. 408 grant. Provides assessment for 2nd and 3rd offenders with cost of treatment to be paid for by defendant.

HB2163 — Relating to penalties for adults allowing possession of alcohol by minors. Not illegal if alcohol is ingredient in medicine, used for religious ceremony, provided with consent of parent and belief that minor would not consume it or only consume it in presence of parent/legal guardian.

Per Se: .10 Drinking Age: 21 yrs. (new 1986) Dram Shop Law: None. Open Container Prohibition: Yes, except 1985 leg. allowing it in limousines (see above). 1986 leg. expands it to include other parts of highway not directly in traffic flow. (see above)

Refusals to Submit:
1st offense: $25–1000, 12 mos. lic. revoc.
2nd offense: 2–5 yr. lic. revoc.

Driving under Revoc. License: $250–1000, mand. 3 day–1 yr. jail.

	Penalties	Jail/CommSvc	LicRevoc/Rehab/ Therapy	Other
1st Offense w/in 5 yrs.	*ONE OR MORE OF:* $1000, 48 hrs. jail, 72 hrs. comm. svc.		14 hr. rehab., 30 days hard lic. revoc., 60 days restricted lic. revoc.	
2nd Offense w/in 5 yrs.	$500–1000	48 hrs. jail or 8 hrs. comm. svc.	1 yr. hard lic. revoc. Assessment, rehab. (costs to be borne by defendant).	
3rd Offense w/in 5 yrs.	$500–1000	10–180 days jail	1–5 yrs. lic. revoc.. Assessment, rehab. (costs to be borne by defendant).	

IDAHO

1986 Legislation: HB451 (CH201) — If eval. indicates treatment, must also indicate type/ cost. Mand if req. by eval. Mand restitution if convicted of aggravated DWI, prev. was at judge's option.

1985 Legislation:
HB102 — Reiterates that legal drug-use is not defense to DWI/Drugs.
HCR13 — Joint resolution authorizing Attny Gen. to sue Congress & DOT over fed'l age 21 law.

1984 Legislation: Nothing enacted.

Per Se: .10 per se, .08 presumptive. Drinking Age: 19 yrs. Dram Shop Law: none. Open Container Prohibition: For wine only.

Refusals to Submit: 120 days admin. lic. revoc.

Driving under Revoc. License:
1st Offense: Max $500, mand. 2 day–6 mos. jail, additional 6 mos. lic. revoc., work-restricted lic. avail.
2nd Offense w/in 5 yrs.: Max. $1000, mand. 20 day–1 yr. jail, additional 1 yr. hard lic. revoc.

3rd Offense w/in 5 yrs.: Felony, max $3000, mand. 30 days–3 yrs. jail, additional 3 yrs. hard lic. revoc.

Youth Offender Legislation: 1 yr. lic. revoc. or until 18th birthday, whichever is longer, for DUI offense. 60 day lic. revoc. for underage (19 yrs.) possession violation (does not have to be DUI).

	Penalties	Jail/CommSvc	LicRevoc/Rehab/ Therapy	Other
1st Offense	Mis-demeanor, max $1000.	Max. 6 mos. jail.	180 days lic. revoc., work-restricted lic. avail.	Be advised by Court, in writing, penalties for subsequent offenses.
2nd Offense w/in 5 yrs.	Mis-demeanor, max $2000.	Mand. 10 days–1 yr. jail.	Mand. 6 mos.–1 yr. lic. revoc., work-restricted lic. avail. after 30 days.	Be advised by Court, in wirting, penalties for subsequent offenses.
3rd Offense w/in 5 yrs.	Felony, max. $5000.	Mand. 30 days–5 yrs. jail.	Mand. 1–5 yrs. lic. revoc.	
Aggravated DUI (injury occured)	Can be charged under Felony (3rd offense) statute.			Also includes restitution.
Vehicular homicide w/ gross negligence	$2000–7000.	and/or 2–7 yrs. jail.	Mand. hard lic. revoc.	

INDIANA

1986 Legislation:

S146 — Relating to admin. lic. procedures for refusals & avail. of restricted licenses.

HB1180 — Defends seller against suits charging patron was illegally denied service, if sellers defense was that patron appeared intoxicated. Also bans "happy hours" eg. reduced prices or 2 for 1's. etc.

SB438 — M.V. Comm. can suspend vehicle registr./plates if owner can't prove $ respon. after 3 yrs.

1984 Legislation:

SB93 — Creates habitual offender statute — 3 or more DWIs or 2 or more DWIs where death occured. 10 yr. admin. lic. revoc.

SB94 — If refuse BAC test, admin. lic. revoc. period (90 days–2 yrs.) is in addition to criminal disposition. If .10, admin. lic. revoc. period is credited toward criminal lic. revoc. sentence. Changes mandatory 2 days jail for 2nd offenders to mandatory 48 hrs.

Per Se: .10 Drinking Age: 21 yrs. Dram Shop Law: No dram shop statute, but prohibition against furnishing alcohol to intoxicated person. Appears to be case law to back up the liability of a seller for injuries caused by intoxicated person. Open Container Prohibition: None. Section 408 Grant: Received $1,206,503 Alcohol/Traffic Safety Grant (Basic and Supplemental).

Refusals to Submit: 1–2 yr. admin. lic. revoc., admissible as evidence. (not mandatory, court may terminate lic. revoc. if in interests of society.

.10 Administrative Revocation: 180 days, but credited against criminal disposition. Restricted lic. avail. for 1st offenders but must prove eligibility.

Driving under Revoc. License: Class D felony, max. $10,000, mand. 5 days–4 yrs. jail. 3 yrs.-permanent lic. revoc.

	Penalties	Jail/CommSvc	LicRevoc/Rehab/ Therapy	Other
1st Offense DWI (not necessarily .10)	Class A mis-demeanor, max. $5000	Max. 1 yr. jail.	90 day lic. revoc. or 180 day probation with 30 day hard and 60 day restricted lic. revoc.	
1st Offense .10	Class C mis-demeanor, max $500	Max. 60 days jail.	90 day lic. revoc. or 180 day probation and 30 day hard and 60 day restricted lic. revoc.	
2nd Offense w/in 5 yrs., or if bodily injury	Class D felony, max. $10,000.	Mand. 5 days jail (48 hrs. consecutive) or 10 days comm. svc.-4 yrs. jail.	1–2 yrs. lic. revoc.	
If death occurs	Class C felony, max. $10,000.	5–8 yrs. jail.	1–2 yrs. lic. revoc.	

Miscellaneous: *Prosecutor must notify victims* of trial date at least 10 days prior.

ILLINOIS

1985 Legislation:

HB1841 — Expands Bill of Rights for Victims & Witness of Violent Crimes to include DWI death/injury. Expands their version of admin. lic. revoc. to include .10 as well as refusals. Req. Sec. of State to suspend IL. d.l. If refuse BAC test in other state. Increase other penalties. New crime: Class A Misd, if lend car to DUI driver.

SB651 — If DUI & personal injury or property damage in excess of $300, Class 4 felony.

HB430 — Distinctive d.l. if under 21 yrs. old.

HB737 — Dram Shop Liability, increases coverage from $20,000 to $100,000, with $300,000 aggregate.

SB993 — Cannot plea down to lesser offense if 2nd offense DWI.

SB341 — Reckless homicide by m.v. (if DWI) from Class 4 to Class 3 felony.

1984 Legislation: SB1484 — if DUI and operating school bus, Class 4 felony.

Per Se: .10 Drinking Age: 21 yrs. Dram Shop Law: Yes, if new law signed (1985), expands maximum liability. (See above HB737). Open Container Prohibition: Yes, driver assessed points for violation, Lic. revoc. for 2nd offense (new)

Refusal to Submit or if .10 per se: (Cannot refuse if death/injury occurs, however cannot use these results for criminal prosecution.) Not technically administrative. If hearing is requested, it is judicial, not administrative hearing, requests for work-restricted lic. go to Circuit Court.d as part of criminal proceedings.

1st refusal: 6 mos. lic. revoc. Restricted lic. avail., but very difficult to get.

.10 BAC: 3 mth. lic. revoc. Restricted lic. avail., but very difficult to get.

2nd refusal or .10BAC: 12 mos. lic. revoc. Restricted lic. avail., but very difficult to get.

Reckless Homicide: Class 3 felony (from weaker Cl.4). Establ. DWI as "reckless act" for purposes of law.

Driving under DUI Revoc. License: Class A misdemeanor. Mand. 7 days jail or 30 days comm. svc. Double orig. liv. revoc. period.

	Penalties	Jail/CommSvc	LicRevoc/Rehab/ Therapy	Other
1st Offense	Class A misdemeanor, max. $1000	Max. 1 yr. jail	Mand. 1 yr. lic. revoc. Restricted lic. avail, but *very* difficult to get.	*OR* court supervision, max $1000, max. 2 yrs. lic. revoc, comm. svc.
2nd Offense w/in 5 yrs.	Class A misdemeanor	Mand. 48 hrs. jail or 10 days comm. svc.	Mand. 1 yr. lic. revoc., hardship lic. avail, but *very* difficult to get. Rehab.	

IOWA

1986 Legislation:

SF97 — Increases drinking age from 19 to 21 yrs. Grandfathered if 19 by 8/1/86. Valid unless fed'l law is overturned or repealed.

HF2493 — Lowers per se from .13 to .10, allows PBTs & roadblocks, increases penalties for driving under revoc. lic., increases lic. revoc. penalties for 1st/2nd offense. No points assessed on speed violations less than 10 mph if posted limit is over 35 mph and less than 2 pts on d.l. in last year.

1985 Legislation: None enacted, bills to raise the drinking age & lower per se will carry over to '86.

1984 Legislation:

HF2486 — Major revision of penalties.

HF2472 — Open container prohibition, parents to be notified of underage drinking violations.

HF2235 — relating to driving under revoc. lic.

Per Se: .13, .10 for administrative revocation. Drinking Age: 21 yrs, new, see 1986 leg above. Dram Shop Law: Yes, §123.92 Open Container Prohibition: yes, parents to be notified of underage drinking violations.

Refusals to Submit (administratively imposed):
1st refusal: 240 days. lic. revoc. (was 180 days).
2nd refusal: 540 days lic. revoc. (was 1 yr.), work-restricted lic. avail. after 365 days.

.10 Admin. Revoc. Penalties (regardless of criminal disposition):
1st Offense: 180 days lic. revoc. (was 120 days), work-restricted lic. avail.
2nd Offense: 1 yr. lic. revoc. (was 240 days), work-restricted lic. avail.

Driving Under Revoc. Lic.: Serious misdm. Double orig. lic. revoc.

	Penalties	Jail/CommSvc	LicRevoc/Rehab/ Therapy	Other
1st Offense	Serious misdemeanor, $500–1000, *OR* 50–200 hrs. comm. svc.	Mand. 48 hrs. jail.	180 days. lic. revoc. ('86 new, was 30–90 days) If .20, mand sub. abuse eval. Inpatient time credited against jail term ('86 new)	If defer. judg. then 30–90 day lic. revoc. ('86 new)
2nd Offense w/in 6 yrs.	Aggravated misdemeanor, min. $750.	Mand. 7 days jail.	1 yr. lic. revoc.	Substance abuse evaluation inpatient time can be credited against sentence.
3rd Offense w/in 6 yrs.	Class D felony, min. $750.	Max. 1 yr. county jail. ('86 new)	Min. 2–6 yr. lic. revoc. Must complete eval; have no subseq convict, abstain from excessive alc. use, not have any other lic. revoc.- to get it back after the 2 yrs.	Substance abuse evaluation inpatient time can be credited against sentence.
If serious injury occured	Class D felony, min. $750.	Max. 1 yr county jail. ('86 new)	Additional 1 yr. lic. revoc., work-restricted lic. avail.	
If death occured	Class D felony, min. $750.	Max. 1 yr county jail. ('86 new)	Addition 6 yrs. lic. revoc.	Restitution.

Miscellaneous: *$100 assessment* (civil penalty) for all lic. revoc.

KANSAS

1986 Legislation:
HB2752 — PBTs allowed.
HB2822 — Expands restrictions on diversion program. See below**

1985 Legislation:
HB2067 — Raises drinking age from 18 yrs. for 3.2 beer to 21 yrs. Grandfather clause if born before 7/1/66. Would revert back to 18 yrs. if fed'l law is nullified. Effective 7/1/85.

HB2570 — Allows previously confidential info. on diversion program to be given to DMV.

HB6071 — Resolution to ask DMV to include DWI info. on lic. tests.

HB2629 — Allows more than 1 BAC test to be given to test for controlled substances.

SB127 — Mand 90 day jail for driving under DWI-revoked lic. Admin. lic. revoc., new revoc. penalties. All lic. revoc. must be consecutive not concurrent. Tightens up diversion program entrance.

SB126 — Increases penalties for underage possession.

HB2614 — Increases fees for diversion program from $85 to $110.

HB2570 — Req. D.A. to keep apprised of status of diversions that have been given & must notify. Dept. of Revenue & DMV so info. is available statewide in future.

HB2142 — Board of Educ. to provide program to identify/resolve drug/alcohol problems in grade school.

SB128 — "Happy Hour Ban" on 2 for 1's, free drinks, 1/2 price drinks etc.

1984 Legislation: None passed.

Per Se: .10 Drinking Age: 21 yrs. for everything (1985 new, see above) Dram Shop Law: No statute, although it is illegal to sell alcohol to intoxicated person. Open Container Prohibition: Misdemeanor, max. $200 and/or 6 mos. jail. PBTs allowed (new 1986 leg. see above).

Refusals to Submit (admissible as evidence): 120 days–1 yr. lic. revoc. NEW: Taken at time of stop, 15 day temp lic. issued, must request hearing within 10 days, revoc. stayed pending hearing.

Driving under DWI Revoc. License:

1st Offense: Class B misd., habitual offender, $100, mand. 90 days jail (was 5 days) double original lic. revoc. period.

2nd Offense: Class A misdemeanor, same penalties as 1st offense.

3rd Offense: Class F felony, same penalties as 1st and 2nd offenses.

	Penalties	Jail/CommSvc	LicRevoc/Rehab/ Therapy	Other
1st Offense	$200–500,*	Mand. 48 hrs. jail or 100 hrs. comm. svc. to 6 mos. jail,	90 days–1 yr. work-restricted lic., pre-sentence evaluation, educ. Must complete treatment before lic. returned.	*OR* Diversion** program, $110 or comm. svc., pre-sentence evaluation, rehab.
2nd Offense w/in 5 yrs.	$500–1000,*	Mand. 90 days–1 yr. jail or 5 days jail and rehab.,	Pre-sentence evaluation, 1 yr. lic. revoc., or 120 day lic. revoc. or until rehab. completed.	
3rd Offense w/in 5 yrs.	Habitual offender, $100–2500,*	Mand. 90 days–1 yr. jail,	Mand. 1 yr. lic. revoc., pre-sentence evaluation.	

**Diversion program not available if: 2nd offense, or if BAC above .20, or if death/injury occured, or if plead no contest to previous alcohol related offense. (last restriction, '86 new)

*Fine provisions can be satisfied by comm. svc. work at $5/hr.

KENTUCKY

1985 Legislation: nothing enacted.

1984 Legislation: SB20 — Major revision of DWI statute, see below.

Per Se: No per se; .10 presumptive; if .15 BAC, person to be detained at least 4 hrs. Drinking Age: 21 yrs. Dram Shop Law: No specific statute, except it is illegal to sell to intoxicated person. May be some weak case law supporting liability of vendor. Open Container Prohibition: None. PBTs: Allowed, refusal not admissible.

Refusals to Submit: 6 mos. admin. lic. revoc. Work-restricted lic. avail. for 1st refusals if enroll in rehab.

Driving under Revoc. License:
1st Offense: Class B misdemeanor, 2x orig. lic. revoc. period.
2nd Offense: Class A misdemeanor, 2x orig. lic. revoc. period.

Youth Offender Legislation: If convicted, lic. to be revoc. until 18th birthday or according to sentence, whichever is longer period.

	Penalties	Jail/CommSvc	LicRevoc/Rehab/ Therapy	Other
1st Offense	$200–500	*&/OR* 48 hrs.–30 days jail (can be served on weekends) *OR* 2–30 days comm. svc. if no injury.	6 mos. lic. revoc. *OR* rehab. and 30 day lic. revoc.	jail mand. if injury occured.
2nd Offense	Mand. $350–500.	Mand. 7 days–6 mos. jail (can be served on weekends) 10 days–6 mos. comm. svc.	Mand. 12 mos. lic. revoc. Max. 1 yr. rehab.	
3rd Offense	Mand. $500–1000.	Mand. 30 days–12 mos. jail. 10 days–12 mos. comm. svc.	Mand. 24 mos. lic. revoc. Mand. 1 yr. rehab.	

Miscellaneous: *Additional $150 assessed* on all convictions, used to fund DWI law.

LOUISIANA

1986 Legislation:

SB30 — Increases drinking age from 18 to 21 yrs. unless fed'l law repealed, expired or unconstitut, $25 fine, earmarked for enforcement, educ. Eff. 9/30/86. As of 6/25 not yet signed by Gov.

HB1356 — If convicted of DWI, court may suspend all/part of sentence & give max. 2 yr. probation, unless prohibited by law.

1985 Legislation:

SCR43 — Resolution for a Joint Committee Study on the impact of allowing refusals to take BAC test.

SB222 (Act579) — Allows morgues, hopsitals e.r. to be used for comm. svce. placements.

SB363 (Act542) — Clarifies Crime Victims Reparation Fund, funded by surcharge imposed upon offenders. Can collect $100–10,000, no minimum for victims over 60 yrs. old.

SB419 (Act746) — Clarifies that "under the influence" also applies to controlled substances.

SB437 (Act747) — Expands crime of vehicular negligent injuring while under the influence to include drugs & controlled substances.

SB1051 (Act572) — Extends time req. for administrative hearings from 45 days to 90 days.

HB127 (Act828) — Allows for the reporting & drug/alcohol testing of students if necessary. Results not admissable in civil/criminal actions.

HB973 (Act382) — Requires defendants who refuse BAC to sign form that stipulates penalties.

HB974 (Act194) — Cannot refuse BAC test if fatality occured.

HB1721 (Act816) — Extends admin. lic. revoc. to include violations of municipal or parish ordinances.

1984 Legislation:

HB1051 (Act511) — Allows exemplary damages (in addition to general and special damages) to be awarded when DWI caused injuries occur.

SB612 (Act409) — Non-substantive technical changes relating to admin. lic. revoc. procedures.

Per Se: .10 Drinking Age: 18 yrs. Dram Shop Law: No statute, except illegal to sell to intoxicated person. Open Container Prohibition: None. Sec. 408 Grant: Received $527,956 (Basic only. Has not yet submitted Supplemental Grant information. Will receive additional $351,971 when that is done.)

Refusals to Submit:
1st refusal: 90 days hard admin. lic. revoc., 90 days restricted lic.
2nd refusal: 545 days hard admin. lic. revoc.

Administrative Lic. Revoc. for .10:
1st Offense: 90 days admin. lic. revoc.
2nd Offense: 365 days hard admin. lic. revoc.

DWI and Driving under Revoc. License: $300–500, mand. 7 days–6 mos. jail.

	Penalties*	Jail/CommSvc	LicRevoc/Rehab/ Therapy	Other
1st Offense	$125–500,	10 days–6 mos. jail,	60 days lic. revoc., restricted lic. avail.	
OR if probation		2 days jail or 32 hrs. comm. svc.,	Rehab., including assessment.	
2nd Offense	$300–500,	30 days–6 mos. jail,	1 yr. hard lic. revoc.	
OR if probation		15 days jail or 30 days comm. svc.,	Rehab., including assessment.	

	Penalties	Jail/CommSvc	LicRevoc/Rehab/ Therapy	Other
3rd Offense	Max. $1000,	6 mos.–5 yrs. jail,	1 yr. hard lic. revoc., rehab. including assessment.	
4th Offense		10–30 yrs. hard labor imprisonment.	1 yr. hard lic. revoc.	
Vehicular Homicide while DWI	$2000–5000,	2–5 yrs. jail		
Vehicular injury while DWI	Max. $500,	and/or 6 mos. jail.		

All penalties are min. mand. unless stated.
Miscellaneous: *Owner of vehicle notified* if car involved in DWI offense.

MAINE

1986 Legislation: HB1571 — Amends the Annual-Operating-Under-the-Influence-Report.

1985 Legislation:

SP332 (Ch402) — Raises drinking age from 20 to 21 yrs. Grandfather clause, 20 yrs. by 6/1/85. Eff. 6/1/85

SP486 (Ch296) — Allows optional reporting of DWI by medical personnel with no personal liability.

SP152 (Ch308) — Allows Sec. of State to revoke restricted lic. for any violation of conditions.

SP614 (Ch331) — Technical relating to license revocation procedures.

HP789 — Prohibits suspending any part of 2nd offense lic. revoc. penalty for underage drinkers even judge did not warn person after the 1st offense.

SP598 — Dram Shop Law: Asserts right to sue 3rd party up to max. of $100,000. Law in effect only until 9/1/87 during which time Legal Affairs Committee will study situation and develop leg.

SP615 — Happy Hour Ban, prohibits free drinks, 2 for 1's, or other practices encouraging excess.

1984 Legislation: Nothing passed.

Per Se: .10 Drinking Age: 21 yrs. (New 1985, see above) Dram Shop Law: Yes, new 1985 see SP598. Open Container Prohibition: None, except if under 20 yrs. old cannot transport liquor at all unless at request of employer or parent. Section 408 Grant: Received $262,000 Alcohol/Traffic Safety Grant (Basic and Supplemental).

Refusals to Submit (administratively imposed and admissible as evidence):
1st refusal: 180 days lic. revoc., work-restricted lic. avail.
2nd refusal w/in 6 yrs: 1 yr. lic. revoc., work-restricted lic. avail.

Driving under Revoc. License: Class D crime, maximum $2500.

Youth Offender Legislation: Provisional lic. until driver is 20 yrs. old. 1 yr. lic. revoc. for DWI, or if .02 BAC or if refusal to submit. Work-restricted lic. avail. after 6 mos. if rehab. is completed.

	Penalties	Jail/CommSvc	LicRevoc/Rehab/ Therapy	Other
1st Offense traffic infraction	Mand. min. $300		Mand. 90 day lic. revoc.	
1st Offense criminal violation if BAC above .15, driving 30 mph over limit, Or if eluded police; Or if 2nd Offense w/in 6 yrs.	Mand. min. $350.	Mand. min. 48 hrs. jail	Mand. 90 day lic. revoc.	
2nd Offense criminal violation	Mand. min. $500.	Mand. 7 days jail.	Mand. 1 yr. lic. revoc.	
3rd Offense criminal violation	Mand. min. $750.	Mand. 30 days jail	Mand. 2 year lic. revoc.	
If homicide occurs			5 yrs. permanent lic. revoc.	

MARYLAND

1986 Legislation: SB85 (Ch652) — Refusal to submit is admissable but does not infer guilt/innocence.

1985 Legislation:

HB245 (Ch599) — Mandatory penalties for 2nd offence, (48 hrs. jail or 80 hrs. comm. svce.)

S871 (Ch584) — Allows DMV to waive lic. revoc. if adversly affects employment/ comm. svce program.

S826 (Ch244) — Technical relating to authority to certify rehab/treatment programs.

HB1150 (Ch681) — Relating to alcohol/driver improvement programs.

SB70 (Ch504) — Prohibits drinking and driving, no fine indicated.

HB491 (Ch758) — Relating to issuance of special i.d. cards to residents of state with no d.l. Will include profile view of person if under 21 yrs. old.

House Joint Resolution 42 — Requests Gov. to establish task force on youth & alcohol.

1984 Legislation:

HB636 — BAC tests are admissible without presence of person who performed test.

HB749 — Relating to time frame for which defendant can notify BAC technician to be present at trial.

HB900 — State's Attorney to be notified if juvenile fails to comply with rehab. or work program.

SB367 — Clarifies that if BAC test required by police, certain equipment standards must be met.

Per Se: No per se; .13 prima facie for DWI, .08 prima facie for DWUI. Drinking Age: 21 yrs. Dram Shop Law: Although statute prohibiting sales to intoxicated people exists, court has ruled that does not expand to include dram shop law. Open Container Prohibition: Yes, new but does not appear to have penalty. PBTs: Allowed.

Refusals to Submit (administratively imposed):
1st refusal: Mand. 60 days–6 mos. lic. revoc. Work-restricted lic. avail.
2nd refusal: Mand. 120 days–1 yr. lic. revoc. Work-restricted lic. avail.

Driving under Revoc. License (12 pts.):
1st Offense: Max. $1000, 1 yr. jail.; 120 day vehicle registration suspension.
2nd Offense: Same as above, except 2 yrs. jail.

DWI .13 BAC	Penalties	Jail/CommSvc	LicRevoc/Rehab/ Therapy	Other
1st Offense	Max. $1000,	1 yr. jail.	6 mos. lic. revoc., if probation then rehab.	
2nd Offense w/in 3 yrs.	Max. $1000,	48 hrs. jail or 80 hrs. commsvce	1 yr. lic. revoc., if probation then rehab.	
3rd Offense w/in 3 yrs.	Max. $1000,	2 yrs. jail.	18 mos. lic. revoc., if probation then rehab.	
DWUI .08 BAC				
1st Offense	Max. $500,	Max. 1 yr. jail.	60 day lic. revoc., if probation then rehab.	
2nd Offense w/in 3 yrs.	Max. $500,	Max. 1 yr. jail.	Max. 129 days lic. revoc., if probation then rehab.	
3rd Offense w/in 3 yrs.	Max. $500,	Max. 1 yr. jail.	Max. 6 mos. lic. revoc. If probation then 6 mos. lic. revoc.	

MASSACHUSETTS

1985 Legislation: HB6508 (Ch223) — Estab. Joint Underwriting Commission for liquor legal liability insurance for alcohol related organizations that are unable to obtain insurance. Provides for claims against establishments arising out of negligence in distributing, selling or serving alcohol. Motor-vehicle related offenses are inclu. but other off-premise offenses are not.

1984 Legislation: HB5952 — Raises drinking age from 20 to 21 yrs. Grandfather clause if 20 yrs. old by effect. date. Effect. 6/1/85 or earlier if ME, NH, CT, NY, & VT adopt 21 yr. law prior to that date.

Per Se: None. Drinking Age: 21 yrs. Dram Shop Law: Illegal to sell to intoxicated person. Case law supports 3rd party (dram shop) liability (138 §69). Open Container Prohibition: $100–500 (adopted 1982).

Refusals to Submit: 90 days admin. lic. revoc. If hearing requested, revoc. not stayed.

Driving under DWI Revoc. License: $200–500, mand. 7 days–2½ yrs. jail.

	Penalties	Jail/CommSvc	LicRevoc/Rehab/ Therapy	Other
1st Offense	$100–1000,	Max. 2 days jail, 36 hrs. comm. svce.	Mand. 1 yr. lic. revoc.	
	OR 2 yrs. probation*, $100–1000,	Max. 2 days jail, 36 hrs. comm. svc.,	Mand. 30 days lic. revoc., 14 day residential treatment program,	Additional $200 assessment to support program.
2nd Offense w/in 6 yrs.	$300–1000,	Mand. 7 days–2 yrs. jail, 36 hrs. comm. svc.	Mand. 1 yr. hard lic. revoc., 1 yr. restricted lic.	
	OR 2 yrs. pro-* if never rec'd before $300–1000.	Mand. 7 days–2 yrs. jail, 36 hrs., comm. svc.	Mand. 1 yr., hard lic. revoc., 2 yrs. restricted lic., 14 day residential treatment program,	Additional $200 assessment.
3rd Offense w/in 6 yrs.	$500–1000,	Mand. 60 days–2 yrs. jail, 36 hrs. comm. svc.,	Mand. 3 yrs. hard lic. revoc., 2 yrs. restricted lic.	
Homicide by M.V. — 1st Offense	Max. $5000,	1–10 yrs. jail,	10 yrs. lic. revoc.	
Homicide by M.V. — 2nd Offense	Max. $5000,	1–10 yrs. jail,	Permanent lic. revoc.	

*No probation available if death/serious injury occured.

Miscellaneous: In all convictions, *court shall obtain name and address of establishment where defendant was served* alcohol prior to the violation.

MICHIGAN

1985 Legislation:

HB4009 — Establishes Victims Rights Act Bills pending include:

HB4018 — Youth offender legislation.

HB4019 — Youth offender legislation, relating to open container violations.

HB4356 — Refusal to submit to BAC is admissable.

HB4374 — 90 day–1 yr. admin. lic. revoc. for .10 BAC

SB123 — Mand. jail/comm. svce. for 2nd offenders (Passed Senate, in House Judl. Comm.)

SB351 — Provides criteria for appeals of lic. revoc. to circuit court.

HB4344 — Provides mand. lic. revoc. for altering d.l. for illegal purposes.

HB4370 — Must make full or partial restitution if convicted of felony or misdm.

1984 Legislation:

HB5804 — Minors d.l. to look different from adults. Eff. 10/1/85.

S877 — Prohibits roadside sobriety checkpoints in state.

H5279 — Adds 1 new member to state Drunk Driving Task Force.

Per Se: .10 Drinking Age: 21 yrs. Dram Shop Law: Yes, §18.993. Open Container Prohibition: Yes.

Refusals to Submit:
1st refusal: 6 mos. admin. lic. revoc.
2nd refusal: 1 yr. admin. lic. revoc.

Driving under Revoc. License:
1st Offense: Max. $100, or 3–90 days jail, registration plates confiscated. Double original lic. revoc.
2nd Offense: Max $500, 5 days–1 yr. jail, other provisions same as above.

	Penalties	Jail/CommSvc	LicRevoc/Rehab/ Therapy	Other
1st Offense DWI .10	Misdemeanor, $100–500,	Max. 90 days jail. Max. 12 days comm. svc.	6 mos.–2 yrs. lic. revoc., restricted lic. avail.	Prosecution costs, pre-sentence assessment/ rehab.
2nd Offense w/in 7 yrs.	Max. $1000	And/or max. 1 yr. jail. Max. 12 days comm. svc.	Mand. lic revoc.	Pre-sentence assessment/ rehab.
3rd Offense w/in 10 yrs.	Felony,	Max. 12 days comm. svc.	Mand. lic. revoc.	Pre-sentence assessment/ rehab.
1st Offense Operating While impaired (.07–.09 BAC)	$300,	Max. 90 days jail. Max. 12 days comm. svc.	90 days–1 yr. lic. revoc.	Pre-sentence assessment/ rehab.
2nd Offense w/in 7 yrs. of either OWI or .10	Max. $1000,	Max. 1 yr. jail. Max. 12 days comm. svc.	Mand. 6–18 mos. lic. revoc., including 60 day hard.	

Miscellaneous: Statute provides for *annual drunk driving audit* to be prepared each year showing number of alcohol-related m.v. accidents, injuries, deaths, arrests made, lic. suspensions, convictions and penalties assessed.

MINNESOTA

1986 Legislation:

SF1014 (Ch435) — Sheriff Contingent Fund reinstated, 25% of county fine $. Victim's Rights language incl. right to demand trial w/60 days & to have separate waiting area at trial.

SF5 (Ch330) — Raises drinking age to 21 yrs., prohibits alcohol industries from sponsoring events on colleges that include alcohol. Application form for d.l. to include DWI pamphlet. Part of lic. revoc. fee to go to school based alcohol educ. programs at all levels.

Legislation:

SF8 (Ch4) — Expands DWI to include violations upon ice of boundary waters. Expands Crime Victim Reparation Fund, Increasing max. amount from $25,000 to 50,000. Estab. Crime Victim & Witness Advisory Council.

SF265 (309) — Relating to Dram Shop. Sets $30,000 as minimum amount if death occured. Stipulates that liquor licensees must submit proof of responsibility before getting license. A showing of dram shop liability insurance of at least $300,00 would be sufficient.

HF1145 (Ch305) — Youth Offender Leg. 30 day lic. revoc. if under 19 yrs. & use d.l. to purchase alcohol.

1984 Legislation:

SF473 (Ch306) — Related to police arrest powers. Can arrest outside jurisdiction if police believe probable cause exists and driver eludes officer. Allows refusal to be admissible as evidence with no restrictions.

SF1642 (Ch430) — Allows use of infrared breath test equipment.

SF1336 (Ch622) — Allows defense to per se law that defend. consumed alcohol after stop but before BAC test given. Defense, if used, must be given to prosec. prior to pre-trial hearing. Youth Offender Legis.: Lic. revoc. for 6 mths or until 18 yrs. (whichever is longer) for DWI viol.; restricted lic. avail. only if needed for school/rehab.; 30 days lic. revoc. for minors purchasing alcohol if d.l. used to do so. Strengthens refusal penalties; was 6 mos, now 1 yr. Expands DWI to include parking lots.

Per Se: .10, .07 recorded on lic., upon 2nd stop of .07, assessment may be required. Drinking Age: 21 yrs., grandfather clause if born before 9/1/67. Eff. 9/1/86, ('86 new) Dram Shop Law: Statute in effect, 1982 amendment deleted maximum dollar amount recoverable (§340.95). Open Container Prohibition: Yes. PBTs: Allowed, not admissible as evidence.

Refusals to Submit: Admiss. as eviden. 1 yr. admin. lic. revoc. Revoc. not stayed even if hearing requested .10 BAC: 90 days admin. lic. revoc. Revoc. not stayed even if hearing is requested.

Driving under Revoc. License: Misd., max. $500, 30 days jail.

DWI and under Revoc. License: Gross Misdemeanor, max. $1000, 90 days jail.

Youth Offender Legislation: If DWI, 6 mos. admin. lic. revoc., or until age 18 yrs., whichever is longer. Also 30 days lic. revoc. for minors purchasing alcohol using drivers lic.

	Penalties	Jail/CommSvc	LicRevoc/Rehab/ Therapy	Other
1st Offense	Max. $500,	90 days jail,	Mand. 30 days lic. revoc.*	
2nd Offense w/in 5 yrs.	Gross misdemeanor, max. $1000,	Max. 1 yr. jail,	Mand. 90 days lic. revoc., and rehab.*	
3rd Offense w/in 5 yrs.	Gross misd. max. $1000.	Max. 1 yr. jail,	Mand. 1 yr. lic. revoc., and rehab.*	

	Penalties	Jail/CommSvc	LicRevoc/Rehab/ Therapy	Other
4th Offense w/in 5 yrs.	Gross misd. max. $1000.	Max. 1 yr. jail,	Mand. 2 yrs. lic. revoc., and rehab.*	
If personal injury	Felony, max $10,000	Max. 5 yrs. jail	Addit'l 90 days lic. revoc.	
DWI death & gross negligence (driver does not stop)	Felony, $5000,	5 yrs. jail.		
DWI injury & gross negligence (driver does not stop)	Felony, $3000,	3 yrs. jail.		

*Restricted lic. avail. immediately except if manslaughter, gross negligence or felony.

MISSISSIPPI

1986 Legislation (vetoed by Governor): HB916 — Would have specifically prohibited dram shop liability, but vetoed.

1985 Legislation:

SB2005 (Ch.431) — Raises drinking age from 18 yrs. beer/lt. wine to 21 yrs. Exception if at least 18 yrs. & in presence of parent/l.g., exception for military bases if allowed by base.

HB703 (Ch346) — Technical, relating to procedures for appealing revocations.

1984 Legislation: Nothing passed.

Per Se: .10 Drinking Age: 21 yrs., 1985 new, see above. Dram Shop Law: No specific statute, but is illegal to sell/furnish alcohol to intoxicated person. '86 leg. vetoed by Gov. would have prohibited dram shop liability by statute. Open Container Prohibition: None. Section 408 Grant: Received $646,055 Alcohol/Traffic Safety Grant (Basic and Supplemental). PBTs: Allowed.

Refusals to Submit (administratively imposed): $500–1000, and/or 1 yr., jail. 90 day lic. revoc., 45 days hard suspension.

Driving under Revoc. License: Misdemeanor, $200–500, 48 hrs.–6 mos. jail. Additional 6 mos. lic. revoc.

	Penalties	Jail/CommSvc	LicRevoc/Rehab/ Therapy	Other
1st Offense	$200–5000,	And/or 24 hrs. jail.	1 yr. lic. revoc. or 90 days and ASAP. Work-restricted lic. avail after 45 days.	

	Penalties	Jail/CommSvc	LicRevoc/Rehab/ Therapy	Other
2nd Offense w/in 5 yrs.	$400–1000,	48 hrs.–1 yr. jail or comm. svc.	2 yrs. lic revoc. or 1 yr. lic. revoc. and rehab.	
3rd Offense w/in 5 yrs.	$500–1000,	30 days–1 yr. jail.	3 yrs. lic. revoc. or 1 yr. and rehab.	
If death occurs	Felony, max. 5 yrs. jail.			

Miscellaneous: *If .10 BAC:* Lic. pulled and 30 day temp. given pending disposition of criminal charges. (Not strictly administrative revoc. because of tie-in to crim. charges.) No *plea bargaining* if .10+ BAC.

MISSOURI

1985 Legislation:

SB345: Specifically prohibits dram shop liability except in case of sale to minor.

SB285: Joins State Drivers Lic. Compact; will suspend lic. of state resident for crimes committed in other states.

1984 Legislation:

SB608/681 — Prohibits imposition of administrative lic. revoc. if arrest was based upon roadblock/checkpoint stop in which there was no probable cause to stop.

HB1226 — Expands Crime Victims Compensation Fund to include DWI victims.

Per Se: .10 per se, administrative lic. revoc. at .13. Drinking Age: 21 yrs. Dram Shop Law: Specifically prohibited by 1985 law, previously there was case law to back up joint negligence of tavern owner and intoxicated person (Carver vs. Schafer (App. 1983) 647 SW.2d 570). Open Container Prohibition: None.

Refusals to Submit (administratively imposed): 1 yr. lic revocation.

Administrative License Revocation for .13 BAC: Cannot be imposed if arrest occured at roadblock/checkpoint (new, see SB60/681). May be credited against later criminal revocation.

1st Offense: 30 day hard lic. revoc., 60 day restricted lic. revoc., rehab.

2nd Offense: 1 yr. hard lic. revoc. and rehab.

Driving under Revoc. License: Class A misdemeanor, $100, mandatory 48 hrs.–1 yr. jail or 10 days (40 hrs.) comm. svc.

	Penalties	Jail/CommSvc	LicRevoc/Rehab/ Therapy	Other
1st Offense DWI (not necessarily .10)	Class B mis-demeanor, $500,	Max. 6 mos. jail.	90 days lic. revoc.	All mandatory unless min. 2 yrs. probation is given.
1st Offense w/.10 BAC	Class C mis-demeanor, $300,	Max. 15 days jail.	No lic. revoc. stipulated.	

	Penalties	Jail/CommSvc	LicRevoc/Rehab/ Therapy	Other
2nd Offense w/in 5 yrs.	Prior offender, Class A mis- demeanor, $1000.	Mand. 48 hrs.– 1 yr. jail or 10 days comm. svc. (40 hrs.)	Mand. 1 yr. lic. revoc.	
3rd Offense w/in 5 yrs.	Persistent offender, Class D felony, $5000,	1–5 yrs. jail, min. mand. ⅓ of jail term must be served.	Mand. 1 yr. lic. revoc.	

MONTANA

1985 Legislation:

SB3 — To submit initiative to voters, removing drinking age (19 yrs.) from the state constitution and allowing age to be established by voter initiative or statute. If approved, eff. 1/1/87.

HB600 — To include other jurisdiction's convictions for purposes of sentence enhancement.

HB210 — Lessens penalties, expands veh. assault to include, under influence of drugs. (see below).

HB390 — Techn. relating to defin. of vehicle in DWI. (expanded to include all veh. except bicycles).

HB246 — Allows court to seize d.l. upon conviction for offense which has mand. lic. revoc/suspen.

HB531 — Clarifies DMV's right to issue probationary lic. & provides for penalties if violate terms.

HB52 — Youth Offender legislat. 90 day lic. revoc., max. $50, and/or complet. of community-based substance abuse program if underage & caught with alcohol while in control of m.v.

HJR22 — Resolution requesting interim study on alcohol regulation and youth.

SJR27 — Resolution endorsing Designated Driver concept & encouraging activity by groups in state.

1984 Legislation: None, did not meet.

Per Se: .10 Drinking Age: 19 yrs. Dram Shop Law: No law, except illegal to sell to intoxicated person. Open Container Prohibition: Yes. Section 408 Grant: Received $363,265 Alcohol/Traffic Safety Grant (Basic and Supplemental).

Refusals to Submit (administratively imposed, refusal admissible as evidence):
1st refusal: 90 days hard lic. revoc.
2nd refusal: 1 yr. hard lic. revoc.

Driving under Revoc. License: Misd., max. $500, 2 days–6 mth jail. 2x/initial revoc. period.

DWI (below .10)	Penalties	Jail/CommSvc	LicRevoc/Rehab/ Therapy	Other
1st Offense	$100–500	Mand. 24 hrs.–60 days jail, unless judge feels imposition poses risk to defendant.	Mand. 6 mos. lic. revoc. Rehab.	
2nd Offense w/in 5 yrs.	$300–500	Mand. 4 days (at least 48 hrs. consec.)–6 mos. jail.	Mand. 1 yr. lic. revoc. Rehab.	
3rd Offense w/in 5 yrs.	$500–1000	Mand 10 days (at least 48 hrs. consec.)–1 yr. jail.	Mand. 1 yr. lic. revoc. Rehab.	
.10				
1st Offense	$100–500	Max. 10 days jail.	Mand. 6 mos. lic. revoc. Rehab.	
2nd Offense w/in 5 yrs.	$300–500	48 hrs.–30 days jail	Mand. 1 yr. lic. revoc. Rehab.	
3rd Offense w/in 5 yrs.	$500–1000	48 hrs.–6 mos. jail.	Mand. 1 yr. lic. revoc. Rehab.	

Vehicular Assault while DWI/Drugs: Max. $1000, and/or 1 yr. county jail. Was max. $20,000 and/or 3 yrs. state prison.

NEBRASKA

1985 Legislation: Nothing enacted, open container law was passed but vetoed by Gov., may have had some drafting problems with it. 1 bill, LB631 regarding penalties will carry over to 1986.

1984 Legislation: LB56 — Raises drinking age from 20 to 21 yrs.

Per Se: .10 Drinking Age: 21 yrs. Dram Shop Law: No statute; illegal to sell to intoxicated person, but no 3rd party (dram shop) liability created. Open Container Prohibition: None.

Refusals to Submit to PBT or .10 BAC:

1st Offense: Class W misdemeanor, 6 mos. hard admin. lic. revoc., or, if probation, 60 days hard. lic. revoc.

2nd Offense: Class W misdemeanor, 1 yr. hard admin. lic. revoc., or, if probation, 6 mos. hard. lic. revoc., 48 hrs. jail.

3rd Offense: Permanent lic. revoc., or, if probation, 1 yr. hard lic. revoc., 7 days jail.

Refusal to submit: 1 yr. hard admin. lic. revoc.

Operating under Revoc. License: Class IV felony

	Penalties	Jail/CommSvc	LicRevoc/Rehab/ Therapy	Other
1st Offense	Class W misdemeanor, $200	Mand. 7 days jail,	Mand. 6 mos. hard lic. revoc.	*OR* probation, mand. 60 days hard lic. revoc.
2nd Offense	Class W misdemeanor, $500,	Mand. 30 days jail.	Mand. 6 mos. hard lic. revoc.	*OR* probation, mand. 48 hrs. jail, mand. 6 mos. hard lic. revoc.
3rd Offense	Class W misdemeanor, $500,	Mand. 6 mos. jail,	Mand. permanent lic. revoc.	*OR* probation, mand. 7 days jail, mand. 1 yr. hard lic. revoc.

NEVADA

1986 Legislation: None, did not meet.

1985 Legislation:

AB85 (Ch359) — Only if 1st offense must defendant be segregated from violent crime offenders.

AB478 (Ch249) — Restricts use of urine tests unless person is hemophiliac/heart condition or unless officer suspects presence of controlled substance.

AB480 (Ch430) — Must obtain 2 breath BAC tests to establish BAC, if person refuses 2nd test, 1st test alone can be used, and lack of 2nd test constitutes refusal.

AB381 (Ch175) — Increases max. jail for DWI/death or serious injury from max. 6 yrs. to max. 20 yrs.

AB318 (Ch416) — Must show $ responsibility for 3 yrs. after restoration of revoc. lic.

AB363 (Ch510) — Fee for lic. reinstatement increased from $50 to $100.

SB181 (Ch175) — Clarifies that DMV can issue restricted lic. for hardship reasons.

1984 Legislation: None, did not meet.

Per Se: .10 Drinking Age: 21 yrs. Dram Shop Law: None. Open Container Prohibition: Partial; illegal to drink while driving. Section 408 Grant: Received $273,488 Alcohol/ Traffic Safety Grant (Basic and Supplemental). PBTs: Allowed, not admissible as evidence.

Refusals to Submit:

1st refusal: 1 yr. lic. revoc.

2nd refusal: 3 yrs. lic. revoc.

Driving under Revoc. License: Mand. $500–1000, mand. 30 days–6 mos. jail does not have to be served consecutively. Double original lic. revoc.

Refusal to submit to PBT or if .10 BAC: 90 day admin. lic. revoc.

	Penalties*	Jail/CommSvc	LicRevoc/Rehab/ Therapy	Other
1st Offense w/in 7 yrs.	Mis-demeanor, $200–1000,	2 days–6 mos. jail or 48 hrs. comm. svc. (dressed in manner to identify as violator of law.)	90 days lic. revoc. 45 days hard.,	Education *OR* prob. max. $200 1 day jail or 24 hrs. comm. svc. 45 day lic. revoc. Prosecutor can request hearing on probation.
2nd Offense w/in 7 yrs.	Mis-demeanor, $500–1000,	10 days–6 mos. jail (at least 48 hrs. consecutive),	1 yr. hard lic. revoc.	*OR* probation. max. $500, 5 days jail (at least 48 hrs. consecutive), rehab., 6 mths lic. revoc. Prosecutor can request hearing on probation.
3rd Offense w/in 7 yrs., or if death/ injury occured	$2000–5000,	1–6 yrs. jail (1–20 yrs if death/serious injury). Must be separ. from violent offen.	3 yrs. hard lic. revoc.	

*All penalties minimum mandatory.

Miscellaneous: Can require more than 1 BAC test. Failure to submit to either or both constitutes failure.

NEW HAMPSHIRE

1986 Legislation:

HB310 (Ch35) — Changes lic. revoc. for aggravated DWI from 1 yr. to 1–2 yrs. lic. revoc.

HB313 (Ch216) — Provides for 3 yrs. probationary lic. if previous DWI revoked lic or probationary lic. until 21st birthday if minor. Illegal to drive if .03 BAC.

1985 Legislation:

Ch3 — Raises drinking age to 21. Grandfather clause if 20 yrs. by 6/1/85. Eff. 6/1/85.

Ch89 — Relating to lic. revocation for implied consent violations.

Ch123 — Allows registered nurses/physicians' assistants to do blood BAC test.

Ch28 — Technical, funding/control of alcohol education program.

Ch162 — Technical, relating to refusal appeals.

Ch242 — Probationary lic. given if lic. previously revoked. BAC of .03 is violation of prob. lic. If have probationary lic. & refuse BAC, 90 day admin. lic. revoc.

Ch290 — Estab. negligence homicide statute for DWI, among other penalties is 7 yr. lic. revoc.

Ch303 — Strengthens penalties for minors who purchase alcohol illegally.

1984 Legislation: None.

Per Se: .10 Drinking Age: 21 yrs. (new 1985). Dram Shop Law: Illegal to serve intoxicated person, act of negligence, but no specific dram shop statute. Open Container Prohibition: Applies only if under 20 yrs. old, traveling without parent/legal guardian. Sec. 408 Grant: Received $262,000 Alcohol/Traffic Safety Grant (Basic and Supplemental).

Refusals to Submit (administratively imposed for refusals, but not .10; admissable as evidence):

1st refusal: 90 days lic. revoc.
2nd refusal: 1 yr. lic. revoc.
This revoc. period to run consecutively with any other periods of lic. revoc.

Driving under Revoc. License: $100, mandatory 7 days jail (to be served consecutively within 6 months). 1 yr. lic. revoc.

	Penalties	Jail/CommSvc	LicRevoc/Rehab/ Therapy	Other
1st Offense	Max. $1000.		Min. Mand. 90 days–2 yrs. lic. revoc.	
2nd Offense w/in 7 yrs.	Mis-demeanor, max. $1000,	Mand. 7 days jail (served consecutively w/in 6 mos.)	Mand. 3 yrs. lic. revoc.	Liable for double damages in civil suit.
3rd Offense			Mand. 3 yrs.-permanent lic. revoc.	
Aggravated DWI — 1) If impaired or .10 BAC and driving 30 mph above posted limit and either — bodily injury occured, or — tried to elude police 2) If BAC above .20	Mis-demeanor, $350–1000.		1–2 yr. lic. revoc. ('86 new, was 1 yr.)	

Miscellaneous:

Plea bargaining from 2nd offense to 1st offense and, to non-alcohol offenses if BAC is .10+, is restricted.

Limits continuation of cases for more than 35 days.

BAC tests taken from all deceased drivers and pedestrians can be used for statistical eveluations or as evidence in trial actions.

NEW JERSEY

1986 Legislation: Bill # not known — Limits 3rd party liability of hosts if guest commits DWI. Guests barred from suing altogether, and other DWI victims must prove strict liability of host. (Not yet signed by Gov. as of 7/1/86).

1985 Legislation:

AB274 (Ch251) — Allows court of deduct up to ⅓ of prisoner's earned income to pay restitution.

SB485 (Ch97) — Estab. offense of assault by auto. Increases penalties for death by auto.

SB2293 (Ch239) — Tech., clarifies implied consent to reiterate inclusion of dangerous substances.

SB2312 (Ch311) — Estab. offense of offering/serving alcohol to minor with exceptions.

SB2679 (Ch113) — Changes penalties for underage purchases or if purchase for minor. Decreases lic. revoc. from 1 yr. to 6 mths.

1984 Legislation:

AB802 (Ch.1) — Surcharge on insurance for DWI convictions and/or increase in points.

AB828 (Ch.4) — Additional $100 assessment for Drunk Driving Enforcement Fund.

Per Se: .10 Drinking Age: 21 yrs. Dram Shop Law: 1986 legislation restricts host liability in direct response to Supreme Court case that extended such liability (see above). In regard to other third party liability, it appears that the legislation does not change it. Seller is liable to both third parties and intoxicated persons themselves. 33:1–39 Note 10. Open Container Prohibition: $200–250, 10 days comm. svc. Section 408 Grant: Received $796,474 Alcohol/Traffic Safety Grant (Basic only. In order to qualify for Supplemental Incentive Grant, state must revoke lic. within 45 days of arrest, or within 90 days of arrest and submit plan to reduce it to 45 days.)

Refusals to Submit:

1st refusal: $250–500, mand. 6 mos. admin. lic. revoc.

2nd refusal: $250–500, mand. 2 yrs. admin. lic. revoc.

Driving under DUI revoc. License: $1000, mand. 30 days jail (45 days if injury occured).

	Penalties	Jail/CommSvc	LicRevoc/Rehab/ Therapy	Other
1st Offense	$250–400,	30 days jail,	6 mos. – 1 yr. lic. revoc.	
2nd Offense w/in 10 yrs.	$500–1000,	Mand. 90 days jail or 30 days comm. svc.	Mand. 2 yrs. lic. revoc., mand. 30 days rehab.	
3rd Offense w/in 10 yrs.	Mand. $1000,	Mand. 180 days jail or 90 days jail/90 days comm. svc.	Mand. 10 yr. lic. revoc.	
Death by m.v. due to DUI	3rd degree,	Mand. 270 days jail or comm. service.		

NEW MEXICO

1985 Legislation:

SB202 (Ch178) — Prohibits granting of work-restricted lic. for refusal to submit, or 2nd offenses. Also reiterates admin. revoc. procedures.

HB198 (Ch23pv) — Court can require community service for DWI conviction.

HB97 (Ch186) — Add'l $150 fine, 2 days–6 mths. jail, double-1 yr. original lic. revoc. for driving under DWI revoc. lic.

SB529 (Ch191) — Dram Shop Liab. Drunk person cannot collect against establishment that served him. No civil liability against establishment by 3rd party unless it can be proven that person was visibly intoxicated. No private host liability unless alcohol was given recklessly. Establishment can be held liable if drunk person was minor.

HB387 (Ch239) — If DWI and injure pregnant woman causing miscarriage/stillbirth, considered felony.

HB481 (Ch187) — Clarifies right of police to determine BAC test to be given and other administrative procedures for DWI arrests, and administrative revocation procedures.

1984 Legislation:

HB67 (Ch72) — Clarifies .10 per se law; adds administrative lic. revoc. for .10. Prohibits work-restricted lic. for refusals and 2nd offenders. Administrative revocations and subsequent criminal revocation penalties to total maximum 1 yr. Prohibits refusals if great bodily injury occured. Youth offender legislation stipulates admin. lic. revoc. if less than 18 yrs old and BAC is .05.

HB75 (Ch73) — Technical amendment appropriates funds for administrative revocation.

Per Se: .10 Drinking Age: 21 yrs. Dram Shop Law: Yes some, see above. Open Container Prohibition: None. Section 408 Grant: Received $389,777 Alcohol/Traffic Safety Grant (Basic and Supplemental)

Refusals to Submit (administratively imposed): 1 yr. lic. revoc., no work-restricted lic. available (1985 new, see SB202 above).

Administrative License Revocation (.10 for over 18 yr. olds, .05 for under 18 yr. olds):
1st Offense: 90 days for 18 yr. olds and older. 6 mos. if under 18 yrs.
2nd Offense: 1 yr. if under 18 yrs. old.
All administrative lic. revoc. penalties to run concurrently with any criminal revocation penalties, if so assessed (new, see HB67).

Driving Under Revoc. Lic.: Misdemeanor, max. $500, 2 days–6 mos. jail, additional revocation.

	Penalties	Jail/CommSvc	LicRevoc/Rehab/ Therapy	Other
1st Offense	$300–500,	30–90 days jail,	Mand. 1 yr. lic. revoc, restricted lic. avail.	*OR* 90 days–3 yrs. probation.
2nd Offense	$1000.	Mand. 48 hrs.–1 yr. jail,	Mand. 1 yr. hard lic. revoc.	*OR* 1–5 yrs. probation and mand. 48 hrs. jail instead of fine.
Homicide or great bodily injury by m.v. while DUI	3rd degree felony,		1 yr. lic. revoc.	

NEW YORK

1986 Legislation:

AB2574 — Raises drinking age to 21 yrs. Effective 12/1/85.

S1592 — Clarifies requ. that more than one type BAC test may be requested.

S2760 — Allows out-of-jurisdiction DWI convictions to be used for purpose of sentence enhancement.

S4801 — Technical, tightens up ability to obtain work-restricted d.l.

S5603 — Tech. Accords felony status to any 2nd offense DWI (Alcohol or drugs). Previously stipulated that it must have been same impairing substance.

S5969 — Increases penalties for leaving scene of accident.

S6430 — Tech. If revoc. due to refusal, lic. cannot be rtned. even after rehab. completed until revoc. period is completed.

S6436 — Increases penalties for vehicular manslaughter/assualt with DWI/revoc. lic.

S2550 — Tech. Bars participation in Drinking Driver Program if 2nd offense occurs within 5 yrs. of earlier participation. Current law stipulated no participation if the conviction occured within 5 yrs. of earlier participation. This encouraged defendants to artificially delay date of conviction.

S4336 — D.L. Must be suspended pending prosecution if DWI-drugs & assualt/homicide or 2nd offense.

S6432 — Increases penalties for driving under DWI suspended/revoked license.

1984 Legislation: S1254D — Deletes provis. allowing completion of rehab. to satisfy ½ of fine or jail penalty.

Per Se: .10 Drinking Age: 21 yrs. (new, 1985 see AB2574, above). Dram Shop Law: Illegal to sell to intoxicated persons, case law supports 3rd party (dram shop) liability based upon this statute. Open Container Prohibition: Yes.

Refusals to Submit: Cannot refuse if accident occurs.
1st refusal: $100, mand. 6 mos. hard lic. revoc.
1st refusal w/ prior conviction w/in 5 yrs.: $250, mand. 1 yr. hard lic. revoc.
2nd refusal w/in 5 yrs.: $250, 1 yr. hard lic. revoc.

Driving under DWI Revoked Lic.: $500, 7–180 days jail or special probation/treatment.

DWI and Driving Under Revoc. Lic.: Class E Felony $500–5000, prison sentence, vehicle impoundment.

Youth Offender Legislation: Lic. revoc. until age 21 for DWI (.10) conviction. $200, and/or 5 days jail for obtaining liquor for underage persons. Also civilly liable for damages caused as a result of that procurement.

DWAI (.06–.09 BAC)	Penalties	Jail/CommSvc	LicRevoc/Rehab/ Therapy	Other
1st Offense	Infraction, mand. $250,	Max. 15 days jail,	Mand. 90 days lic. revoc.	*OR* Drinking driver program, same penalties except restricted lic. avail.
2nd Offense w/in 5 yrs.	Infraction, mand. $350–500,	Max. 30 days jail,	Mand. 6 mos. hard lic. revoc.	

	Penalties	Jail/CommSvc	LicRevoc/Rehab/ Therapy	Other
3rd Offense w/in 5 yrs.	Infraction, mand. $500–1500,	Max. 90 days jail,	Mand. 6 mos. hard lic. revoc.	
DWI (.10)				
1st Offense	Misdemeanor, mand. $350–500,	Max. 1 yr. jail,	Mand. 6 mos. hard lic. revoc.	
2nd Offense w/in 10 yrs.	Felony, mand. $500–5000,	Max. 4 yrs. jail,	Mand. 1 yr. lic. revoc.	
2nd offense w/in 10 yrs., personal injury	Felony, mand. $500–5000,	Max. 4 yrs. jail,	Mand. permanent lic. revoc.	
Vehicular Assault	Class E felony,	Max. 4 yrs. jail,	Mand. 6 mos. lic. revoc.	
Vehicular Manslaughter	Class D felony,	Max. 7 yrs. jail,	Mand. 6 mos. lic. revoc.	

Miscellaneous:

STOP-DWI (Special Traffic Options Program for DWI): 1981 legislation created funding mechanism for local drunk driving programs approved by state. Provides return of fines from state to county, earmarked for DWI. Prohibits plea barganing from DWI to non-alcohol offense.

Insurance companies to provide clients with info. on current NY DWI-DWAI laws on an annual basis.

NORTH CAROLINA

1985 Legislation: HB101 (Ch141) — Raises drinking age for beer/table wine from 19 to 21 yrs. (spirits already were 21 yrs.) under fed'l pressure. Would be repealed upon repeal or finding that fed'l law is unconstitutional. Eff. 9/1/86.

1984 Legislation: HB1660 (Ch1101) — Technical changes to last yr.'s bill.

Per Se: .10 Drinking Age: 21 yrs. (1985 new, see above). Dram Shop Law: Limited to minors, $500,000 limit of liability. Must prove that furnishing beverage was negligent, if minor misrepresented himself this is evidence of non-negligence. Open Container Prohibition: Yes. PBTs: Allowed, not admissible as evidence.

Refusals to Submit: 10 days + 12 mos. lic. revoc. Work-restricted lic. avail. after 6 mos., if 1st offense and no death/injury occured. .10 BAC: 10 day admin. lic. revoc.

Driving under Revoc. License: Level 2, max $100, mand. 7 days–12 mos. jail, mand. 1 yr. lic. revoc.

If 1st offense and no serious injury occured, judge must review aggravating and mitigating factors:

Aggravating include:
.20 BAC
$500+ property damage
personal injury
eluded police
passed stopped school bus
drove 30+ mph over limit

Mitigating include:
under .11 BAC
driving safe/lawful other than DWI
due to lawfully prescribed drug
voluntary rehab. after charge

	Penalties	Jail/CommSvc	LicRevoc/Rehab/ Therapy	Other
1 st Offense (mitigating outweigh aggra- vating)	Level 5, max. $100,	Mand. 24 hrs.–60 days jail, rehab., *OR* combination of 24 hrs jail, 24 hrs. comm. svc. w/in 30 days, 30 days lic. revoc., rehab.		
1st Offense (counter- balanced)	Level 4, max. $250,	Mand. 48 hrs.–120 days jail, rehab., *OR* combination of 48 hrs. jail, 48 hrs. comm. svc. w/in 60 days, 60 days lic. revoc., rehab.		
1st Offense (aggra- vating outweigh mitigating)	Level 3, max. $500,	Mand. 72 hrs.–6 mos. jail, rehab., *OR* combination of 72 hrs. jail, 72 hrs. comm. svc. w/in 90 days, 90 days lic. revoc., rehab.		
2nd Offense w/in 7 yrs. or if 1st Offense/ serious injury	Level 2, max. $1000,	Mand. 7 days–12 mos. jail,	Rehab, mand. 1 yr. lic. revoc. if serious injury. Otherwise 2 yrs. hard lic. revoc., 2 yrs. restricted.	
3rd offense w/in 7 yrs, or if 2 out of 3: serious injury, driving under DWI revoc. lic., 2nd Offense	Level 1, max. $1000,	Mand. 7 days–12 mos. jail,	Rehab. Mand. 4 yrs. lic. revoc. (2 yrs. hard).	
3rd Offense w/in 5 yrs.	Same as above 3rd offense,		3 yrs.-permanent lic. revoc.	
If death occurs	Class 1 felony,		3 yrs.-permanent lic. revoc.	

Miscellaneous:

Roadblocks allowed by statute, plan must be developed in advance.

Pre-trial release of impaired driver: Held in custody until no longer impaired, or if can be released to sober responsible adult.

NORTH DAKOTA

1986 Legislation: None, did not meet.

1985 Legislation:
HB1140 (Ch443) — Blood test done on persons killed in mv's, results submitted to NHTSA.
SB2086 (Ch82) — Tech. wording change "claim for relief" from "right of action" for civil liab.
SB2301 (Ch110) — Raises fine for open container violation from $20 to $50.
SB2373 (Ch429) — Reduces mandatory jail for driving under revoc. lic. from 15 days to 4 consec. days. Recog. admin. lic. revoc. procedures from other states, need certfd. cc of record. Increases lic. reinstatement fee from $25 to $50 if DWI-related. Strengthens, clarifies admin. revoc./refusal penalties & issuance of restricted lic.

1984 Legislation: None, did not meet.

Per Se: .10 Drinking Age: 21 yrs. Dram Shop Law: NDCC5-01-06, recently revised (1983) to also allow damages if death occurs. Open Container Prohibition: $50 fine, no points on d.l. unless offense was on driver. Section 408 Funds: Received $387,264 Alcohol/Traffic Safety Grant (Basic and Supplemental). PBTs: Allowed.

Refusals to Submit:
1st offense: 1 yr.
2nd offense: 2 yrs.
3rd offense: 3 yrs. All admissable as evidence.

Driving under Revoc. License: Class B misdemeanor, mand. 15 days jail, mand. fine (amount not specified). Possible m.v. plates impounded. Minimum 6 mos.-double original lic. revoc.

.10 BAC Administrative License Revocation (separate from criminal disposition):
1st Offense: 91 days lic. revoc., 30 days hard.
2nd Offense: 364 days hard. lic. revoc.
3rd Offense: 2 yrs. hard lic. revoc.

	Penalties	Jail/CommSvc	LicRevoc/Rehab/ Therapy	Other
1st Offense	Class B misdemeanor, min. mand. $250.		Addiction evaluation.	In-patient rehab. can be credited against jail sentence.
2nd Offense w/in 5 yrs.	Class B misdemeanor, min. mand. $500	Mand. 4 days jail (at least 48 hrs. consecutive) or 10 days comm. svc.	Addiction evaluation.	In-patient rehab. can be credited against jail sentence.
3rd Offense w/in 5 yrs.	Class A misdemeanor, mand. $1000 115 points on d.l.	Mand. 60 days jail (48 hrs. must be consecutive)	Addiction evaluation. Rehab + 2 yrs. before lic. will be returned.	In-patient rehab. can be credited against jail sentence.

	Penalties	Jail/CommSvc	LicRevoc/Rehab/ Therapy	Other
4th Offense w/in 7 yrs.	Class A misdemeanor, mand. $1000 115 points on d.l.	Mand. 180 days jail (48 hrs. must be consecutive).	Addiction evaluation. Rehab + 2 yrs. before lic. will be returned.	In-patient rehab. can be credited against jail sentence.
If death occurs	Manslaughter or negligent homicide	Mand. 1 yr. jail	Mand. 1 yr. hard lic. revoc.	In-patient rehab. can be credited against jail sentence.

Miscellaneous: *Failure to complete rehab:*
1st Failure: Additional 180 days lic. revoc.
2nd Failure: Additional 1 yr. lic. revoc.
Work-restricted lic. avail. for both after 7 days.

OHIO

1986 Legislation: Bills pending on number of issues includ. raising drinking age. Will probably not be considered until after November election.

1985 Legislation:
HB252 — 4th degree felony if 4th offense DWI.
HB460 — Court can send DWI to intervention program or jail but must total at least 3 days.

1984 Legislation: SB74 — Allows 19 yrs. olds to serve distilled spirits in capacity of waiter/waitress, but *not* as bartender.

Per Se: .10 Drinking Age: 19 yrs. for beer, 21 yrs. for wine/spirits. Dram Shop Law: None, except illegal to sell to intoxicated person, and can sue restaurant if damages occured on premises but not DWI.

Refusals to Submit or .10 BAC: Administratively imposed but, if plead guilty or convicted on DWI this revoc. is terminated. 1 yr. lic. revoc., work restricted lic. avail. If defendant appeals and loses, must pay cost of hearing.

Driving under Revoc. License: 1st degree misdemeanor max. $500 and/or 1 yr. jail, additional lic. revoc. and possible vehicle impoundment.

	Penalties	Jail/CommSvc	LicRevoc/Rehab/ Therapy	Other
1st Offense	$150–1000,	Mand. 3 days jail (being interpreted as 3 days in-house rehab.)	Mand. 60 days–3 yrs. lic revoc. (work-restricted lic. avail.), rehab.	

	Penalties	Jail/CommSvc	LicRevoc/Rehab/ Therapy	Other
2nd Offense w/in 5 yrs.	$150–1000,	Mand. 10 consecutive days jail.	Mand. 120 days–5 yrs. lic. revoc. (work-restricted lic. avail.), rehab.	
3rd Offense w/in 5 yrs.	$150–1000,	Mand. 30 consecutive days jail.	180 days–50 yrs. lic. revoc. (work-restricted lic. not avail. until after 180 days), rehab.	
Vehicular Homicide — 1st Offense	1st degree mis-demeanor, no probation.		Permanent lic. revoc.	
Vehicular Homicide — 2nd Offense	4th degree felony, no probation.			
Aggravated Vehicular Homicide — 1st Offense	3rd degree felony.		Permanent lic. revoc.	
Aggravated Vehicular Homicide — 2nd Offense	No probation.			

OKLAHOMA

1985 Legislation:

HB1393 — Req. special design d.l. for under 21 yr. old drivers. Defines 2nd offense as within 10 yrs. Pre-screening assessment fee increased from $50 to $75. Requ. defendent to reim. all/part of actual rehab cost.

HB1368 — Technical as it relates to DWI.

SB336 — Technical relating to Alcohol & Drug Abuse courses.

HB1480 — Cannot refuse BAC if death/serious injury occurred.

SB111 — Raises age for consumption/possession to 21 yrs. (previous law only dealt with purchase.) Pending bills will carry over to 1986 include, youth offender; requ. special plates for DWI offenders, new penalties.

1984 Legislation:

SB403 — Increases fee from $50 to $75 for DUI school.

HB1034 — Increases mand. lic. revoc. from 2 yrs. to 3 yrs. for 3rd offenders. Increases penalties for driving under DUI revoc. lic. from $100–500 and 10 days–2 mos. jail to min. $500 and 60 days–1 yr. jail. Discusses treatment/assessment program.

HB1432 — Refusal to submit is admissible as evidence.

Per Se: .10 Drinking Age: 21 yrs. Dram Shop Law: No statute, although illegal to sell to intoxicated person. Open Container Prohibition: $50–250, max. 6 mos. jail.

Refusals to Submit: 90 days admin. lic. revoc., admissible as evidence.

Driving under Revoc. License (due to .10 or prior refusal): $100–500, 10 days–2 mos. jail.

	Penalties	Jail/CommSvc	LicRevoc/Rehab/ Therapy	Other
1st Offense	Misdemeanor, max. $1000	10 days–1 yr. jail	Mand. 6 mos. lic. revoc. & alcohol/ drug abuse course.	Pre-sentence
1st Offense w/injury	Misdemeanor, max. $2500	90 days–1 yr. jail	Mand. 6 mos. lic. revoc.	Pre-sentence screening $75.
2nd Offense w/10 yrs.	Felony, max. $2500	1–5 yrs. jail	Mand. 1 yr. lic. revoc.	May have to reimburse state for some/all of rehab/educ. costs.
2nd Offense w/injury w/10 yrs.	Felony, max. $5000	1–5 yrs. jail	Mand. 1 yr. lic. revoc.	
3rd Offense	Felony, max. $2500	1–5 yrs. jail	Mand. 3 yr. lic. revoc. (new)	
Negligent Homicide	$100–1000	Max. 1 yr. jail	Mand. 6 mos. lic. revoc.	

Miscellaneous: *If defendant pleads guilty, no contest, or convicted before judgement entered*, judge can suspend execution of sentence upon condition that rehab. be completed.

OREGON

1986 Legislation: None, did not meet.

1985 Legislation:

SB203 — Specifies procedures for appeals of license revocation.

SB148 — Removes authority of Hlth Dept. to issue BAC testing permits.

SB123 — Clarifies & revises lic. revoc. procedures.

SB726 — Estab. Alcohol Server Educ. Advisory Comm. to develop educ. & testing programs that will be required of Class A, B, & C restaurants, as of 1/1/87.

HB2073 — $5 DWI assessment to pay cost of D.A. obtaining m.v. records.

HB2513 — Clarifies that 5 yr. lic. revoc. for habitual offenders applies to all habitual offenders.

1984 Legislation: None, did not meet.

Per Se: .08 Drinking Age: 21 yrs. Dram Shop Law: Revamped in 1979, liability extends to tavern-keepers and private hosts if defendant was visibly intoxicated. Defendant cannot recover, only 3rd party can recover (ORS 30.950). Open Container Prohibition: Class B misdemeanor, max. $250.

Refusals to Submit (administratively imposed, admissible as evidence):
1st refusal: 1 yr. lic. revoc., 90 days hard
2nd refusal: 3 yrs. lic. revoc., 1 yr. hard.

.08 BAC Administrative Penalties (separate from criminal disposition):
1st Offense: 90 days lic. revoc., 30 days hard.
2nd Offense: 1 yr. lic. revoc., 90 days hard.

Driving under Revoc. License due to Prior Homicide/Assault Charge: Class C Felony, max. $100,000, 5 yrs. state prison.

Driving under Revoc. License due to Prior Refusal: Class F misdemeanor.

Youth Offender Legislation for any alcohol-related offense (does not have to be DWI): 90 days lic. revoc. and 1 yr. admin. lic. revoc. or until age 17, whichever is longer.

	Penalties	Jail/CommSvc	LicRevoc/Rehab/ Therapy	Other
1st Offense, no crash				Eligible for pre-trial diversion prog. $282, agree not to DWI, rehab. + costs.
1st Offense	Class A misdemeanor, max. $2500	Mand. 48 hrs.–1 yr. jail or 80–250 hrs. comm. svc.	1 yr. lic. revoc., work-restricted lic. avail. Mand. rehab.	
2nd Offense w/in 5 yrs	Class A misdemeanor, max. $2500	Mand. 48 hrs.–1 yr. jail or 80–250 hrs. comm. svc.	3 yrs. lic. revoc., 90 days hard. Mand. rehab.	
3rd Offense w/in 5 yrs.	Class A misdemeanor, max. $2500	Mand. 48 hrs.–1 yr. jail or 80–250 hrs. comm. svc.	3 yrs. lic. revoc., 1 yr. hard. Mand. rehab.	
If death occurs			Mand. 5 yrs. hard lic. revoc.	

Miscellaneous: Restitution can be recovered in DWI cases. Requires *pre-sentence investigation reports* to include Victim Impact information.

PENNSYLVANIA

1985 Legislation: First year of two year session. Nothing passed to date, approximately 20 bills pending.

1984 Legislation: SB1239 (Act99) — Relating to Work Release Program (Comm. Svce) for DWI Offenders.

Per Se: .10 Drinking Age: 21 yrs. Dram Shop Law: Yes, 47 §4–493. Open Container Prohibition: Yes. PBTs: Allowed, refusal not admissible as evidence.

Refusals to Submit: 12 mos. lic. revoc.

Driving under Revoc. License: $1000, 1 yr. jail, 6–12 mos. additional lic. revoc.

	Penalties	Jail/CommSvc	LicRevoc/Rehab/ Therapy	Other
1st Offense	2nd degree mis-demeanor, min. $300,	Min. 48 hrs. jail,	Max. 6 mos. lic. revoc., pre-sentence assessment.	*OR* Accelerated Rehab Disposition Program if no injury/death. Counts as conviction, must pay own fees, mand. 30 days–12 mos. lic. revoc. restitution.
2nd Offense w/in 7 yrs.	Min. $300,	Min. 30 days jail,	1 yr. lic. revoc., pre-sentence assessment.	
3rd Offense w/in 7 yrs.	Habitual offender, min. $300,	Min. 90 days jail,	5 yr. lic. revoc, pre-sentence assessment.	
4th Offense w/in 7 yrs.	Habitual offender, min. $300,	Min. 1 yr. jail,	Min. 5 yr. lic. revoc., pre-sentence assessment.	
Homicide by m.v.	3rd degree felony,	Min. 3 yr. jail.		

RHODE ISLAND

1985 Legislation:

H6189 — Penalties for underage consumption/age misrepresentation, $100–500. (Was $250–500)

H5537 — Limits dram shop liability to $200,000.

H5170 — Banning happy hours.

S394 — Allows 2BAC tests to be given to ascertain alcohol & toulene, or other controlled substances.

S398 — Expands Criminal Injuries Compensation Fund to include offense of refusing to submit to BAC test after collision. Previously, all other traffic offenses except DWI were exempt from collecting, and if defendant refused BAC, could hinder ability to obtain DWI conviction and technically victim could collect under Compensation Fund.

S399 — Estab. separate penalties for offenders under 18 yrs. See penalty section for info.

1984 Legislation:

S373 — Establishes flat maximum $500 fine for underage possession (was staggered from $100–500 according to prior offenses).

H7050 — Resolution asking U.S. Congress to ban alcohol advertising on radio and TV.

H7662 — Techn. change clarifying admin. adjudication of drinking and driving (not DWI) offenses.

H7041 — Raises drinking age from 20 to 21 yrs.

Per Se: .10 Drinking Age: 21 yrs. (raised in 1984). Open Container Prohibition: Only illegal for minors and extends to with open or closed containers. Dram Shop Law: Rev. 1985. H5537 estab. max. $200,000 if server can prove defendant not visibly intox. Section 408 Grant: Received $262,000 Alcohol/Traffic Safety Grant (Basic and Supplemental) . Procurement of Alcohol for Minors: Felony, max. $1000 &/or 6 mos. jail.

Drinking and Driving (not DWI):
1st offense: max. $200 &/or max. 6 mos. lic. revoc.
2nd offense: max. $500 &/or max. 1 yr. lic. revoc.

Refusals to Submit (Administrative Revocation):
1st refusal: $200 minimum and $150 assessment, 10–60 hrs. comm. svc., 3–6 mos. lic. revoc.
2nd refusal: $500 minimum and $150 assessment, 1–2 yr. lic. revoc.
3rd refusal: $800 minimum and $150 assessment, 2–3 yrs. lic. revoc.

Driving under Revoc. License:
1st Offense: Misdemeanor, $500, 10 days jail, additional 3 mos. lic. revoc.
2nd Offense: $500, 6 mos.–1 yr. jail, additional 6 mos. lic. revoc.
3rd Offense: felony, $1000, min. 1 yr. jail, permanent lic. revoc.

	Penalties	Jail/CommSvc	LicRevoc/Rehab/ Therapy	Other
1st Offense	$200,*	10–60 hrs. comm. svc. &/or 1 yr. jail.		If under 18 yrs., 6 mth. lic. revoc. educ., comm. svc. no jail. New '85
2nd Offense	$500,*	10 days jail.	1–2 yrs. lic. revoc. and treatment ($150).	Under 18 yrs., 1 yr. lic. revoc., max.
3rd Offense	$500,*	6 mos.–1 yr. jail.	2–3 yrs. lic. revoc. and treatment ($150).	1 yr. training school and/or max. $500. New '85
If death occurs — 1st Offense	Felony, $500–1000,	6 mos.–10 yrs. jail,	1 yr. lic. revoc.	
If death occurs — 2nd Offense	Felony, $800–5000,	5–20 yrs. jail,	3 yrs. lic. revoc.	

*All penalties are minimum mandatory.

SOUTH CAROLINA

1986 Legislation: Nothing enacted

1985 Legislation:
HB2261 — Raised drinking age to 21 yrs., effective 9/14/86.
HB2640 — $50 fee assessed against defendants for ASAP program.
HB2025 — Increases penalties for minors who misrepresent age for purposes of purchasing alcohol.
Other legislation pending will carry over to next year (2nd year of session).

1984 Legislation:

H2080 — Raises drinking age for beer/wine from 18 yrs. to 20 yrs. with grandfather clause.

S106 — Open container prohibition, misdemeanor, max $100 or max. 30 days jail.

Per Se: none. Drinking Age: 21 yrs. (new, see above). Dram Shop Law: None, except illegal to sell to intoxicated persons. Open container Prohibition: 1984, misd. max $100 or max. 30 days jail.

Refusals to Submit: 90 day lic. revoc.

Driving under Revoc. License:
1st Offense: $100 or 30 days jail, additional revocation.
2nd Offense: $500 and/or max. 60 days jail, additional lic, revoc.
3rd Offense: 45 days–6 mos. jail, additional lic. revoc.

	Penalties	Jail/CommSvc	LicRevoc/Rehab/ Therapy	Other
1st Offense	Mand. $200,	Mand. 48 hrs.–30 days jail (comm. svc. can be substituted for jail).	6 mos. lic. revoc.	
2nd Offense w/in 5 yrs.	Min. $1000,	Mand. 48 hrs. jail or 10 days comm. svc.	1 yr. lic. revoc., restricted lic. avail. if enroll in ASAP.	
3rd Offense w/in 5 yrs.	Min. $2000,	Mand. 60 days–3 yrs. jail.	2 yr. lic. revoc., restricted lic. avail. if enroll in ASAP.	
4th Offense w/in 5 yrs.	Min. $3000,	Mand. 90 days–4 yrs. jail.	3 yr. lic. revoc., restricted lic. avail. if enroll in ASAP.	
5th Offense w/in 5 yrs.		1–5 yrs. jail.	5 yr.–perm. lic. revoc., restricted lic. avail. if enroll in ASAP.	
DWI-Great bodily injury	Felony, mand. $5000–10,000,	Mand. 30 days–1 yr. jail.		
DWI-Death	Felony, mand. $10,000–25,000,	Mand. 1–15 yrs. jail.		

Miscellaneous: Names/Addresses of all DWI's released to public each month.

SOUTH DAKOTA

1985 Legislation:

SB72 (Ch253) — Clarifies language regarding timeframe of lic. suspension.

SB73 (Ch263) — 1st offense, min. 30 days–1 yr. lic revoc., with work restricted lic. available. 3rd offense, unconditionally revoke lic. for minimum 1 yr. If caught driving without license during that period, then mandatory minimum 10 days jail.

SB240 (Ch.295) — Dram Shop: Although reiterates that it is illegal to sell to intoxicated person, law prohibits any civil liability for both licensees and social hosts.

1984 Legislation: HB1026 — Raised drinking age for 3.2 beer from 18 yrs. to 19 yrs.

Per Se: .10 Drinking Age: 19 yrs. for 3.2 beer, 21 yrs. for everything else. Dram Shop Law: See above, new 1985 legislation. Open Container Prohibition: Class 2 misdemeanor.

Refusals to Submit: Administratively imposed but penalty can be canceled if plead guilty to criminal charges before revoc. order is issued. Refusal admissible into evidence. Work restricted lic available. 1 yr. lic. revoc.

Driving under Revoc. License: Class 2 misdemeanor, $100 and/or 30 days jail.

	Penalties	Jail/CommSvc	LicRevoc/Rehab/ Therapy	Other
1st Offense	Class 1 misdemeanor, max. $1000	*&/OR* 1 yr. jail.	30 day–1 yr. lic. revoc., work-restricted lic. avail.	
2nd Offense w/in 5 yrs.	Class 1 misdemeanor, max. $1000	*&/OR* 1 yr. jail.	Mand. 1 yr. hard lic. revoc.	
2nd Offense DWI & driving under revoked lic.		Mand. 3 days jail.		
3rd Offense w/in 5 yrs.	Class 6 felony, $2000	*&/OR* 2 yrs. jail.	Mand. 1 yr.-permanent hard lic. revoc.	
3rd Offense DWI & driving under revoked lic.		Mand. 10 days jail.		
Vehicular homicide (while DWI	Class 4 felony, $10,000	*&/OR* 2 yrs. jail.		

Miscellaneous: *Prosecutor must state, or record, reasons* for reducing or dismissing .10 BAC chargeable offense.

TENNESSEE

1986 Legislation: HB1199 (PC519) — Restricts dram shop liability. See below section.

1985 Legislation: No legislation passed.

1984 Legislation:
SB4 (PC1005) — Raises drinking age to 21 yrs. Exempts active duty military personnel. Exempts 18–19 yr. olds accompanied by parents/legal guardians, however, parents/l.g. are civilly liable for damages caused.

HB1633 (PC695) — Driver must be told that refusal to submit to BAC test will result in license suspension.
SB1598 (PC653) — Relates to fees for drug analysis.
HB1402 (PC597) — Technical amendment relating to fees collected for BAC tests.

Per Se: None. Drinking Age: 21 yrs. (1984, see above). Open Container Prohibition: None. Dram Shop Law: Illegal to sell to intoxicated persons. Recent Nashville case (Aug. 1984) support (Wheeler v Nashville Palace, & Road Venture Inn). 1986 leg. appears to overide court case by specifying that as matter of course, consumption not sale is proximate cause. Jury must find that sale was proximate cause, and that sale was to underage or drunk person.

Refusals to Submit (administratively imposed): License revoked, no specific penalty set forth in statute.

Driving under Revoc. License:
1st Offense: Misd., 2 days–6 mths. jail, max. $500.
2nd Offense: Misd., 45 days–1 yr. jail, $500–1000 felonies.

	Penalties	Jail/CommSvc	LicRevoc/Rehab/ Therapy	Other
1st Offense	$250–500,*	48 hrs.–1 yr. jail *(48 hrs. can be served on week ends, remain. jail time, if any, can be satisf. by comm. svce. work.*)	1 yr. lic. revoc., restricted lic. avail.	DUI school.
2nd Offense w/in 10 yrs.	$500–2500,*	45 day–1 yr. jail	2 yrs. lic. revoc., rehab.	Restit. for injuries/losses.
3rd Offense w/in 10 yrs.	$1000–5000,*	120 day–1 yr. jail	3–10 yrs. lic. revoc., rehab.	Restitution.
Habitual Offender (3 or more offenses w/ in 3 yr. period.)	3 yrs.-permanent lic. revoc. in addition to other penalties.			

*All penalties are minimum mandatory.

Miscellaneous: DUI fines are retained at local level. $10 BAC charge earmarked to each county to cover costs.

TEXAS

1985 Legislation:
SB21 — Raised drinking age from 19 to 21 yrs. Effective 9/1/86.
SB598 — Add'l assessment for DWI/Homicide.
HB51 — Relating to the term intoxicated.

1984 Legislation: None, did not meet.

Per Se: .10 Drinking Age: 21 yrs. (New, see above). Dram Shop Law: No specific statute giving right of action against 3rd party. There is a statute prohibiting sales to intoxicated persons. Open Container Prohibition: None.

Refusals to Submit: Admissible as evidence. Administratively imposed although lic. revoc. period would be credited against any criminal DWI conviction (would run concurrently, not separately). 90 day lic. revoc.

Driving under Revoc. License: Misdemeanor, $25–500 and 72 hrs.–6 mos. jail. If allow m.v. to be used by DWI revoc. lic. holder: class b misd., max. $1000 & 180 days jail.

Youth Offender Legislation: Between 14–17 yrs. old, if caught DWI, misdemeanor, max. $100 fine.

	Penalties	Jail/CommSvc	LicRevoc/Rehab/ Therapy	Other
1st Offense	$100–2000.	75 hrs.–2 yrs. jail.	90–365 days lic. suspension	*OR* probation assessment (if county has funds) and rehab.
2nd Offense w/in 10 yrs.	$300–2000.	15 days–2 yrs. jail.	180 days lic. revoc.	*OR* probation and mand. 72 hrs. jail, and assessment (if county has funds) and rehab.
3rd Offense w/in 10 yrs.	$500–2000.	30 days–5 yrs. jail.	180 days–2 yrs. lic revoc.	*OR* probation, mand. 10 days jail and assessment (if county has funds) and rehab.
If bodily injury	Additional $500	*AND* additional 60 days jail.		*OR* probation, mand. 30 days jail, assessment (if county has funds) and rehab.

Miscellaneous: 3 yr. insurance premium surcharge per DWI offense. Mandates *videotaping* of DWI arrests in certain counties. Refusal admiss. as evidence.

UTAH

1985 Legislation:

HB124 — Technical, clarifies funding mechanism for DUI Victim Restitution Fund.

HB3 — Technical, standardizes the offense of negligent homicide with auto.

HB193 — Technical, stipulates that officer can arrest for DWI without warrent even if he/she did not see offense committed.

1984 Legislation: HB125 — Allows impounded vehicle to be released if another registered owner is present at time of arrest.

Per Se: .08 Drinking Age: 21 yrs. Dram Shop Law: No statute, except illegal to sell to intoxicated persons. Open Container Prohibition: Exists. Section 408 Grant: Received $383,915 Alcohol/Traffic Safety Grant (Basic and Supplemental).

Refusals to Submit or .08 BAC: Admissible, 1 yr. admin. lic. revoc. and $25 reinstatement. Possible vehicle impoundment.

Driving under DWI Revoc. License: $299–1000 and/or max. 1 yr. jail. Double orig. lic. revoc. period.

	Penalties	Jail/CommSvc	LicRevoc/Rehab/ Therapy	Other
1st Offense	$299 and/or min. 60 days jail.	Mand. 48 hrs.–10 days drunk tank jail or 2–10 days comm. svc.	90 days hard lic. revoc.	Mand. assessment and educ.
2nd Offense w/in 5 yrs.	$299 and/or min. 60 days jail.	Mand. 48 hrs.–10 days drunk tank jail or 10–30 days comm. svc.	1 yr. hard lic. revoc.	Mand. assessment and educ.
3rd Offense w/in 5 yrs.	$299 and/or min. 60 days jail.	Mand. 30–90 days drunk tank jail, or 30–90 days comm. svc.	1 yr. hard lic. revoc.	Mand. assessment, educ. and rehab.
Bodily Injury	Max. $1000 and 1 yr. jail.			
Homicide by m.v.	3rd degree felony.			

VERMONT

1985 Legislation: H380 (PA85): Non-residents lic. can be revoc/suspen for same cause as residents. Court to notify resident's state.

1984 Legislation: HB387 (ACT134) — Increases fines, including maximum assessment charged for rehab. from $125 to $175. Simplifies jail and license revocation penalties by deleting either/or options relating to rehab. Adds mandatory 48 hrs. jail or 10 day community service for 2nd offenders. Adds mandatory therapy (in addition to rehab.) for repeat offenders.

Per Se: .10 Drinking Age: 18 yrs. Dram Shop Law: Yes; Ch. 17, Title 7 §501. Open Container Prohibition: None. Admin. Lic. Revoc.: No, but if plead Not Guilty DWI, judge can rev. lic. before pre-trail release. PBTs: Allowed, but not admissible as evidence.

Refusals to Submit (not administrative revocation):
1st refusal: 6 mos. lic. revoc. & rehab. (was 1 yr. *or* 6 mos. & rehab.).
2nd refusal: 18 mos. lic. revoc. & rehab. & therapy (was 3 yrs. *or* 18 mos. & rehab.).
3rd refusal: 3 yrs. lic. revoc. & rehab. & therapy (was 6 yrs. *or* 3 yrs. & rehab.).
4th refusal: 6 yrs. lic. revoc. & rehab. (new).
4th refusal w/in 15 yrs.: Permanent lic. revoc.

Driving under Revoc. License:
1st Offense: $500 &/or 30 days jail
2nd Offense: $500 &/or 90 days jail
3rd Offense: $1000 &/or 6 mos. jail
4th Offense: $1000 &/or 2 yrs. jail

	Penalties	Jail/CommSvc	LicRevoc/Rehab/ Therapy	Other
1st Offense	$200–750 (was $50–500),	And/or max. 1 yr. jail (was max. 2 yrs. jail)	90 days lic. revoc. & rehab. (was 1 yr. lic. revoc. *OR* 90 days & rehab.). 1 yr. lic. revoc. & rehab. if fatality occured.	
2nd Offense w/in 5 yrs.	$250–1000 (was $500)	Mand. 48 hrs.–1 yr. jail or 10 days comm. svc. (new; was max. 2 mos.–2 yrs. jail).	18 mos. lic. revoc. & rehab. & therapy (paid for by defendant) (was 3 yrs. lic. revoc. *OR* 18 mos. & rehab.)	
3rd Offense w/in 15 yrs.	$500–1500 (was $500)	Mand. 48 hrs.–1 yr. jail or 10 days comm. svc. (new; was 2 mos.–2 yrs. jail).	3 yrs. lic. revoc. & rehab. & therapy.	If lic. is suspended for 3 yrs.+, can apply for reinstatement after 2 yrs. if defendant can prove total abstinence from drugs &/or alcohol. If death/injury can also prose. manslaughter.
4th Offense w/in 15 yrs.	Same penalties as 2nd and 3rd offense except permanent lic. revoc.			
If death or injury	Max. $3000,	1–15 yrs. jail.		

VIRGINIA

1986 Legislation:
H326 (Ch379) — Conform. language, specif. implied consent applies to public highways.
H502 (Ch635) — Lowers per se from .15 to .10
H797 (Ch475) — Relating to regulations for legal withdrawal of blood for BAC test.
S49 (Ch552) — Relating to distribution of fine money between state/county ASAP.

1985 Legislation:

Ch559 — Raises drinking age to 21 yrs., grandfather clause if 19 yrs. by July 1, 1985

Ch292, Ch355, Ch393, Ch597 — All technical bills.

Ch609 — Defendant entitled to observe BAC analysis process. May elect blood/breath BAC but not both. Fee increased from $15 to $25.

1984 Legislation:

S306 (Ch623) — Increases penalties for refusal to submit to BAC test. Stipulates that revoc. period does not begin until lic. is surrendered to Court or DMV.

H958 (Ch666) — Establishes .15 per se, allows police officer, not defendant, to choose type of BAC test given.

Per Se: Was .15 now .10 (new 1986 law) Drinking Age: 21 yrs. (1985 new, was 19 yrs. for beer, 21 for wine & spirits) Eff. 7/1/85. Dram Shop Law: Misdemeanor to sell to intoxicated person (§4–1112). 2 recent cases, 1 judge ruled in favor of liability, another judge prohibited it which will be appealed. Open Container Prohibition: None.

Refusals to Submit to BAC test (imposed by Court but independent of criminal sanctions):

1st refusal: 6 mos. (was 90 days) lic. revoc.

2nd refusal: 1 yr. (was 6 mos.) lic. revoc.

Driving under Revoc. License: Misdemeanor, max. $500, 10 days–6 mos. jail.

	Penalties	Jail/CommSvc	LicRevoc/Rehab/ Therapy	Other
1st Offense			6 mos. lic. revoc., may be suspended if rehab.	
2nd Offense w/in 5 yrs.	$200–1000,	Mand. 48 hrs.– 1 yr. jail.	Mand. 2–3 yr. lic. revoc. and rehab.	
2nd Offense w/in 5– 10 yrs.	$200–1000,	1 mo.–1 yr. jail.	Mand. 1–3 yrs. lic. revoc. and rehab.	
3rd Offense w/in 5 yrs.	$500–1000,	Mand. 30 days– 1 yr. jail.	Perm. lic. revoc., ineligible to participate in special rehab. program to regain lic. quickly.	
3rd Offense w/in 5– 10 yrs.	$500–1000,	Mand. 10 days– 1 yr. jail.	Perm. lic. revoc., ineligible to participate in special rehab. program to regain lic. quickly.	
3rd Offense w/in 10 yrs.	$500–1000,	2 mos.–1 yr. jail.	Perm. lic. revoc., ineligible to participate in special rehab. program to regain lic. quickly.	

WASHINGTON

1986 Legislation: HB1499 (Ch153) — Relates to definition of BAC

1985 Legislation:

HB163 (Ch101) — Alcohol related lic. revoc. can be stayed if undergo treatment.

SB3267 (Ch302) — Standardizing & increases penalties for driving under revoc. lic.

SB3230 (Ch352) — Min. mand. fines, clarifies DWI Deferred Prosecution Program, & prohibits alcohol industry (at any level) to conduct promotional activities involving direct alcohol consumption.

HB593 (Ch407) — Repealed .10 admin. per se lic. revoc. (had not yet gone into effect). Can still revoke for refusal to submit to BAC. Can only get 1 work-restricted lic. per 5 yrs.

1984 Legislation:

HB1582 — $3 million appropriation to counties to help pay enforcement (primarily adjudication) of DWI. Needed because many cities are refusing to prosecute because of state Supreme Court case requiring speedy jury trials be offered to traffic infraction violators (DWI). The cases are being heard at county level instead.

SB4362 — Exempts vehicles for hire from open container law. Illegal to mislabel alcohol container or add alcohol to non-alcoholic container while in m.v.

Per Se: .10 Drinking Age: 21 yrs. Dram Shop Law: Illegal to sell to intoxicated person, but no clear 3rd party liability established. Open Container Prohibition: Yes.

Refusals to Submit: Criminal and admin. lic. revoc. penalties run concurrently; longer period to prevail.
1st refusal: 1 yr. admin. lic. revoc.
2nd refusal: 2 yrs. admin. lic. revoc.

Admin. Lic. Revoc. for .10: Repealed in 1985 (see above)

Driving under Revoc. License: (If DWI, jail time is minimum mandatory)
1st Offense: 10 days–6 mths jail, $500 fine, 2x original lic. revoc. period.
2nd Offense: 90 days–1 yr. jail, $500 fine, 2x original lic. revoc. period.
3rd Offense: Minimum 1 yr. jail, $500 fine, 2x original lic. revoc. period.

Youthful Offender Legislation: If under 19 yrs. old and charges with DWI license suspended until 19th birthday, or for 90 days, whichever is longer.

	Penalties	Jail/CommSvc	LicRevoc/Rehab/ Therapy	Other
1st Offense	Mand. $250–$1000 (unless indigent)	Mand. 24 hr.–1 yr. jail unless judge finds it poses phys. mental risk.	60 days hard lic. revoc., 30 days restricted. Diagnostic evaluation and rehab.	or Deferred Prosecution Program avail. (2 yr. program) Abstinence, inpatient & outpatient counseling.
2nd Offense w/in 5 yrs.	Mand. $500–$2000 (unless indigent)	Mand. 7 day–1 yr. jail unless judge finds it poses	1 yr. hard lic. revoc. Diagnostic evaluation and rehab.	Additional 180 days–1 yr. jail levied if terms are violated.

	Penalties	Jail/CommSvc	LicRevoc/Rehab/ Therapy	Other
3rd Offense w/in 5 yrs.		physical or mental risk	2yrs. hard lic. revoc. Diagnostic evaluation and rehab.	Additional 180 days–1 yr. jail levied if terms are violated.

WASHINGTON, D.C.

1986 Legislation: Drinking age raised to 21 yrs. old.

1985 Legislation: Nothing passed, 21 yrs. old drinking age bill failed.

1984 Legislation: Nothing passed.

Per Se: .10 Drinking Age: 21 yrs. for all. (new see 1986 legislation). Dram Shop Law: Illegal to sell to intoxicated persons. Case law supports 3rd party (dram shop) liability. Specifically forbids dram shop liability of private host. 25§121. Open Container Prohibition: None.

Refusals to Submit: 12 mos. lic. revoc. admissible as evidence.

Driving under Revoc. License: Max. $5000 and/or max. 1 yr. jail.

	Penalties	Jail/CommSvc	LicRevoc/Rehab/ Therapy	Other
1st Offense .10	Max. $300,	90 days jail,	Yes.	*OR* probation if BAC less than .20, rehab, must pay own fees.
2nd Offense w/in 5 yrs. .10	$5000	And/or 1 yr. jail.	Yes.	
3rd Offense w/in 5 yrs. .10	$10,000	And/or 1 yr. jail.	Yes.	
1st Offense DUI (less than .10)	$300	And/or 30 days jail.	Yes.	
2nd Offense DUI w/in 5 yrs.	$300	And/or 90 days jail.	Yes.	
3rd Offense DUI w/in 5 yrs.	Max. $5000	Max. 1 yr. jail.	Yes.	
Negligent homicide	Felony, max. $5000	And/or 5 yrs. jail	Yes.	

License can be revoked for all offenses, no statutory limits given. If BAC is .10+, practice is to suspend lic. pending outcome of criminal proceedings.
Miscellaneous: *Implied consent law* provides that 2 tests can be given, both chosen by police. All *fine monies go to Ofc. of Alcohol Countermeasures.*

WEST VIRGINIA

1986 Legislation: SB339 — Raises the purchase age for residents from 19 to 21 yrs. Still unclear if this also includes the *drinking* age, although leg. introduction appears to include it, actual legislative language may not.

1985 Legislation: Nothing passed.

1984 Legislation: Nothing passed.

Per Se: No .10 criminal per se. .10 prima facie and .10 administrative per se (for license revocations only). Drinking Age: Unclear, new legislation passed in 1986 (see above) with intent to raise to 21 yrs. but language of law may only relate to purchase, not consumption. Originally was 21 yrs. for non-residents and 19 yrs. for residents. PBT's: Allowed, but not admissible as evidence. Dram Shop Law: Illegal to sell to intoxicated person but no dram shop liability against seller (§60.3-22). Open Container Prohibition: Misdemeanor $5–100 and/or max. 60 days jail.

Refusals to Submit (Administratively imposed but to run concurrently with any other sentence imposed.):
- 1st refusal: 1 yr. admin. lic. revoc.
- 2nd refusal: 5–10 yrs. admin. lic. revoc.
- 3rd refusal: 10 yrs.-permanent admin. lic. revoc.

Driving under Revoc. License & Refusing BAC (both):
- 1st Offense: misdemeanor, $100–500, 48 hrs.–6 mos. jail.
- 2nd Offense: misdemeanor, $1000–3000, 6 mos.–1 yr. jail.
- 3rd Offense: felony, $3000–5000, 1–3 yrs. jail.

	Penalties	Jail/CommSvc	LicRevoc/Rehab/ Therapy	Other
1st Offense	Misdemeanor, $100–500.	Mand. 24 hrs.–6 mos. jail or comm. svc.	6 mos. admin. lic. revoc. or 90 days & rehab.	
1st Offense w/injury	Misdemeanor, $200–1000.	Mand. 24 hrs.–6 mos. jail or comm. svc.	2 yrs. admin. lic. revoc. or 1 yr. & rehab.	
1st Offense w/death	Misdemeanor, $500–1000.	Mand. 90 days–1 yr. jail or comm. svc.	5 yrs. admin. lic. revoc. or 2½ yrs. and rehab.	
1st Offense of giving car to DUI driver	Misdemeanor, $100–500.	Max. 6 mos. jail.	6 mos. admin. lic. revoc. or 90 days and rehab.	
2nd Offense	Misdemeanor, $1000–3000.	Mand. 6 mos.–1 yr. jail or comm. svc.	10 yrs.-permanent admin. lic. revoc. or 5 yrs. and rehab.	
3rd Offense	Felony, $3000–5000.	Mand. 1–3 yrs. jail or comm. svc.	Permanent lic. revoc. or 10 yrs. and rehab.	
If DUI and death occurs due to DUI	Felony, $100–3000.	Mand. 1–3 yr. jail or comm. svc.	10 yrs. lic. revoc. or 5 yrs. and rehab.	

Miscellaneous: Blood tests req. for all drivers and pedestrians killed in m.v. crashes. Infor can only be used for statistical purposes.

WISCONSIN

1986 Legislation: SB1 (special session): Raises drinking age from 19 to 21 yrs.

1985 Legislation:

(Act28) — Allows minors to possess alcohol in limited circumstances relating to employment.

(Act32) — Youth Offender legislation: Cannot drive with BAC +01. If refuse BAC, 6 mth lic. revoc.

(Act29) — Increases mand. assess. from $150 to $200.

(Act71) — Creates statute relating to habitual offenders. If 2nd offense w/1 yr. or 4 w/ 3 yrs., then habitual offender w/max 180 days jail, $5000 and/or 5 yr. lic. revoc.

(Act80) — Prior convict. in other states/local ordin. to be consid. prior for sentence enhancement.

1984 Legislation:

AB169 (Act472) — Expands restrictions on alcoh. consump. by minors by forbidding adults to allow underage consumption on premises owned/under adult control except for relig. svce.

SB232 (Act535) — Prior convict. of similar local ordin. of driving under revoc. lic. to be consid. prior offense. Increases penalties for habitual offenders (4+). Tech. changes.

Per Se: .10 Drinking Age: 21 yrs. (raised from 18 to 19 yrs. in 1983, and 21 yrs. in 1986). Open Container Prohibition: Yes. Dram Shop Law: Limited only if server was prev. notified not to serve person (not revised; 176.30). PBTs: Allowed, not admissible as evidence.

Refusals to Submit (Administrative Revocation) or if .20 BAC: 2hr confinement or until BAC <.05 or if released into custody.

1st refusal: 6 mths lic. revoc. and assessment, 15 days hard revoc. included.
2nd refusal: 1 yr. lic. revoc. and assessment, 60 days hard revoc. included.
3rd refusal: 2 yrs. lic. revoc. and assessment, 90 days hard revoc. included.

Driving under Revoc. License:

1st Offense: $150–600, max. 6 mos. jail, 6 mos. hard lic. revoc.
2nd Offense: $300–1000, 10 days–6 mos. jail, 6 mos. hard lic. revoc.
3rd Offense: $1000–2000, 30 days–9 mos. jail, 6 mos. hard lic. revoc.
4th Offense: $1500–2000, 60 days–1 yr. jail, 6 mos. hard lic. revoc.
5th Offense: $2000–2500, 6 mos.–1 yr. jail, 6 mos. hard lic. revoc.

	Penalties	Jail/CommSvc	LicRevoc/Rehab/ Therapy	Other
1st Offense	$150–300.*		3–6 mos. lic. revoc. Work restricted lic. avail. Alcohol assess./neces. treatment	
2nd Offense	$300–1000,*	5 days–6 mos. jail.	6–12 mos. lic. revoc.; 30 days hard. Alcohol assessment/ necessary treatment.	

	Penalties	Jail/CommSvc	LicRevoc/Rehab/ Therapy	Other
3rd Offense	$600–2000,*	30 day–1 yr. jail	1–2 yrs. lic. revoc.; 60 days hard.	
4th Offense	Habitual offen $5000.*	180 days jail.	Lic. revoc.	
If injury while OWI	$300–2000,*	30 day–1 yr. jail.	1–2 yrs. lic. revoc; 60 day hard. Alcoh. assess/treatment.	
If great bodily harm while OWI	Max. $10,000, max. 2 yrs. jail*		2 yrs. lic. revoc.; 120 days hard.	
Homicide while OWI	Same as great bodily harm except max. 5 yrs. jail and 5 yrs. lic. revoc.*			

*All penalties are minimum mandatory.

Miscellaneous:

Mandatory $200 highway assessment added to all OWI's and refusals.

Restrictions on plea bargains, prosecutor must apply to court for permission.

WYOMING

1986 Legislation: Bill to raise drinking age defeated.

1985 Legislation:

S101 (Ch211) — Admin. lic. revoc. for .10 per se. (not strictly admin. because penalty will be in lieu of criminal revoc.) Increases penalty for refusal.

SB243A — Similar to S101

S250 (Ch39) — Clarifies penalties for DWI-serious bodily injury occurring.

S47 (Ch107) — Clarifies penalties for driving under revoked license.

HB390 — Dram Shop liability: prohibits liability of private host & limits it unless can be proven that licensee knew patron was intoxicated.

HB345 — Increase lic. revoc. penalties for refusal to submit.

1984 Legislation: SF46 (Ch41) — Provides for admin. lic. revoc. if arrested for DWI. Lic. surrendered to police at time of stop. Changes lic. revoc. period for 3rd Offender from permanent to 3 yrs.

Per Se: No per se, .10 presumptive only. Drinking Age: 19 yrs. Dram Shop Law: Statute gives right of action only to those related to habitual drunkard who gave bar owner notice not to sell to person (§12-5-502). Prohibits liab. against private host. Open Container Prohibition: None. Admin. Lic. Revoc.: (1985, new see above) 90 day for .10, not strictly admin., can count toward crim. lic. revoc. penalty (if any).

Refusals to Submit: 6 mths lic. revoc., (was 30 days) if hearing requested, revoc. stayed.

Driving under Suspended Lic.: Max. $750, 6 mos. jail.

	Penalties	Jail/CommSvc	LicRevoc/Rehab/ Therapy	Other
1st Offense	$750,	*OR* 6 mos. jail.	3 mos. lic. revoc.	
2nd Offense	$200–750,	Mand. 7 days–6 mos. jail,	1 yr. lic. revoc. Rehab.	
3rd Offense	$200–750,	Mand. 7 days–6 mos. jail,	3 yrs. lic. revoc. (new) Rehab.	
Serious bodily injury—1st Offense	Max. $5000,	And/or 1 yr. jail,	2 yrs. lic. revoc.	
Serious bodily injury—2nd Offense	Max. $5000,	20 yrs. jail,	2 yrs. lic. revoc.	
Homicide by M.V.	Felony,	Max. 20 yrs. jail,	Permanent lic. revoc.	

12

Epidemiologic Basis of Alcohol Psychomotor Performance Impairment

Barbara R. Manno
Joseph E. Manno

The occurrence of impaired psychomotor performance (PMP) after humans drink alcoholic beverages is commonly accepted among the lay public, forensic, and medical communities. Additionally, it is accepted that PMP tasks are impaired in a dose-related manner. This serious finding has been derived by a series of seemingly unrelated studies rather than through well-integrated scientific investigations. With the recent emphasis on alcohol's impact on motor vehicle accidents, health care delivery, and the general economy, the impairment of PMP should be well researched and carefully documented. Therefore it is of importance to understand how the multitude of individual studies can be related to one another in order to support the concept of alcohol-induced impairment of PMP.

ESTABLISHING THE RELATIONSHIP

The general format for seeking the relationship of alcohol PMP impairment is outlined in Figure 12-1. The initiation of such documentation usually begins with the casual observation that alcohol appears to be a common factor associated with changes in an individual's ability to perform psychomotor tasks, for example, driving an automobile. Figure 12-1 defines the process as a five-step procedure. The first step of necessity asks the question: How many events (crashes, mishaps, accidents, etc) in the target population involve drinking drivers? If the answer is "few," then there obviously need be no further expenditure of effort on the problem. If, on the other hand, many events involve drinking

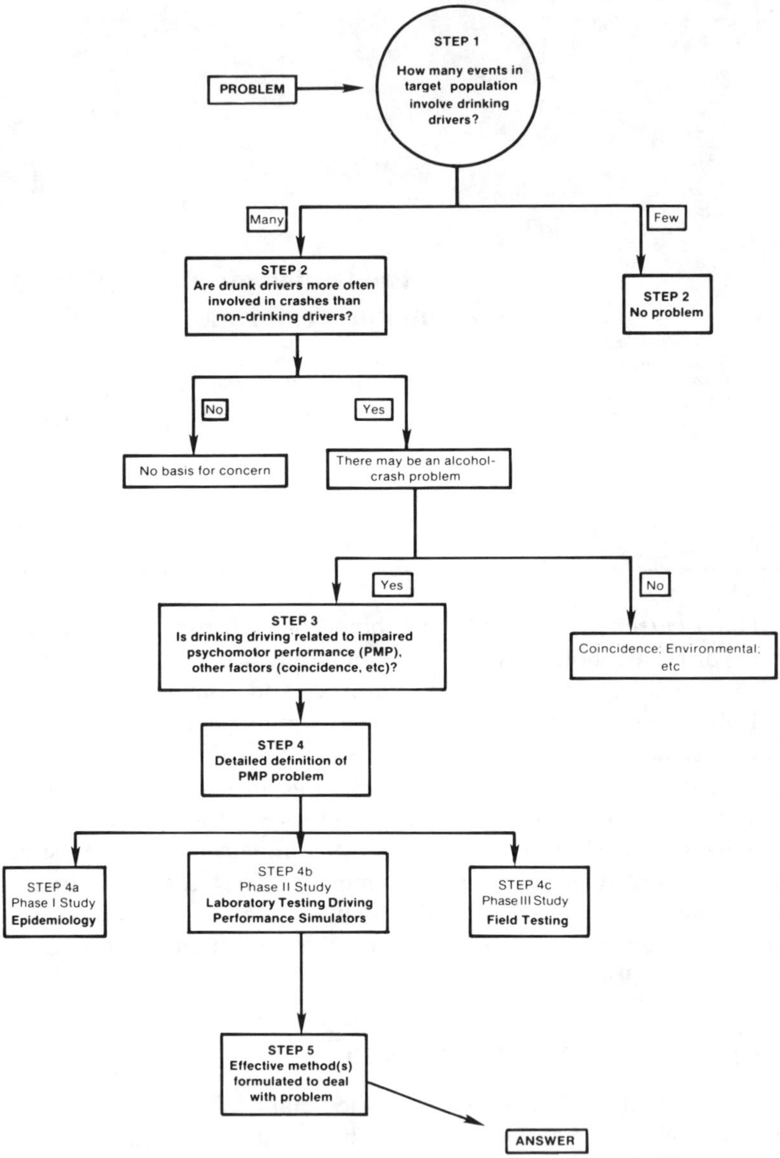

Figure 12-1 Paradigm seeking the relationship of alcohol to impairment of pyschomotor performance.

drivers, then the population and events involving drinking drivers should be compared with a comparable population of nondrinking drivers. If no difference in the two groups is shown, then no problem exists. If a positive response is attained, further investigation is required. Fortunately, initial investigators (Holcomb, 1938) chose automobile (personal injury) accident cases to study and found that 25% of the drivers had blood alcohol concentrations greater than or equal to 0.10% wt/vol. He also showed that sample populations of noncrash drivers were positive for alcohol in only 2% of the cases. More recent studies (Pendleton et al, 1986) explored the circumstances of 1260 driver fatalities and found that 51% of the drivers were legally intoxicated (blood alcohol concentration [BAC] = 0.10% wt/vol).

While the end result may be the same, that is, a vehicular personal injury, distinction between the *drinking driver* and *drunk driver* may be necessary. This may be required in order to describe cause-and-effect relationships surrounding the accident for legal aspects of the event. While "drinking driver" and "drunk driver" quite often can be described based on such things as BAC, behavior, drinking pattern, and other issues, the terms are often used synonymously.

In our situation we are concerned in step 3 of Figure 12-1 with the question: Is the alcohol consumption pattern of the drinking driver the cause of impaired PMP or can it be due to other factors, such as vehicular, environmental, or human? Examples of other factors are defined in Table 12-1. If other factors are contributory to accident causation, it may serve the purpose of the accident researcher to pursue these at another time. In our case we are limited to discussion of alcohol-induced PMP impairment and will proceed to step 4 of Figure 12-1. This general approach obviously could serve to direct many avenues of study.

Once the relationship has been superficially established that alcohol may be involved as a causative factor in vehicular accidents, the problem must be defined with as much detail as is feasible. This may be approached as shown in Figure 12-1, steps 4a–c. In general, the studies may be grouped into three phases: Phase I consists of epidemiologic

Table 12-1
Variables in Accident Research

Categories	Definition
Vehicular	Relationship to design, construction, operating characteristics of vehicle
Environmental	Operating conditions, traffic conditions, time of day, etc
Human	Characteristics of driver, eg, physical, social, psychological, etc, which may affect and performance of driving tasks

studies of accidents, where a correlation may be drawn between the presence or absence of alcohol in accident cases. Phase II is composed of laboratory testing in animals and/or humans using testing devices. The purpose of this phase is to provide an environment where controlled studies may be performed utilizing selected variables which may be included or excluded during testing. Included in phase II would be drinking simulation as well as individual response and/or behavior testing devices. Phase III consists of testing under controlled conditions using actual driving experiments or field tests. Step 5 addresses the formulation of methods to deal with the problem and will not be discussed here since it is beyond the scope of the present chapter.

It may be generalized that the incidence of alcohol-related accidents is underreported. In the United States and to a lesser extent in other countries, there is no uniform reporting responsibility, either by official agency or reporting format. Many times the arresting officer or investigating official does not question the presence of alcohol in either the accident victim or vehicle operator until hours after the incident occurs, by which time the alcohol has disappeared from the blood of the subject. In many instances, the presence of alcohol is never questioned (Jones and Joscelyn, 1978; Pendleton et al, 1986). These problems in reporting would suggest that, due to the nonhomogeneous nature of data collection, a distinct underestimation of the magnitude of alcohol-treated mishaps exists. This is not a new suggestion but tends to be lost when reading epidemiologic studies of hundreds or even thousands of accidents.

DEFINING LIMITATIONS OF INTERPRETATION

"Accidents," for a long period of time, referred only to automobile accidents. Interestingly enough, with technological developments in the more recent past, additional data are becoming available on both passenger and operators of motor vehicles, aircraft, motorcycles, bicycles, as well as industrial and pedestrian accidents and alcohol. Operation of mechanical devices, however simple, requires psychomotor control as well as maintenance of behavioral control.

Both retrospective and prospective epidemiologic reports indicate that a strong relationship exists between alcohol consumption and the occurrence of automobile accidents. Correlation of these observations have been made more reliable with the advent of tests for alcohol in human body fluids and tissues (Widmark, 1914, 1932; Heise, 1934; Harger et al, 1938; Jones and Joscelyn, 1978). Application of the data in the first two appellate court decisions upholding the admissibility of evidence on a charge of operating a motor vehicle while under the influence of alcoholic liquor were recorded in 1937 in *State v Duquad*

(1937), and *People v Henry* (1937). The first state law establishing the admissibility in evidence of alcohol tests in driving offenses was enacted in Indiana in 1939 (American Medical Association, 1970).

Closer examination of epidemiologic reports indicates that prospective studies would most likely yield more useful information because uniform questions concerning the accident circumstances would be asked at the time of the accident investigation. Retrospective studies, on the other hand, require addressing a battery of standard questions from multiple nonhomogeneous sources at a future point in time, often far removed from the accident event. This obviously leaves interpretation of data open to question in many instances, or at best restricted within very narrow limits.

A strong case exists for the need to understand how the epidemiologic studies are germane to impaired PMP. This need is implied when reference to these same epidemiologic studies is made with increased emphasis on alcohol's impact on the human and financial consequences of accidents and health care delivery, and the general economy, as well as as its ramifications in the law enforcement and judicial systems. Close examination of epidemiologic studies leaves one with the impression that the customary cohesiveness of the scientific method is lacking when assessing the contribution of alcohol to impaired PMP. This literature is represented, with few exceptions, by a series of mostly isolate, noncontrolled collections of demographic information concerning accidents and alcohol. The notable exceptions are summarized in Table 12-2. The format of Table 12-2 was selected because there were not sufficient commonalities between the studies to use a more traditional tabular comparison.

Before proceeding, it is necessary that certain key terms used throughout the epidemiology literature be defined. *Epidemiology* is the study of the incidence, distribution, and control of disease in a population, or the sum of the factors controlling the presence or absence of a disease or pathogen. An *epidemic* is a disease or the number of cases of a disease, that affects or tends to affect many persons within a community, area, or region at one time. In the strict sense, epidemiology would not readily apply to the study of the alcohol impairment of PMP. However, the principles established by investigators in epidemic research may be applied to problems in other areas. Retrospectively, *demography* may better define the type of study reported concerning the alcohol PMP work. Predominantly, the reports are statistical studies of the characteristics of human populations, especially with reference to size and density, growth, distribution, migration, and vital statistics, and the effect of all of these on social and economic conditions, which are *demographic data.*

All reports center around a common point, that is, the occurrence of an *accident*. Here it is interpreted as a sudden event or change occur-

Table 12-2
Major Epidemiology Studies

Original Citation	Geographic Origin	Highlights of Reports and Comments
	North American	
Heise (1934)	Pennsylvania	BAC of drivers, passengers, pedestrians including "hit-and-run" drivers. Analysis of 199 consecutive automobile accidents where victims required hospitalization. Alcohol accidents were more numerous than those without alcohol. Alcohol was present in accidents involving injury or death of two people per accident *v* one person per accident in nonalcohol crashes. Average BAC = 0.21% (wt/vol); pedestrian accidents, driver BAC = 0.14% (wt/vol); drinking pedestrian accidents, BAC = 0.20% (wt/vol); majority of accidents involving young and old people were alcohol-involved. If driver was sober in series then passenger usually sober; those with high BAC also had passenger with equally elevated BAC. Weekend showed peak in alcohol-related accidents (Sunday showed 3:1 increase with alcohol with number of injuries per death increasing to 8:1.) This disproportion not observed on weekdays. Higher accident rate during early evening (dark) overall. Alcohol user–related cases peaked higher at 6–7 PM. Correlation is between alcohol and accident not darkness and accident. Early morning accidents nonalcohol-related. Conclusions: (1) Considering a person sober if he can walk and talk is of little value in assessing alcohol-related statistics, (2) high incidence of weekend and night, male alcohol-related accidents, (3) drinking pedestrian often involved while children and old people are struck often by sober drivers.

Original Citation	Geographic Origin	Highlights of Reports and Comments
Holcomb (1938)*	Evanston, Ill.	BAC of drivers involved in personal injury crashes *v* drivers (control) using same roadways: 2% of noncrash compared to 25% of crash drivers were legally drunk. BAC performed at crash scene.
Lucas et al (1955)*	Toronto (1951–1952)	Study conducted from approximately 6:30–10:30 PM, daily except Sundays from Dec 1951 through Nov 1952. Involved 433 drivers of nonfatal crashes, personal injury, or property damage crashes: 15% of drivers were legally intoxicated by US standards, ie, BAC of ≥ 0.10% (wt/vol). One of three controlled North American Studies showing data from nonfatal crashes.
Haddon and Braddess (1959)	Westchester Co, New York (1950–1953)	About 70% of driver fatalities in single vehicle crash had BAC ≥ 0.10% (wt/vol). 55%–65% of sample were too intoxicated to drive, 35%–54% had BAC ≥ 0.15% (wt/vol).
Haddon et al (1961)	New York City (Manhattan)	Studied 50 cases of pedestrians 18 years and older fatally injured compared to similarly exposed nonaccident involved persons. Controls were obtained at accident site, same day of week and time of day, same age and sex as accident cases (200 subjects). Descriptive results: accidents tended to occur in major shopping and business districts. Time: 6–12 PM — 51%; 3 PM — 3 AM — 73%; 6–9 AM — smallest % involved in accidents; 41% died within 6 h of accidents. Weather (rain) not a significant factor. Mean age of fatality: 58.8 yr, nonfatal injury age 48.4 yr, control 41.6 yr. There is an age-associated risk of involvement as well as age-related risk of fatal outcome if involved. Data also suggest correlation of increased risk to the elderly with little or no BAC and middle-aged, high BAC persons. Those

Table 12-2 cont'd

Original Citation	Geographic Origin	Highlights of Reports and Comments
		involved were more often foreign-born, not married, lower socioeconomic level as compared with matched control. Involved persons were within short distance of their homes. BAC of cases first becomes evident in the 10%–40 mg% BAC range. Surviving less than 6 h: 0 mg% = 26%; 50 mg% = 47%; 100 mg% = 42%; 150 mg% = 32%. Control BAC: 0 mg% = 67%; 50 mg% = 16%; 100 mg% = 8%; 150 mg% = 6%. BAC fatalities were significantly different whether compared to site-matched or age and sex–matched controls.
McCarroll and Haddon (1962)*	New York City (Manhattan)	Matched control taken at times and places of fatal crashes. 73% accident-responsible drivers had been drinking to some degree compared with 26% similarly exposed but noninvolved drivers. 46% of accident-responsible group (86) had BAC ≥ 250 mg% contrasted to negative BAC of larger control groups (N = 516). Fatalities were closer to home than noninvolved drivers but no fatally injured subject lived outside city. Males were overly represented in case group; nonmarried cases had higher BAC than married cases. Fatally injured cases and controls were age- and socioeconomic-matched. No association between accident involvement and vehicle age was evident. Suggest relationship of alcoholism may be a factor in involved cases with very high BAC.
Borkenstein et al (1964)*	Grand Rapids, Mich (1962–1963)	Nonfatal crashes; on-scene BAC. Daily all hours. Random selection of controls using road at times and places of crashes. Most extensive study of nonfatal crashes conducted through 1978. Data

Original Citation	Geographic Origin	Highlights of Reports and Comments
		collected at scene for period July 1962–June 1963. Data collected 7 d/wk, 24 hours a day on 5985 drivers. Randomly selected control groups (N = 7590 drivers), from drivers using roadway at times and places of all types of crashes. Approximately 6% of drivers had BAC ≥ 0.10% (wt/vol). Note value lower than Lucas et al (1955) reported probably because Lucas et al study done during evening hours. Data on 300 crashes classified as "fatals and driver injured" and 404 crashes labeled "other visible injury" show that approximately 9% of drivers had BAC ≥ 0.10% (wt/vol). Results from this controlled study show that higher BAC were much less prevalent among noncrash drivers than crash-involved drivers. One of three controlled nonfatal crash studies.
Neilson (1969)*	California (1962–1968)	Single and multivehicle crashes; BAC on motor vehicle fatalities. 45% of all fatally injured drivers in crashes had BAC ≥ 0.10% (wt/vol). About 60% of fatalities had BAC of 0.10% (wt/vol) when involved in single vehicle crashes. 30%–35% of multivehicle crash drivers had BAC ≥ 0.10% (wt/vol). Pedestrian data show 40% of fatalities had BAC ≥ 0.10% (wt/vol). Data of Waller et al (1970) and Neilson (1969) consistent with this report.
Waller et al (1970)*	California (1950–1967)	BAC on motor vehicle fatalities; single and multivehicle crashes. Approximately 50% of all fatally injured drivers involved in crashes had BAC ≥ 0.10% (wt/vol). 60% of single vehicle fatalities had BAC ≥ 0.10% (wt/vol); 30%–35% multivehicle fatalities had BAC ≥ 0.10% (wt/vol). Data summary excludes deaths occurring more than 6 h after

Table 12-2 cont'd

Original Citation	Geographic Origin	Highlights of Reports and Comments
		accident. Pedestrian data: 35% of fatalities had BAC ≥ 0.10% (wt/vol). Data consistent with data of Neilson (1969).
Baker and Spitz (1970)*	United States	Study based upon autopsy and police reports. Considers control or cause of bias of BAC in drinking driving crash study. Period studied Jan 1, 1964 through Dec 31, 1968, 328 subjects (305 auto drivers, 22 truck drivers, 1 taxi driver). No limit placed upon length of time between crash and death. Variety of road conditions (urban, rural roads, highways). BAC done on all drivers who died within 6 h of crash. Results analyzed according to driver responsibility, age of driver killed *v* surviving, multivehicle collisions, length of survival, microscopic liver findings by age and BAC, presence of arteriosclerotic heart disease. Found no correlation between driver responsibility and disease or physical disability. Decreased ability of older drivers to survive crashes caused them to be overrepresented in fatality crash statistics. Delayed death resulting from crashes occurred more often among older drivers (60 + yr) than younger drivers.
Perrine et al (1971)*; Haddon et al (1961)*; Jones and Joscelyn (1976)*	United States	Pedestrian fatalities: 31%–43% of subjects tested had BAC in excess of 0.10% (wt/vol). 25%–37% had BAC in excess of 0.15% (wt/vol).
Perrine et al (1971)*	Vermont (1967–1969)	Single and multivehicle crash; BAC on motor vehicle fatalities. Bias of study considered. Controls used roads at times and places of fatal crashes. About 65%–70% of drivers fatally injured in single vehicle accidents had BAC ≥ 0.10% (wt/vol). About 40% of

Original Citation	Geographic Origin	Highlights of Reports and Comments
		fatalities in multivehicle accidents had BAC ≥ 0.10% (wt/vol). Less than 4% of control or noncrash drivers had BAC ≥ 0.10% (wt/vol). High BAC rarely observed in noncrash drivers compared with crash-involved drivers.
Waller (1972)*; Zylman (1974)*	United States	Retrospective data from police reports: 40% of "responsible" drivers in multivehicle crash had BAC ≥ 0.10% (wt/vol); only 10% of "nonresponsible" drivers ≥ 0.10% (wt/vol); 64% of drivers with BAC of 0% found responsible for crash.
Joscelyn and Treat (1973)*	United States	Multidiscipline team approach to study accident causes. Lists alcohol impairment as the prime cause of 7% of all types of accidents investigated and a prime or contributing cause of 16% of crashes studied by them. They consider impairment to be at BAC ≥ 0.08% (wt/vol).
Clark and Clark (1973)*	Washtenan, Mich (1968–1973)	Fatal crashes studied. Statistics on drivers and adult pedestrian crashes; 50%–60% of fatally injured adult drivers had BAC ≥ 0.10% (wt/vol); 40% of fatally injured adult pedestrians had BAC ≥ 0.10% (wt/vol).
Filkins et al (1970)*; Zylman et al (1975)*	Detroit, Wayne Co, Mich (1967–1969)	Single and multivehicle crash; BAC on motor vehicle fatalities. BAC on 309 subjects; 96% survived less than 6 h; 40%–50% of drivers tested had BAC ≥ 0.10% (wt/vol); 29%–43% of drivers had BAC of ≥ 0.15% (wt/vol); 16%–28% had BAC of ≥ 0.20% (wt/vol).
Ellingstad and Westra (1974)*	South Dakota (1972–1973)	Fatal crashes studied: 40%–45% of driver fatalities had BAC ≥ 0.10% (wt/vol).
Jones and Jocelyn, (1976)*	New Orleans (1972–1973)	Fatal crashes studied: 50%–55% of driver fatalities had BAC ≥ 0.10% (wt/vol). 25%–30% of pedestrian fatalities had BAC ≥ 0.10% (wt/vol).

Table 12-2 cont'd

Original Citation	Geographic Origin	Highlights of Reports and Comments
Jones and Josceyln (1976)*; Hurst (1970; 1974)*; Lucas et al (1955)	United States	Review of crash predictability based on presence of alcohol. Lucas et al (1955) introduced a risk term called *hazard*; defined as the involvement of drivers in any BAC interval *relative* to the drivers in the lowest BAC interval measured. Hurst (1970; 1974) applied this term to controlled studies in conjunction with probability theory (ie, Bayes law) to calculation of probability of drivers being involved in a crash if a given BAC is reached relative to probability of crash involvement at zero (or lowest measured) BAC. Risk begins to increase very rapidly at BAC near 0.08% (wt/vol) and increases rapidly at high BAC, ie, BAC $\geq$ 0.15% (wt/vol).
Florendo (1975)*	Los Angeles (1972–1974)	Fatal crashes studied. About 50% of driver fatalities had BAC $\geq$ 0.10% (wt/vol).
Spencer and Ferguson (1975)*	Fairfax, Va (1974)	Fatal crashes studied: 60% of driver fatalities had BAC $\geq$ 0.10% (wt/vol).
Farris et al (1976)*	Huntsville, Ala	Nonfatal, personal injury crashes, daily all hours; BAC on scene (⅔) or hospital (⅓). Controls used road at same time and place as crashes. 13% of 596 drivers in nonfatal, personal injury crashes had BAC $\geq$ 0.10% (wt/vol). 804 noncrash drivers (control) using roadway at times and places of 314 personal injury crashes. ⅓ controlled nonfatal crash studies.
Baker and Fisher (1977)	United States	Retrospective study of 99 fatal motorcycle crashes from police and medical examiner records. BAC determined in 62 motorcycle drivers; ⅔ had measurable amount of alcohol, ½ had 100 mg%, high concentrations

Original Citation	Geographic Origin	Highlights of Reports and Comments
		most commonly found in 20–34 yr age group. Police mentioned alcohol in only 9 cases. BAC distribution of motorcycle drivers was similar to those in fatally injured drivers of cars and trucks in Maryland.
Jones and Joscelyn (1978)*; Traffic Injury Research Foundation of Canada (1975)*	Canadian National Survey (1973)	BAC on motor vehicle fatalities. BAC on 1111 subjects; 1006 died within 6 h of crash; 44% had BAC ≥ 0.11% (wt/vol). 49% had BAC equal to Canadian legal limit for impairment [0.08% (wt/vol)].
Riddick and Luke (1978)	District of Columbia	Postmortem study, noncontrolled; 604 cases examined from Medical Examiner's office, District of Columbia. Study has a population bias because cases included death by natural causes, homicide, suicide, traffic accidents, nontraffic accidents, cause of death unknown. In the 44 traffic accidents 12 had positive BAC, 22 deaths or 50% were alcohol-associated. Cases were biased because death due to trauma and younger age groups included.
McGuire (1978)	United States	Controlled behavioral study; classroom and behind-the-wheel with alcohol: 1-yr record of 876 court-referred, first-offender, drinking drivers who graduated from a "Don't Drink and Drive" Program compared with 802 drivers exposed to usual court procedures of probation and fine (control group). Control group had 78% more alcohol-related violations, 23% more moving violations, 40% more license suspensions, and 34% more accidents. Discusses importance of study design in accident research.
Jalazo et al (1978)	Pennsylvania	Noncontrolled; arrested relationship between BAC at time of screening with self-reported alcohol use and clinical judgment of recent drinking. Showed moderate

Table 12-2 cont'd

Original Citation	Geographic Origin	Highlights of Reports and Comments
		correlation with Breathalayzer measurements of BAC; self-reports and clinical judgment of alcohol consumption are unreliable.
Shultz and Layne (1979)	Arkansas	Study of DWI and public drunkeness offenses in "dry" rural setting; noncontrolled. BAC tended to be higher in young persons arrested for DWI and public drunkeness than in older people.
Maistro et al (1979)	Tennessee	Retrospective evaluation, controlled; single and multiple offenders. Control group: random sample of all drivers in state; other group: random samples of single and multiple DWI offenders. Some demographic data, eg, race, sex, type of offense. Concluded average interval decreases between convictions for DWI offenses (first and second, 2 yr; second and third, 17 mo; third and fourth, 11 mo; fourth and fifth, 8 mo).
Soderstrom et al (1979)	Maryland	Difficulties in diagnosis and management of roadway trauma involving presence of alcohol; noncontrolled. 48% of roadway trauma patients had positive BAC; 78% of positive BAC were ≥ 0.10% (wt/vol) ie, prima facie or presumptive evidence of DWI in most states.
Lundberg et al (1979)	California	Prospective and retrospective portions of study. Includes drug and/or alcohol; controlled study. Behavior of driver observed and recorded. Compared observed alcohol odor on subject against analysis of BAC, only 56% of odor-detected cases were positive on analysis. Pooled data from 13 labs. Conclusions: Data include observations on persons with psychoactive drugs and/or alcohol

Original Citation	Geographic Origin	Highlights of Reports and Comments
		present in blood. Data not well separated in order to draw conclusions on alcohol alone; otherwise study well presented. Observation notes rarely included in literature reports to substantiate "impaired function" change.
Weston (1980)	New Mexico	Psychological autopsy; noncontrolled: 39% of automobile driver fatalities and 40% of pedestrian fatalities had some blood alcohol present. Alcohol was involved in 39%–74% of several types of violent crime. Psychological autopsy was used to prepare profiles of drivers in vehicular accidents. Drivers were grouped by behavioral characteristics likely to contribute to accident. Behavioral disorders where alcohol played a role were judged to be present in 28% of serious and fatal accidents studied.
Patterns of alcohol use among teenage drivers in fatal motor vehicle accidents — United States 1977–1981 (1982)	United States	1981 data analysis from Fatal Accident Reporting System (FARS). Based on crude death rate. In 1981 FARS shows alcohol played important role in highway fatalities in young drivers. Young driver fatalities (DWI): 4738. Persons in accidents involving young drivers: 9310. 49% of young drivers with known alcohol involvement were more likely to be killed than those with zero or unknown alcohol involvement. Also shows data on distribution of crashes by BAC age.
Lloyd and Venus (1983)	Texas	Noncontrolled study. Speeding accounted for 24% of fatalities. 40% of fatally injured people were nondrivers. This decrease occurred with enactment of 55 mph speed limit. DWI was a contributing factor in 24% of all fatal accidents and 28% of all rural fatalities. An increase of young fatalities and DWI was observed in the 10-yr period 1970–1980.

Table 12-2 cont'd

Original Citation	Geographic Origin	Highlights of Reports and Comments
Pendleton et al (1986)	Texas	Results of study comparing medical examiners findings with investigating officer's conclusion concerning alcohol as a contributing factor to accidents involving 1260 fatally injured drivers. 51% of DWIs had BAC ≥ 0.10%. Data collection covered 15 Texas counties for period Jan 1, 1983–Dec 31, 1984. Legal limit for intoxication in Texas is ≥ 0.10% BAC. Average BAC = 0.114% in 1260 driver fatalities studied; 80% of accident reports did not cite alcohol as contributing factor to accident; however, average BAC of these was 0.96% (wt/vol). Statistics cited: driver age — 26–30-yr age group most involved. Males more involved than females; most accidents occurred between 11 PM–3 AM on Sunday, Saturday, and Thursday. State police reported alcohol involvement in fatal accidents more often than local authorities. Data consistent with national statistics.
	National Origin	
Plueckhahn (1978)	Australia	Noncontrolled, retrospective study; 344 vehicular fatalities studied for period Jan 1967–June 1978: 344 deaths of persons, 17 + years of age within 4 h of accident. 147 victim drivers were 17–50 yr old. 54% of 147 victims had BAC ≥ 0.1 g%; autopsy of 35 male pedestrians; 60% had BAC ≥ 0.15 g% and 80% of pedestrian accidents occurred between 6–10 PM. Fewer women road traffic victims observed.
Brown (1978)	New Zealand	Comparison of alcohol crash statistics with availability of alcohol. Noncontrolled study of the effects of a beer distribution strike on occurrence of alcohol-

Original Citation	Geographic Origin	Highlights of Reports and Comments
		related incidents. Reduction in number of incidents on weekends and on total number; however, no long-term effects observed.
McDermott and Strang (1978)	New Zealand	Historical review. Experience over 3 yr postlegislation on compulsory blood alcohol tests: 21.7% of 21,863 male driver casualties had BAC legal limit (0.05 g%) and 13.7% had BAC ≥ 0.15 g%. BAC of 9187 female driver casualties ≥ 0.05 g% with 3.7% ≥ 0.15 g%. Nondrivers had a slightly lower incidence of elevated BAC. Again confirmed greater drinking involvement of males and city *v* country driving data.
McDermott (1978)	Australia	Discusses alcohol-driving legislation; BAC — driving incidence; relates BAC incidents to variables of sex, geography, religion, ethnicity, recidivism; role of medical community in prevention program.
Robinson (1979)	Ireland	Survey deals with presence of drugs in specimens of impaired driver cases. Impaired driver defined in law. Includes primarily drugs of abuse, alone or in combination with alcohol. Diazepam was most common of all drugs detected.
Honkanen et al (1980)	Finland	Controlled, prospective study. Blood serum drug screen and BAC on 201 drivers within 6 h of road accident. 325 control drivers randomly selected at service stations. Questionnaire on subject's health and use of drugs completed. 15% of drivers and 13% of controls admitted taking drugs during previous 24 h. 2% of both drivers and controls had taken psychotropic drugs; however, analysis revealed 5% of patients and 2.5% of controls were positive for this type of drug. Diazepam was found in 16/18 subjects positive for psychotropic drugs. 15% of drivers and 1% of

Table 12-2 cont'd

Original Citation	Geographic Origin	Highlights of Reports and Comments
		controls positive for alcohol. Conclusions: drug use in Finland lower than other Western Countries; illness appears to be a greater risk hazard. Interview not reliable method to determine psychotropic drug use. Diazepam may increase accident risk but alcohol still most important risk factor.
Landauer (1981)	Australia	Literature review. Study involves diazepam literature; however, some alcohol information surfaced.
Galloway and Patel (1981)	Scotland	Prospective study: 1566 road traffic victims studied. 41% were drivers, 36% passengers and 23% were pedestrians. 76% were discharged after treatment and 24% required additional inpatient care. 46% of accidents occurred between 12 midnight and 8AM ⅓ occurred on Saturdays and Sundays. Men < 35 yr old were overrepresented as drivers and passengers. ¾ of male drivers were between 17–35 yr old. Age of pedestrians and women passengers were similar. ½ of pedestrian total were > 35 yr old. Automobile crashes were more frequent than motorcycle and bus crashes, in that order. 19% of road accident victims and 19% of other accident victims had detectable levels of ethanol. Data show male pedestrians were often highly intoxicated; also large number of road accident cases in general showed presence of intoxicating levels of alcohol.
Simpson et al (1982)	Canada (Ontario)	Review with emphasis on young people and alcohol crashes. Good presentations of variables in epidemiologic studies and the state of existing alcohol data.
Cromptom (1982)	England	Autopsy study. 208 cases, type vehicle, age, sex, alcoholic data.

Original Citation	Geographic Origin	Highlights of Reports and Comments
		Data suggest that majority of fatal accidents occur before the alcohol levels in the urine and blood have reached equilibrium, ie, during the phase of rising blood alcohol. Evidence also shows that young chronic alcoholics rather than occassional drinker are at cause in road accidents. Passenger with BAC approximately 100 mg% is at great risk especially if driver is also drinking. Accidents appear to occur within half-hour of drinking. Suggest an hour "sobering period" thereby bypassing rising BAC phase and the overconfident and impulsive phase because drinker would be on falling side of BAC curve.
Cimbura et al (1982)	Canada (Ontario)	484 fatally injured drivers and pedestrians studied for presence of drugs and alcohol in blood and urine, occasionally on vitreous humor, stomach contents, liver. Alcohol was found in 57% of drivers, and other drugs in 26% of the drivers. 9.5% of drivers had psychoactive drugs present in blood in concentrations which could adversely affect driving ability. Δ-9-THC and diazepam accounted for the majority of psychoactive drugs present.
McDermott and Hughes (1982)	Australia	Driver-nondriver accident casualties; noncontrolled. Country has compulsory alcohol testing for all road crashes. 20.5% of driver and 20.5% of nondriver fatalities had alcohol levels in excess of legal driver limit (0.05 g%). 9.8% driver and 6.4% nondriver samples had BAC ≥0.15 g%; 27.4% male and 9.2% female drivers exceeded the BAC limit. 18.7% city and 25% of country drivers exceeded BAC limit. Greatest decrease in DWI immediately implementing increased penalities for DWI.

*Synopsis in Jones and Josceyln (1978).

ring without intent or volition through carelessness, unawareness, ignorance, or a combination of causes and producing a negative or detrimental result. The keys to this definition are "sudden event" or "change...without intent" and "producing a negative or detrimental result." This permits us to include data other than automobile accidents since alcohol accident research is now including use of other vehicles or means of locomotion and other equipment, for example, pedestrians, industrial accidents, airplanes, motorcycles, snowmobiles, bicycles (Baker and Fisher, 1977; Birrell, 1971, Davis and Smith, 1982; Dietz and Baker, 1974; Eriksson and Bjornstig, 1982; Haddon et al, 1961; McCarroll et al, 1962; Plueckhahn, 1982; and Irwin, 1983). These new inclusions in alcohol PMP reports are applicable to understanding alcohol PMP because of their involvement in forensic cases other than automobile drunk driving and impact a larger population of accident perpetrators and victims.

It soon becomes apparent to readers with a background in toxicology or pharmacology that even the word *impairment*, as utilized in alcohol PMP reports, can be ambiguous. "Impairment" in common and scientific usage refers to something being made worse or diminished in value, quality, etc. Alcohol accident epidemiology uniformly applies a legal definition of impairment or one defined by law. *Legal impairment* states that at a given blood concentration of alcohol the individual is considered to be *impaired*. "Impaired" is further described by descriptive terms such as "drunk," "driving while intoxicated" (DWI), or "driving under the influence." The blood alcohol value will vary with the state or country in which the law is applicable. On the other hand, pharmacologic impairment refers to the blood concentration of alcohol whereby certain body functions, behavioral patterns, or as in our work here, PMP, is altered.

The blood concentrations at which alcohol produces legal and pharmacologic impairment may differ significantly. For example, the legal impairment level in most states in the United States is established at 0.10% wt/vol blood alcohol concentration (BAC) whereas in Great Britain and Sweden it is set at 0.08% wt/vol. The blood alcohol level for threshold pharmacologic impairment may be as low as 0.02% wt/vol. According to some researchers neuromuscular responses are impaired at 0.04% to 0.05% wt/vol; vision at levels below 0.10% wt/vol, simple and complex tracking at levels between 0.05% and 0.10% wt/vol, and attention at levels as low as 0.03% wt/vol (Jones and Joscelyn, 1978). The basis for impairment in epidemiologic literature pivots around the various states' (national) legal definitions of BAC. Impairment therefore is implied rather than explicit because data collection has been subjective rather than objective in nature.

Psychomotor performance can be influenced by a number of variables. A term commonly confused and even interchanged with PMP is "behavior." *Psychomotor performance* refers to performance of tasks involving muscular action believed to ensue from prior conscious mental activity. Behavior is a less tangible variable, is more encompassing, and has several definitions depending upon its direct application. A general meaning of *behavior* is the manner in which a person responds in reaction to social stimuli, or to inner need, or to a combination thereof. An operant psychologist may define behavior as an activity of a defined organism (eg, man in this case), especially observable activity when measurable in terms of quantifiable effects on the environment whether arising from internal or external stimuli. A yet more general meaning that applies is anything which an organism does involving action and response to stimulation. A grossly general definition broadly states that behavior is the response of an individual, group, or species to a broad range of factors constituting its environment. An officer of the law or court may choose to depend upon the meaning of behavior which states that it is the treatment shown by a person toward another or others, especially in his conformity with or divergence from the norms of good manners or social decorum.

In the final analysis it is very difficult in alcohol PMP epidemiologic research to completely isolate any given variable discussed above. The interplay of major variables upon the drunk or drinking driver is illustrated in Figure 12-2. In carefully reviewing existing epidemiologic reports it becomes readily evident that all variables shown in Figure 12-2 impinge upon each other to produce their respective and collective

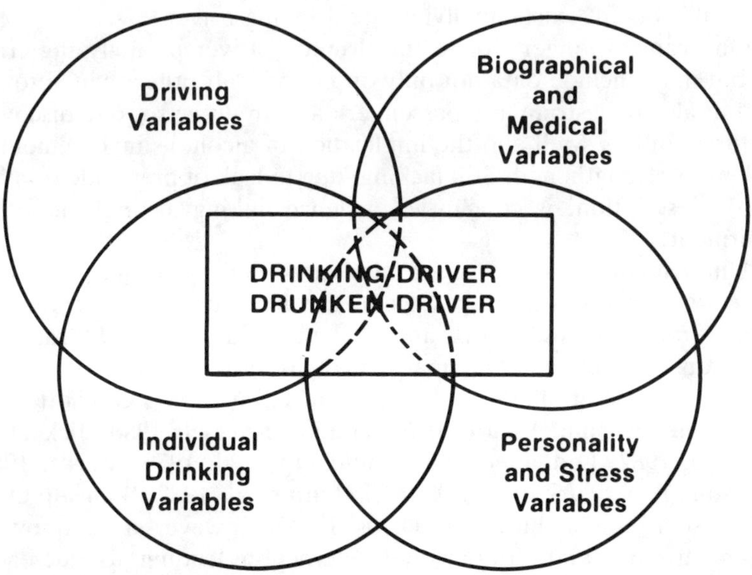

Figure 12-2 Major variables impinging upon interpretation of drunken driver assessment.

alterations in the drinking or drunk driver, as does alcohol. In addition, the impact of sociological and demographic variables such as alcohol consumption patterns, recidivism, repeated DWI offenses, driving records, age of drivers, and effects of DWI treatment programs must be given consideration (Baker and Spitz, 1970; Bako et al, 1977; Brown, 1978; Filkins et al, 1970; Hagger and Dax, 1977; McGuire, 1978; Maisto et al, 1979; Maki and Linnoila, 1976; Rosenberg et al, 1974; Shaffer et al, 1977; Shultz and Layne, 1979; Whitlock et al, 1971; Davis, 1974; Pelz et al, 1975; Perrine, 1975, 1976; Waller, 1972, 1973). Recidivism and repeated DWI offenses are referred to separately. Recidivism is a tendency to return to bad habits after some intervening attempt to alter one's habits through a learning or alcohol treatment program. It is therefore critical that laboratory and field testing be performed in addition to epidemiologic research in studying alcohol PMP impairment of humans who drive or ride in motor vehicles or who walk near where motor vehicles are operated.

After discussing the variables which may influence the drinking driver and the multiple, sometimes confusing definitions of the parameters to be studied, a commonality can be found which strongly indicts alcohol as an offending variable in impaired PMP. The fact remains that after investigation of thousands of motor vehicle accidents, alcohol has been present in the blood of many drivers in amounts greater than described as the minimum concentration for legal PMP impairment. Since legal impairment is demonstrated at blood alcohol concentrations higher than are described for pharmacologic impairment, it follows that a societal problem exists involving the drinking driver.

One can no longer isolate the drinking driver in analyzing crash data but must include data not only on motor craft other than automobiles but also pedestrian and passenger data. In doing so, one discovers that the numbers swell and the implication of alcohol's involvement in accidents is strengthened. Still lacking, due to lack of preaccident investigative description, is conclusive evidence linking alcohol and PMP impairment.

Unfortunately, as the use of mind-altering drugs of all pharmacologic classes becomes more prevalent, this literature must also be surveyed. A relatively few reports appear in the epidemiologic literature at present on drug-related as compared with alcohol-related motor vehicle accidents (Finkle et al, 1968; Mason and McBay, 1984; Garriott et al, 1977; Honkanen and Visuri, 1976; Honkanen et al, 1980; Jick et al, 1981; Job, 1982; Landauer, 1981; Lundberg et al, 1979; Marks, 1982; Robinson, 1979; Turk et al, 1974; Cimbura et al, 1982; Simpson et al, 1982; Bastos and Galante, 1976; Davis, 1974). However, a trend toward drug-impairment and drug-alcohol interaction leading to decreased PMP is emerging.

SUMMARY

There is conspicuous lack of descriptive material, such as erratic driving or unsteadiness in drivers' ability to walk soon after an accident, which supports any measure of PMP alteration. We can only say that alcohol is present in a large number of arrested drivers in amounts greater than legally permissible, especially in driver populations involved in accidents. In the majority of these persons, alcohol is present in amounts exceeding the legally and pharmacologically accepted limits for PMP impairment. However, this fact alone does not solely support the argument that a strong relationship exists between the presence of alcohol and the occurrence of accidents whether one studies drivers, passengers, or pedestrians. The proof of actual PMP impairment remains with the phase II and III studies where other variables such as environment can be controlled. These laboratory and field investigations will also permit prospective design and standardization of testing procedures. These data may be used to correlate blood alcohol concentration with general and functional impairment which may occur. In the absence of such thorough investigations, were we to base our interpretation of alcohol PMP impairment solely upon existing epidemiologic data, we would be forced to conclude that the case has not yet been conclusively proved that alcohol impairs PMP. Nevertheless, the simple correlation of the high incidence of BAC above legal limits in drivers having accidents indicates that a significant problem exists which cannot be disregarded by society.

The authors express their appreciation for the assistance given by Mrs Sharon Farrar in the preparation of this manuscript.

REFERENCES

American Medical Association Committee on Medicolegal Problems. *Alcohol and the Impaired Driver. A Manual on the Medicolegal Aspects of Chemical Tests for Intoxication*, American Medical Association, Chicago, 1970.

Baker, S.P., and Fisher, R.S. Alcohol and motorcycle fatalities. *Am. J. Public Health* 67:246–249, 1977.

Baker, S.P., and Spitz, W.M. Age effects and autopsy evidence of disease in fatally injured drivers. *JAMA* 214:1079–1088, 1970.

Bako, G., MacKenzie, W.C., and Smith, E.S.O. Case-control study of recidivist drivers involved in fatal highway accidents in Alberta in 1970–72. *Can. Med. Assoc. J.* 116:149–151, 1977.

Bastos, M.L., and Galante, L. Toxicological findings in victims of traumatic deaths. *J. Forensic Sci.* 21:176–186, 1976.

Birrell, J.H.W. A comparison of the post-mortem blood-alcohol levels of drivers and passengers compared with those of drinking drivers who killed pedestrians. *Med. J. Aust.* 2:945–948, 1971.

Borkenstein, R.F., Crowther, R.F., Shumate, R.P., et al. *The Role of Drinking*

Driver in Traffic Accidents, Indiana University, Dept. of Police Administration, Bloomington, 1964.

Brown, R.A. Some social consequences of partial prohibition in Auckland, New Zealand. *Drug Alcohol Depend.* 3:377–382, 1978.

Cimbura, G., Lucas, D.M., Bennett, R.C., et al. Incidence and toxicological aspects of drugs detected in 484 fatally injured drivers and pedestrians in Ontario. *J. Forensic Sci.* 27:855–867, 1982.

Clark, D.C., and Clark, F.A. *Analyses of Washtenaw County Alcohol Safety Action Program Crash Criteria Measures*, University of Michigan, Highway Safety Research Institute, Ann Arbor, 1973.

Crompton, M.R. Alcohol and fatal road traffic accidents. *Med. Sci. Law* 22: 189–194, 1982.

Davis, J.H. Carbon monoxide, alcohol, and drugs in fatal accidents in Dade County, Florida, 1956–1968. *Clin. Toxicol.* 7:597–613, 1974.

Davis, S., and Smith, L.S. Alcohol and drowning in Cape Town: A preliminary report. *S. Afr. Med. Tydskr.* 62:931–933, 1982.

Dietz, P.E., and Baker, S.P. Drowning: Epidemiology and prevention. *Am. J. Public Health* 64:303–312, 1974.

Ellingstad, V.S., and Westra, D.P. *Analytic Study. I: An Analysis of Total Project Impact*, University of South Dakota, Department of Psychology, Vermillion, 1974.

Eriksson, A., and Bjornstig, U. Fatal snow mobile accidents in Northern Sweden. *J. Trauma* 22:977–982, 1982.

Farris, R., Malone, T.B., and Lilliefors, H. *A Comparison of Alcohol Involvement in Exposed and Injured Drivers. Phases I and II*, National Highway Traffic Safety Administration Technical Report DOT-HS-801-826, 1976.

Filkins, L.D., Clark, C.D., Rosenblatt, C.A., et al. *Alcohol Abuse and Traffic Study: A Study of Fatalities, DWI Offender, Alcoholics and Court-Related Treatment Approaches*, Final Report U.S. Dept. of Transport, National Highway Safety Bureau Contract No. FH-11-6555 and FH-11-7129, 1970.

Finkle, B.S., Biasotti, A.A., and Bradford, L.W. The occurrence of some drugs and toxic agents encountered in drinking driver investigation. *J. Forensic Sci.* 13:236–245, 1968.

Florendo, R.M. *An Analysis of Ultimate Performance Measures: 1974*, County of Los Angeles, Alcohol Safety Action Project, Los Angeles, 1975.

Galloway, D.J., and Patel, A.R. Road traffic accident–related morbidity as seen in an accident and emergency department. *Scot. Med. J.* 26:121–124, 1981.

Garriott, J.C., Di Maio, V.J.M., Zumwalt, R.A., et al. Incidence of drugs and alcohol in fatally injured motor vehicle drivers. *J. Forensic Sci.* 22:383–389, 1977.

Haddon, W., Jr., and Bradess, V.A. Alcohol in the single vehicle fatal accident. *JAMA* 169:1587–1593, 1959.

Haddon, W., Valien, P., McCarroll, J., et al. A controlled investigation of the characteristics of adult pedestrians fatally injured by motor vehicles in Manhattan. *J. Chron. Dis.* 14:655–678, 1961.

Hagger, R. and Dax, E.C., The driving records of mutli-problem families. *Soc. Sci. Med. (A)* 11:121–127, 1977.

Harger R.N., Lamb, E.B., and Hulpieu, H.R. Rapid chemical test for intoxication employing breath; new reagent for alcohol and procedure for estimating concentration of alcohol in body from ratio of alcohol to carbon dioxide in breath. *JAMA* 110:779–785, 1938.

Heise, H. Alcohol and automobile accidents. *JAMA* 103:739–741, 1934.

Holcomb, R.L. Alcohol in relation to traffic accidents. *JAMA* 3:1076–1085, 1938.

Honkanen, R., and Visuri, T. Blood alcohol levels in a series of injured patients with special references to accident and type of injury. *Ann. Chir. Gynecol.* 65:287–294, 1976.

Honkanen, R.L., Ertama, L., Linnoila, M., et al. Role of drugs in traffic accidents. *Br. Med. J.* 281:1309–1312, 1980.

Hurst, P.M. Estimating the effectiveness of blood alcohol limits. *Behav. Res. Hwy. Safe.* 1:87–99, 1970.

Hurst, P.M. Epidemiology aspects of alcohol and driver crashes and citations. In *Alcohol, Drugs and Driving* (M.W. Perrine, ed.), National Highway Traffic Safety Administration Technical Report DOT-HS-801-096, 1974.

Irwin, S.T., Patterson, C.C. and Rutherford, W.H. Association between alcohol consumption and adult pedestrians who sustain injuries in road traffic accidents. *Br. Med. J.* 286:522, 1983.

Jalazo, J., Steer, R.A., and Fine, E.W. Use of breathalyzer scores in the evaluation of persons arrested for driving while intoxicated. *J. Stud. Alcohol* 39:1304–1307, 1978.

Jick, H., Hunter, J.R., Denan, B.J., et al. Sedating drugs and automobile accidents leading to hospitalization. *Am. J. Public Health* 71:1399–1400, 1981.

Job, R.F.S. Does diazepam affect driving ability? *Med. J. Aust.* 1:89–91, 1982.

Jones, R.K. and Joscelyn, K.B. A systems approach to the analysis of transportation law. *Transp. Law J.* 8:71–89, 1976.

Jones, R.K., and Joscelyn, K.B. *Alcohol and Highway Safety 1978: A Review of the State of Knowledge*, National Highway Traffic Safety Administration Final Report DOT-HS-5-01217, 1978.

Joscelyn, K.B., and Treat, J.R. *A Study to Determine the Relationship Between Vehicle Defects and Crashes*. Indiana University, Institute for Research in Public Safety, Bloomington, 1973.

Landauer, A.A. Diazepam and driving ability. *Med. J. Aust.* L; 624–626, 1981.

Lloyd, L.E., and Venus, P. Death on Texas roads: The picture worsens for young adults. *Tex. Med.* 79:53–56, 1983.

Lucas, G.W.H., Kalow, W., McColl, J.D., et al. Quantitative studies of the relationship between alcohol levels and motor vehicle accidents. In *Proceedings of the Second International Conference on Alcohol and Road Traffic*. Garden City Press Cooperative, Toronto, 1955.

Lundberg, G.D., White, J.M., and Hoffman, K.I. Drugs (other than or in addition to ethyl alcohol) and driving behavior: A collaborative study of the California Association of Toxicologists. *J. Forensic Sci.* 24:207–215, 1979.

McCarroll, J.R., and Haddon, W., Jr. A controlled study of fatal automobile accidents in New York City. *J. Chron. Dis.* 15:811–826, 1962.

McCarroll, J., Braunstein, P., Cooper, W., et al. Fatal pedestrian automotive accidents. *JAMA* 180:127–133, 1962.

McDermott, F. Control of road trauma epidemic in Australia. *Ann. R. Coll. Surg. Eng.* 60:437–450, 1978.

McDermott, F.T., and Hughes, E.S.R. Compulsory blood alcohol testing of road crash casualties in Victoria. The second three years (1978–1980). *Med. J. Aust.* 1:294–296, 1982.

McDermott, F., and Strang, P. Compulsory blood alcohol testing of road crash casualties in Victoria: The first three years. *Med. J. Aust.* 2:612–615, 1978.

McGuire, F.L. The effectiveness of a treatment program for the alcohol-involved driver. *Am. J. Alcohol Abuse* 5:517–525, 1978.

Maisto, S.A., Sobell, L.C., Zelhart, P.F., et al. Driving records of persons convicted of driving under the influence of alcohol. *J. Stud. Alcohol* 40: 70–77, 1979.

Maki, M., and Linnoila, M. Characteristics of driving in relation to the drug and alcohol use of Finnish outpatients. *Mod. Probl. Pharmacopsychiatry* 11: 11–21, 1976.

Marks, V. Drugs and driving. *R. Soc. Health J.* 102:205–210, 1982.

Mason, A.P., and McBay, A.J. Ethanol, marijuana, and other drug use in 600 drivers killed in single-vehicle crashes in North Carolina, 1978–1981. *J. Forensic Sci.* 29:987–1026, 1984.

Neilson, R.A. *Alcohol Involvement in Fatal Motor Vehicle Accidents.* California 1962–1968, California Traffic Safety Foundation, San Francisco, 1969.

Patterns of alcohol use among teenage drivers in fatal motor vehicle accidents — United States 1977–1981. *MMWR* 32:344–347, 1982.

Pelz, D.C., McDole, T.L., and Schuman, S.H. Drinking-driving behavior of young men in relation to accidents. *J. Stud. Alcohol* 36:956–972, 1975.

Pendleton, O.J., Hatfield, N.J., and Bremer, R. *Alcohol Involvement in Texas Driver Fatalities: Accident Reports Versus Blood Alcohol Concentration*, Texas Transportation Institute, Texas A & M University System, College Station, 1986.

People v Henry 72 P2d 915 (Cal 1937).

Perrine, M.W. Alcohol involvement in highway crashes: A review of the epidemiologic evidence. *Clin. Plast. Surg.* 2:11–34, 1975.

Perrine, M.W. Alcohol and highway crashes. *Mod. Probl. Pharmacopsychiatry* 11:22–41, 1976.

Perrine, M.W., and Huntley, M.S., Jr. *Influences of Alcohol Upon Driving Behavior in an Instrumental Car,* National Highway Traffic Safety Administration Technical Report DOT-HS-800-625, 1971.

Perrine, M.W., Waller, J.A. and Harris, L.S. *Alcohol and Highway Safety: Behavioral and Medical Aspects.* National Highway Safety Administration Technical Report DOT-HS-800-599, 1971.

Plueckhahn, V.D. Alcohol consumption and death by drowning in adults: A 24-year epidemiological analysis. *J. Stud. Alcohol* 43:445–452, 1982.

Plueckhahn, V.D. Alcohol and road safety: Geelong experience 1967 to 1978. *Med. J. Aust.* 2:615–625, 1978.

Riddick, L.R., and Luke, J.C. Alcohol-associated deaths in the District of Columbia — A postmortem study. *J. Forensic Sci.* 23:493–501, 1978.

Robinson, T.A. The incidence of drugs in impaired driving specimens in Northern Ireland. *J. Forensic Sci. Soc.* 19:237–244, 1979.

Rosenberg, N., Laessig, R.H., and Rawlings, R.R. Alcohol, age and fatal traffic accidents. *Q. J. Stud. Alcohol* 35:473–489, 1974.

Shaffer, J.W., Schmidt, C.W., Zlotowitz, H.I., et al. Social adjustment profiles of female drivers involved in fatal and non-fatal accidents. *Am. J. Psychiatr.* 134:801–804, 1977.

Shultz, S.D., and Jayne, N.R., Jr. Age and BAC when arrested for drunken driving and public drunkenness. *J. Stud. Alcohol* 40:492–495, 1979.

Simpson, H.M., Mayhew, D.R., and Warren, R.A. Epidemiology of road accidents involving young adults: Alcohol, drugs and other factors. *Drug Alcohol Depend.* 10:35–63, 1982.

Soderstrom, C.A., DuPriest, R.W., Benner, C., et al. Alcohol and roadway trauma: Problems of diagnosis and management. *Am. Surg.* 45:129–137, 1979.

Spencer, J.A., and Ferguson, W.S. *An Analysis of Ultimate Performance*

Measures to Determine Total Project Impact of the Fairfax County Alcohol Safety Action Project. Highway Safety Division of Virginia, Virginia Highway Traffic Research Council, 76-R29, Richmond, 1975.)

State v Duquad 72 P2d 435 (Ar 1937).

Traffic Injury Research Foundation of Canada. *Analysis of Fatal Traffic Crashes in Canada, 1973. Focus: The Impaired Driver.* Ottawa, 1975.

Turk, R.F., McBay, A.J., and Hudson, P. Drug involvement in automobile driver and pedestrian fatalities. *J. Forensic Sci.* 19:90–97, 1974.

Waller, J.A. Factors associated with alcohol and responsibility for fatal highway crashes. *Q. J. Stud. Alcohol* 33:160–170, 1972.

Waller, J.A. Current issues in the epidemiology of injury. *Am. J. Epidemiol.* 98:72–76, 1973.

Waller, J.A., King, E.M., Nielson, G. et al. Alcohol and other factors in California highway fatalities. In *Proceedings of the 11th Annual Meeting of the American Association for Automotive Medicine.* Charles C Thomas, Springfield, Ill. 1970.

Weston, J.T. Alcohol's impact on man's activity: Its role in unnatural death. *Am. J. Clin. Pathol.* 74:755–758, 1980.

Whitlock, F.A., Armstrong, J.L., Longe, J.I., et al. The drinking driver or the driving drinker? Alcohol, alcoholism and other factors in road accidents. *Med. J. Aust.* 2:5–16, 1971.

Widmark, E.M.P., Alcoholic excretion in urine and a simple clinically applicable method for diagnosing alcoholic intoxication in drivers. *Ups. Lakaref. Forh.* 19:241–273, 1914.

Widmark, E.M.P. *Die theoretischen Grundlagen und die praktische Verwendbarkeit der gerichtlich-meizinischen Alkoholbestimmung*, Urban and Schwarzenberg, Berlin, 1932.

Zylman, R. A critical evaluation of the literature on "alcohol involvement" in highway deaths. *Accid. Anal. Prevent.* 6:163–204, 1974.

Zylman, R., Blomberg, R.D., and Preusser, D.F. *A Review of the Literature on the Involvement of Alcohol in Pedestrian Collision Resulting in Death and Injury.* National Highway Traffic Safety Administration Technical Report DOT-HS-801-413, 1975.

13

Report of Laboratory Findings

James C. Garriott

Results of analyses for ethyl alcohol are used regularly in the courts for various types of litigation (as in prosecution of the drinking driver), in medicine, for evaluation and treatment of the patient, and in other forensic settings, such as evaluation of cause of death in autopsy cases.

Since legal limits for driving under the influence are defined by the concentration of alcohol in the blood, it is essential to report findings uniformly and accurately, as well as to include adequate documentation of chain of custody for acceptability in courts of law.

ANALYSIS SPECIFICITY

Any forensic analysis for ethyl alcohol must be performed by a procedure that is specific for ethyl alcohol, to the exclusion of any other interfering substances. Methods and methodologic considerations have been discussed in chapters 7 and 8. Although oxidation and enzyme procedures have long been used for ethyl alcohol determinations, and are currently used in many clinical laboratories, these methods do not involve separation of the analyte prior to measurement, and are not totally exclusive.

The methods now uniformly accepted for forensic alcohol analysis utilize gas liquid chromatography. It is generally accepted that the only other volatile substances present in the blood of human subjects at concentrations similar to those encountered for ethyl alcohol, and with the potential for eluting from the column in the same retention time range as ethyl alcohol or with sufficient volatility to potentially interfere with breath analysis are: acetone, acetaldehyde, methanol, isopropanol, and paraldehyde (Mason and Dubowski, 1974). Thus any forensic methodology for ethyl alcohol must properly separate these potentially interfering agents, to rule out any possible coelution in gas chromatography or interference by cross-reactivity when using enzyme or oxidation techniques.

UNIFORMITY OF REPORTING

In the United States, designation of ethyl alcohol concentrations in the blood is usually in conformance with state laws. Since most statutes express alcohol concentration in "percent weight/volume" concentration units, the blood concentration is expressed as grams (of ethyl alcohol) per 100 milliliters of blood, and often, "wt/vol" is written after this result. Another commonly used concentration unit is milligrams per deciliter, or mg/dL. This unit is easily converted to grams by dividing by 1000.

If the units are to be expressed as weight/weight (wt/wt), a slight correction must be made to convert the volume in milliliters to weight in grams. Thus one divides the figure in wt/vol by 1.055, the average specific gravity of blood (American Medical Association, 1968).

In Europe, the concentration unit *per mille* is often used. This designation is by weight, and refers to milligrams of alcohol per gram of blood, or grams of alcohol per 1000 grams of blood. This unit is approximately equivalent to the percent wt/vol when the former is divided by 10 (eg, 0.10% wt/vol = 1.00‰) (Widmark, 1981).

The units discussed above utilize conventional metric units. Since July 1, 1986, the *Journal of the American Medical Association*, following recommendations of the American National Metric Council, has reported all drug concentrations in conformance with the Système International d'Unités (SI) (International System of Units). Presumably, other journals will follow. The SI unit for alcohol (as with other drugs) bears no resemblance to the conventional metric units now used. The SI unit for alcohol is expressed as millimoles per liter (mmol/L) and expresses the number of molecular weight units of alcohol (1 mole) per liter of volume. (mol wt of alcohol = 46.07.) The conversion factor becomes 217.1. Thus, 0.10% (wt/vol) of ethyl alcohol in blood is equivalent to 21.71 mmol/L (See Table 13-1) (Lundberg, 1986).

Table 13-1
Units for Expressing Ethyl Alcohol Concentrations

Conventional metric units
0.10% (wt/vol) = 0.10 g/100 mL of blood = 100 mg% = 100 mg/dL = 1000 ppm = 0.0948% (wt/wt) = 1‰ (per mille, mg/g, wt/wt) = 1.00 g/L
SI units
0.10% (wt/vol) = 21.71 mmol/L (46.07 = mol wt of ethyl alcohol)

CHAIN OF CUSTODY

Principles of chain of custody of evidence will be discussed in chapter 14. The chain of custody must be clearly documented when reporting results of forensic alcohol examinations. Generally, the laboratory's official chain of custody begins with the arrival of the sample in the laboratory. The report of the analysis should include the date and time of arrival of the sample (most conveniently by a date stamp on the report form); the deliverer's signature or initials, the receiving person's signature, a brief description of the evidence, date of completion, and results. Of course, the units of measurement should be clearly indicated (eg, "the blood contained 0.15% wt/vol ethyl alcohol").

OTHER CONSIDERATIONS FOR REPORTING RESULTS

It is often desirable to further elucidate the criteria used for alcohol analysis. The method used for the analysis can be referred to simply as "gas chromatography" or, "headspace gas chromatography." Since many laboratories use their own procedures or their own modifications of published procedures, it is not practical to refer to a specific procedure in reporting results. However, the laboratory should always be prepared and willing to provide a copy of the actual procedure used, if the laboratory analysis is used in litigation. The accuracy and confidence limits of the procedure used should also be known. For example, if a laboratory reports a blood alcohol of 0.11 g/100 mL, and the method is accurate only to ±11%, this single blood alcohol analysis may not be sufficient prima facie evidence for conviction of driving while intoxicated, in a state whose limit for intoxication is 0.10 g/100 mL.

It also may be desirable to define the limits of detectability for the analyte, alcohol. A negative result may be reported if the amount found was less than 0.01 g/mL or in some cases 0.02 g/100 mL. If such limits are used as laboratory policy, this should also be stated.

REFERENCES

American Medical Association Committee on Medicolegal Problems. *Alcohol and the Impaired Driver. A Manual on the Medicolegal Aspects of Chemical Tests for Intoxication*, American Medical Association, Chicago, 1968.

Lundberg, G.D., Iverson, C., and Radulescu, G. Now read this: The SI Units are here. *JAMA* 255:2329–2338, 1986.

Mason, M.F., and Dubowski, K.M. Alcohol, traffic, and chemical testing in the United States: A resume and some remaining problems. *Clin. Chem.* 20: 126–140, 1974.

Widmark, E.M.P. *Principles and Applications of Medicolegal Alcohol Determination*. 1932, Biomedical Publications, Davis Calif., 1981.

14

The Expert Witness

Patricia H. Field
Barbara Basteyns

Presenting one's results or opinions in a court of law is a challenging experience. Often, one side in the case has an interest in demonstrating one's results to be accurate and one's opinion credible, while the other side may want to show that the results are erroneous and the opinion worthless. The adversary system of law practiced in the United States allows counsel for both sides to examine and question the witness in order to present their viewpoints for the judge or jury's consideration.

THE ROLE OF THE EXPERT WITNESS

There are two kinds of witnesses: witnesses to fact, and expert witnesses. Fact witnesses must confine their testimony to what they themselves saw or did, and cannot venture opinions. Expert witnesses may form and voice opinions based on their experience and the prevailing wisdom in their area of expertise. Most witnesses presenting the results of alcohol tests or interpreting them will be considered expert witnesses. Often, they are contacted by the prosecutor or the lawyer for the plaintiff or defendant and asked to render an opinion. After discussing the case with the expert, the lawyer will decide whether or not to use that expert's testimony at trial. Persons who collect and analyze samples for alcohol may be treated as fact witnesses, however, and the first notice of a case may be a subpoena commanding them, "laying aside all other business," to appear at court at a certain time.

If they are not already familiar with the case, they will need to know why they were subpoenaed and what testimony is expected of them. The process server may be able to tell who issued the subpoena.

If it came in the mail, the envelope should give the return address. The agency or law firm issuing the subpoena should be contacted and the witness should ask to speak to the person handling the case (often, the person who signed the subpoena) in order to determine the witness's part in the case. In some cases, for example, preliminary hearings, a certified copy of the test result or other document may be used in place of an appearance.

If testimony is required, a conference should be scheduled to allow the witness and the lawyer to review the witness's qualifications, the information he or she can provide, any documentation pertinent to the case, and the scope and limitations of his or her expertise. This is the time to inform the attorney of possible problems with the specimen, analysis, or interpretation, and to discuss what questions should be asked at trial to guard against or rebut anticipated questions or opposing testimony which could cast doubt on the evidence and opinions to be presented. All documents related to the case should be brought to this conference.

If the witness performed an alcohol analysis, it is likely that some of the documents will be part of the laboratory's permanent records, and the danger exists that they could be entered into evidence as exhibits at trial. If this would present a problem for the laboratory, the attorney should be alerted and asked to enter only photocopies. In depositions or at trial, the witness may be required to produce all notes and materials relevant to the case, so one should be judicious as to what notes are kept. Calculations should be clear and legible. The notes should be limited to the facts of the case, not opinions. The information should be accurate and unbiased, so that it will not embarrass the witness or indicate that assumptions were made about the case before reviewing the evidence.

Preparation for Court

In those cases where a specimen has been or will be analyzed for alcohol content, preparation for court begins with specimen collection and analysis. The specimen should be collected from an appropriate anatomical location and analyzed promptly or preserved and stored properly. All persons who were responsible for the custody of the sample should be known, and these should be few, if possible. The chain of custody (evidence) linking the sample analyzed with the subject is proper material for challenge in court, and it may be necessary to demonstrate the integrity of the chain and admissibility of the result by requiring testimony of each person who had access to the specimen. The method of analysis should be specific and accurate. Its limits of variability should be known, and quality control records documenting precision and accuracy should be available. Records of the test itself (gas chromatograms, for example, and the work sheet showing the test or tests, standards, and controls run that day) should be preserved for as long as it is likely that the results may be relevant in court. This can be several years for civil cases in many jurisdictions.

Records may be stored off-site or microfilmed, but it is essential to have an efficient location and retrieval system in order to avoid lengthy and laborious searches when stored information becomes needed. Specimen collection, analysis, and quality control are discussed in chapters 9 and 10. Standard operating procedures should be followed faithfully. Inevitably, the question, "But you don't really remember what you did with *this* sample, do you?" will be raised, and unless the analyst has an excellent memory or analyzes very few samples, the only way to be able to answer "Yes, I do" is to be able to add, "because that is my invariable procedure, and any irregularities that may occur are always documented."

Standard operating procedures make it possible for the laboratory director or section supervisor to introduce in court results produced by people working under his or her supervision. This is an exception to the hearsay rule for records kept in the normal conduct of business, and becomes especially important if the employee is no longer available. The process is facilitated if the supervisor has a policy of reviewing all data and signing all reports before they leave the laboratory. If the alcohol result is prima facie evidence of the offense (eg, driving under the influence when a certain alcohol concentration is illegal per se), the constitutional right to confront one's accuser (the person who performed the test which alone is evidence of guilt) may require the analyst himself to testify. The supervisor will have personal knowledge of the alcohol content only if he or she has reanalyzed a portion of the sample.

The person who testifies about an alcohol result from a laboratory not under his or her control may wish to investigate the laboratory's specimen handling, analytical, and quality control procedures before deciding how much confidence to place in the reliability of the result. It is possible, of course, that a qualified expert may be asked to make calculations or form opinions about alcohol and its effects even when no analysis was performed.

Types of Testimony Related to Alcohol

The expert witness may be called for a number of different kinds of cases in which alcohol is involved. In a coroner's inquest, he may be asked how much alcohol was present and whether this amount, alone or in the presence of other drugs or debilitating conditions, would be sufficient to cause death. In a worker's or prisoner's hearing, the mere presence of alcohol may be sufficient to show an infraction. Given a person's alcohol concentration, gender, and body weight, the expert may be asked to calculate how much alcohol was consumed. A minimum amount can usually be given with some confidence, but factors affecting absorption and metabolism make precise calculations of the total amount of alcohol consumed more difficult. A witness may be asked to substantiate the idea that if the subject consumed alcohol after or immediately before the event in question, the blood alcohol content at that time would have been less than the amount measured at a later time.

If no tests were done, the witness may be asked to calculate the probable blood alcohol concentration or range of concentrations from the subject's statements about what he or she was drinking. This request may be made by the prosecution or the defense (usually depending on whether the subject claims to have been drinking a lot or a little). A defendant who had a high blood alcohol test but claims to have been drinking only a little or not at all may seek an expert to calculate and testify about the probable blood alcohol based on his story, and perhaps to give other testimony to attempt to discredit the test. Experts may be called in any adversary proceeding to discredit any test unfavorable to one side or the other.

In civil suits, the defendant may retain an expert to show that the plaintiff was impaired by alcohol at the time the accident or injury occurred ("contributory negligence"). This is not uncommon in product liability suits against insurance companies and the manufacturers of vehicles and recreational equipment. The basis for the expert's testimony may be either a blood alcohol test, or statements about what the plaintiff was drinking prior to the accident. Some civil suits are brought against drinking drivers by injured passengers or other drivers. In suits with multiple defendants, one defendant may call an expert to show that another defendant's drinking was a major factor in the accident, thus reducing the liability of the first defendant. Finally, the presence of alcohol may be used in an attempt to defend persons accused of crimes such as homicide. While the expert cannot determine the person's intent to commit the crime, he or she may describe the adverse effect of alcohol on a person's judgment, and the release of inhibitions which can potentially lead to aggresive or violent behavior.

In contrast to the fact witness, who has no choice, the expert should use discretion in deciding whether to assist in a case. The presence of a competent expert lends credibility to that side of the case, and may suggest to the jury that the expert is convinced of the guilt or innocence of the defendant, or of the merits of the side that called him or her in a civil case. This may well be true. But if the expert testifies to a scientific truth that supports one side of a case when there is information available that clearly supports the merits of the other side, he will make it harder for the jury to make a sound decision. Common examples are experts who limit their testimony to the possibilites for errors in tests, without acknowledging that most alcohol tests are accurate, and experts who discourse at length on the numerous organic substances that could react with breath tests, without considering or stating that most of the substances described are not going to be present in human breath in sufficient quantity to react under normal test conditions (Dubowski and Essary, 1984; Coldwell and Grant, 1963). These "experts" are, at best, misleading the courts with their one-sided testimony (Figure 14-1).

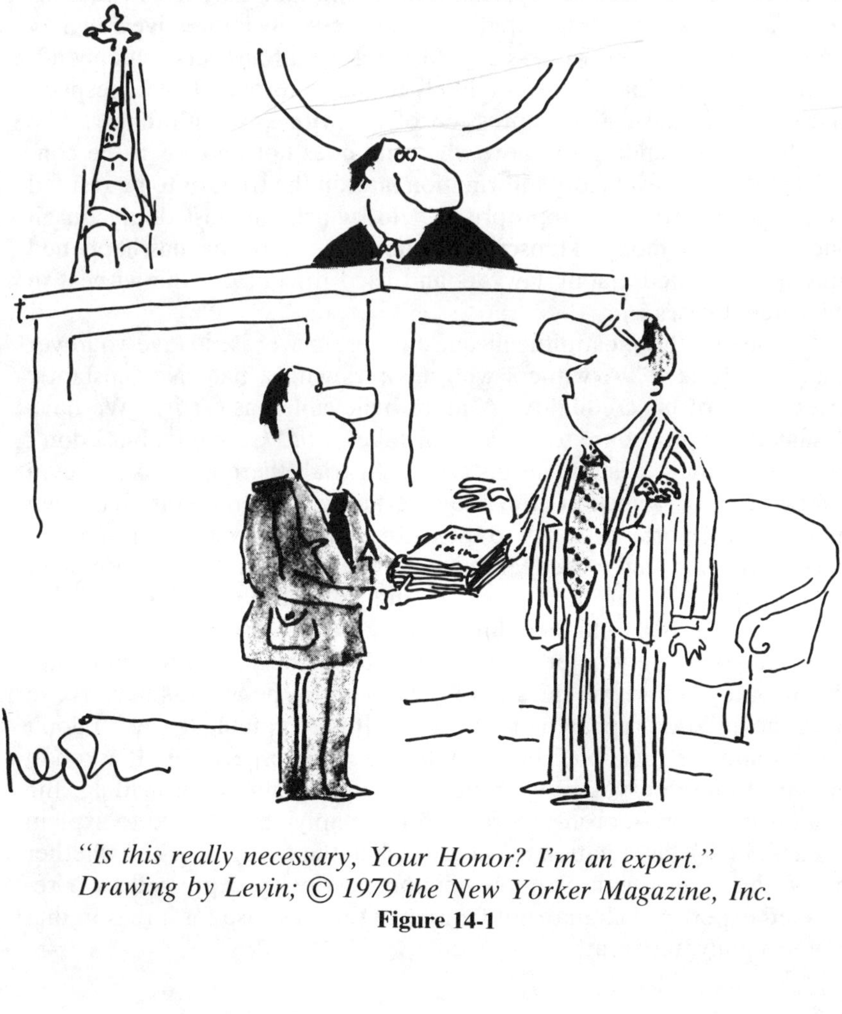

"Is this really necessary, Your Honor? I'm an expert."
Drawing by Levin; © 1979 the New Yorker Magazine, Inc.
Figure 14-1

Testimony and Demeanor

The expert's opinion should be based on extensive and current knowledge in his or her field. In some jurisdictions, the expert must have personal knowledge (by having performed research or observed tests) of each fact he or she testifies about. More commonly, appropriate education and employment, membership in professional organizations, and extensive reading are sufficient to permit the expert to testify about the work of other scientists in the field.

Being accepted by the court as an expert witness may suggest that a person should know everything, or at least everything about his or her field. This is not likely to be true, but the witness can get into trouble by thinking that it should be true. The expert witness should not stray beyond his or her area of expertise and should take time to consider his or her answers. Answering rapidly is not necessarily impressive and may lead to mistakes. The witness should not guess at answers. Openly admitting, "I don't know" is more likely to evoke respect than disrespect, and conveys a favorable impression of the witness's truthfulness. The penalty for pretending to know what one does not know is to be confronted with contradictory information later in the trial, or to be refuted by an expert from the appropriate field, which can cast doubt on all one's prior testimony. Transcripts from trials where this has happened may be circulated among lawyers and used to confront the witness in subsequent cases.

Probably the most difficult question to answer is, "Have you ever made a mistake?" A witness who answers with a flat "No" instantly loses much of his credibility. A more believable answer is, "We have designed our procedure to prevent mistakes," or "Certainly, but I don't believe I made a mistake in this case." At trial, there is likely to be an interruption or objection after the "Certainly," but the point has been made. It is important to stick to the truth. A witness who has committed perjury (been found to deliberately lie under oath) will find subsequent juries instructed that they are not bound to believe anything she says.

The witness should take time to be sure he or she understands each question completely before answering. He or she should not interrupt the attorney before the question is completed. The witness may ask to have the question repeated or rephrased. It is acceptable to say, "I don't understand the question," but it should be done respectfully. If asked to answer a question yes or no, when to do so would be misleading, the witness may say so, or interpose (before complying), "I need to explain my answer." This situation may occur when the expert is asked whether he or she agrees with a sound opinion previously expressed by a respected expert, which may not be relevant to this case for a reason that is not readily apparent.

Since the judge and jury have only a short time to evaluate the credibility and competence of the witness, appearance, demeanor, and vocabulary take on unusual importance. The witness should dress neatly and conservatively. His or her bearing and attitude, on the stand and whenever in or near the courtroom, should convey an understanding of and respect for the importance of the matter at trial. Observers should be able to see that the witness is serious about his or her work. The language used should be grammatically and technically correct, but not stilted, confusing, or obscure. Technical jargon should be avoided. If one has little or no courtroom experience, it is useful to practice explaining the information one needs to convey to an intelligent adult who is not well acquainted with the field. It may take a while to find language which is natural and comfortable, neither unduly technical nor so oversimplified that the listener doubts the witness's expertise. On the stand, the witness's truthfulness and sincerity should be evident in his or her answers, facial expressions, and body language. The jury is expected to observe the witness and judge his or her credibility and competence by these signs.

Circumstances in Which Testimony May be Required

Testimony may be needed in a coroner's inquest, employment or parole hearing, deposition, military or civilian court. Civilian courts are generally divided into two areas: trial courts and appellate or review courts. Review courts do not hear the testimony of witnesses, although interested parties may assist those who prepare the briefs for appeal. Coroner's inquests do not operate strictly on the adversary system, since the intent is to determine the cause of death and to discover whether there is sufficient information to charge someone with responsibility for it. Although a lawyer may contact relevant witnesses and question them at the inquest, the coroner and/or the coroner's jury may also question the witness in an effort to elicit sufficient information to make their decision. A preliminary hearing, in which a judge determines whether there is sufficient evidence to proceed with a trial, is a similar situation.

Sworn depositions may be requested prior to or instead of trial testimony. At depositions, two or more opposing attorneys and a court reporter are present. The attorney who requested the deposition will conduct the initial questioning. In a discovery deposition, this will be the attorney for one of the opposing parties in the case who wishes to learn the witness's opinions and conclusions. After he or she has finished, the attorney who intends to present the witness at trial may then ask questions for clarification. In a deposition taken in lieu of testimony at trial, which may be videotaped and shown at trial or merely read, the initial questioning is conducted by the attorney who has requested the witness to testify. Then the opposing attorney or attorneys may cross-examine the witness. Since there is no judge to rule on objections, the witness must answer all questions asked. Later, a judge will rule on whether questions which have been objected to at the deposition may be read at trial or become part of the official records in the case. Parole board, licensing body, and other hearings may be much less formal, with questions asked by anyone present. At any hearing, the witness should maintain the seriousness of demeanor and purpose appropriate to the courtroom.

TRIAL COURTS

Systems and Structure

Most states have two levels of trial courts: local or municipal courts for violations of municipal ordinances, and district or circuit (superior) courts for statutory violations and civil cases. The names will vary from jurisdiction to jurisdiction. First offense driving under the influence of an intoxicant (DUI) cases, if the penalty does not include jail time, may be heard at the local court level. In this situation, the rules of evidence are somewhat different. For instance, the defendant may be called adversely (by the prosecutor) to give his own accounting of what he drank and ate on the date in question. This can be useful if alcohol absorption is in question. In any criminal action, the constitutional right against self-incrimination prevails, and the defendant's testimony is usually not available. DUI cases against American Indians for offenses occurring on reservations, and civil suits against foreign corporations may be held in Federal court. Since procedures vary from state to state, a reader who has need for specific information on the local court system should consult legal counsel.

WHAT TO EXPECT AT TRIAL

Personnel

In courts in the United States, there will always be a judge presiding. The judge's role is to ensure orderly proceedings and to rule on matters of law. The judge may also be the trier of fact who makes the decision in the case if there is no jury. In preliminary hearings, which are used to decide whether there is enough evidence to proceed with a trial, or to rule on pretrial motions which require testimony, there is usually no jury. Juries usually consist of six or 12 persons, often with one or two alternates who hear the entire case but do not participate in the decision unless one of the other jurors becomes unavailable due to illness or other very serious commitments. Since the jurors are responsible for deciding the case, testimony should be addressed to them, and the witness should watch their expressions to be sure that they are not puzzled, confused, or bored by the testimony.

A court reporter will record the entire proceedings, including the witness's testimony, questions and objections by the attorneys, and the judge's rulings. It is important to speak slowly and distinctly for the court reporter. This has the added advantage that the jury will have a much easier time following the testimony of someone who is speaking slowly and distinctly than one who is rushing and mumbling using complicated scientific terminology. It is a good idea to keep an eye on the court reporter. If he is looking exasperated, the witness should slow down. It is helpful to provide the court reporter with a list of frequently used scientific terms, to aid him or her in preparing an accurate transcript.

There will be an attorney for the plaintiff. In a criminal case, the plaintiff is the state or federal government, and the attorney is called the prosecutor. The prosecutor may also be a city attorney, a district attorney, a state attorney general, or a United States attorney. The defendant may hire an attorney or may represent himself. In criminal cases, he has a constitutional right to be defended by counsel, and may request the court to appoint counsel if indigent. The defendant is usually present in criminal cases. In civil cases, the defendant is usually represented by an attorney or attorneys, and need not be present.

The other personnel present vary from court to court. There may be a guard near the courtroom entrance who can advise witnesses whether they are sequestered and when their testimony is expected to occur. The jury may have an attendant to escort them to and from the courtroom and remain with them during their breaks, meals, and deliberations. There may be a clerk present. This is usually the person who swears the witness in. If the witness is unwilling to swear for religious or ethical reasons, he or she should so inform the attorney before trial, and ask that the traditional oath be altered to: "Do you solemnly swear *or affirm* that you will tell the truth, the whole truth, and nothing but the truth (so help you God)?"

Sequence

Jury trial begins with the jury selection, which can be a time-consuming process. All witnesses may be subpoenaed for the beginning of the trial, so it is wise to check with the attorney who requires the testimony to find out what time one is really needed.

At trial, witnesses may be sequestered. This means that they must remain outside the courtroom until called, and must not discuss the case with other witnesses. Sequestration is more commonly required for fact witnesses than for expert witnesses. At any trial, discussing the case with a juror or in the presence of a juror outside the court proceeding may result in a mistrial, so it is vital to use discretion about conversations in hallways, rest rooms, and common eating areas during breaks. Discussions with the attorney will usually take place in a conference room or other area removed from the courtroom. Discussions with all others should not be about the case, unless the attorney gives permission in advance.

After opening statements in which first the attorney for the plaintiff and then the attorney for the defendant summarizes the merits of his side of the case and what he expects to show, the plaintiff or prosecution presents its witnesses, and then the defense presents its witnesses. There may be rebuttal testimony by witnesses for the plaintiff, followed by more rebuttal by witnesses for the defense, but this is unusual. If an expert is asked to be a rebuttal witness, he or she is usually allowed to hear the testimony of the witness he or she is expected to rebut.

Each witness testifies according to the following pattern: The judge asks the lawyer to call the next witness. The witness goes to the front of the courtroom. The clerk or other designated person administers the oath. The witness is seated. If there is a microphone, the witness should adjust it so he or she is speaking into it. The lawyer who called the witness begins by asking the witness questions. This is called the "direct" examination. These questions cannot be "leading," that is, the lawyer should not formulate concepts and ask the witness to agree with them; rather the questions should be open-ended.

The first questions establish the witness's qualifications as an expert. It is helpful to have a current resume for the lawyer to refer to. This may be entered into evidence. The opposing attorney may request voir dire, or an opportunity to question the witness about his qualifications and experience before the judge rules on whether the witness is an expert in his or her field. This may be done out of the presence of the jury. Later, if the testimony goes beyond the field in which the expert is qualified, there is likely to be an objection. Whenever there is an objection, the witness should remain silent until the judge makes a ruling. Often, the basis for the objection is a point of law which does not concern the witness. Even when the question is one on which the witness could offer information (for instance, why the witness is qualified to answer the question that was asked), it is the responsibility of the attorney to ask the proper questions to draw the information out. If the witness continues to answer after an objection has been raised, the jury may hear information which the judge may rule is not pertinent to the case, and this can cause a mistrial, since juries are not presumed to be able to forget important information which they should not have heard.

After the witness's credentials are established, the direct examination continues. If pretrial preparation and discussions with the attorney have been thorough, there should be no surprises. Testimony should be natural and forthright, not "rehearsed." However, it would be unwise to go into a trial without having discussed what questions will be asked and, in general, what the answers will be. Questions and answers should be simple, direct, and brief. The witness should not wander from the topic of the specific question which has been asked. If an issue is complicated and some explanation is required, it is a good idea to preface the answer with a statement to that effect, in order to prepare all parties for the length and complexity of the answer. In general, the more that is said on direct examination, the more material there will be for cross-examination, and the more opportunities there will be to slip up, misspeak, or go beyond one's area of expertise. Furthermore, lengthy explanations may divert the jury from the point of the trial, so volunteering information is to be avoided as a general rule (Figure 14-2).

After the direct examination is completed, the opposing attorney has an opportunity to cross-examine the witness. He or she is allowed to ask leading questions on cross-examination. In general, the scope of the

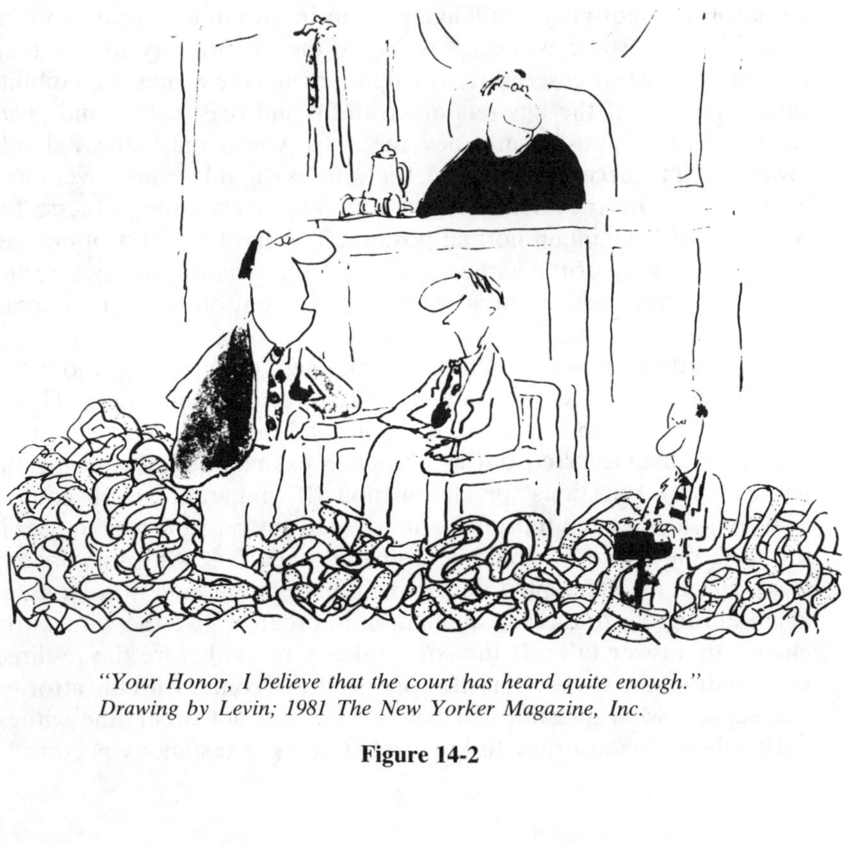

"Your Honor, I believe that the court has heard quite enough."
Drawing by Levin; 1981 The New Yorker Magazine, Inc.

Figure 14-2

cross-examination is limited to the material covered in the direct examination and the witness's area of expertise, but many judges allow broad latitude, and many attorneys fail to object when an opposing attorney strays beyond the strict limits of the direct examination. If the witness has been qualified as an expert on alcohol metabolism, for instance, any question related to alcohol metabolism may be permitted.

The cross-examination may be brief and low-key, merely an opportunity to clear up any points that seemed unclear in the direct examination. Or, it may be an attempt to undermine the witness's credibility and the basis for his or her opinions. If the analysis seems accurate, the opposing attorney may attack the source of the sample, the manner of collection and storage, or the chain of custody.

If all these seem secure, the opposing attorney may try to attack the witness himself. As scientists and professionals, we may quite naturally become indignant at this approach. However, the jury is likely to interpret any emotional reaction as detracting from the witness's appearance of unbiased truthfulness. They may wonder, "Why is he/she so upset? What is he/she trying to hide? Is the opposing attorney coming uncomfortably close to a problem area?" If the witness is sure of his/her data and opinions, there should be no reason to become upset by the opposing attorney rigorously challenging them in an attempt to defend his client. In fact, some witnesses welcome the opportunity to test their opinions against strict scrutiny. The opinions and the witness's credibility should hold up if the answers are truthful and reasonable, and given calmly. If the opposing attorney raises his voice, the witness should lower his. If he becomes bellicose, the witness should become ever more calm. If the attorney leans forward or approaches the witness, the witness should maintain normal posture. This has the effect of increasing the credibility of the witness and decreasing that of the lawyer, and tends to greatly reduce the amount of time spent on belligerent cross-examination.

After the cross-examination is completed, the attorney who called the witness has an opportunity for "re-direct" examination. This is the time to clear up any misconceptions and unfavorable or confusing testimony that occurred during the cross-examination, by asking the witness more questions for clarification. If preparation with counsel prior to trial has been thorough and covered any possible weaknesses in the case, the attorney should be prepared to do this. Any answers that were cut off or interrupted during the cross-examination may be asked again during the re-direct examination in order to give the witness the chance to answer fully. If the court takes a recess before the re-direct examination, the witness has the opportunity to confer with the attorney and suggest what questions to ask. If this does not occur, the witness must rely on the attorney to know what areas of testimony need to be

laboratories and other laboratories throughout the country? Could a transcription error have been made when recording the result? Do the actual records of the analysis demonstrate that this did not occur?

Breath tests Were a standard and room air blank run with the subject's test? This rules out external contamination and assures that the instrument was capable of giving accurate results at the time. If the subject alleges interference due to compounds in his mouth, was a waiting period observed before the test during which the subject was observed for regurgitation and food or objects in the mouth? If liquids (eg, saliva) are alleged to have reacted, could they reasonably have traveled through the mouthpiece and the instrument to the analytical chamber? If volatiles are alleged, could they reasonably be found in human breath in sufficient quantities to react? (Not likely; see Coldwell and Grant [1963] and Dubowski and Essary [1984].) If the alleged volatiles were on the subject's skin and clothing, does the room air blank give evidence that they did not react appreciably? If the compounds react with dichromate more slowly than ethanol does, does a high final test show unexpected delayed reactivity? If not, does this rule out the contamination in question? If the subject's analysis was run in duplicate and the results were comparable, does this not rule out the likelihood of most of the alleged problems, since they are unlikely to occur reproducibly?

Metabolism calculations The expert should avoid making assumptions about when the subject's blood alcohol concentration peaked, if there is insufficient information about the eating and drinking on the day in question. However, if absorption and elimination of alcohol are treated as separate processes, the blood alcohol level at a certain time may be approximated by first using standard clearance rates, stating that an assumption was made that there was no unabsorbed alcohol in the gastrointestinal tract for the purpose of the calculation, then subtracting the effect of a hypothetical amount or amounts of unabsorbed alcohol that may have been present. If beer is the beverage that was consumed, for example, it would be very unusual to have more than a quart unabsorbed.

If the measured blood alcohol concentration is very small, the standard clearance rate may not apply for the last hour or hours (Bogusz et al, 1977). One may question the validity of reports of trace alcohol concentrations. Factors that can affect the metabolic rate, such as liver disease, history of exposure to alcohol, barbiturates and pesticides, and fructose ingestion, should be considered in selecting an appropriate clearance rate or range of rates for calculations. If samples collected at two times were analyzed by different laboratories or different analytical techniques, the expert should refrain from drawing conclusions about a metabolism "curve," since method variability may far exceed the metabolic rate over short periods of time.

Drugs and stress are among the factos that can affect gastric emptying. However, alcohol will be fully absorbed from the stomach itself, even if the gastric emptying rate is slowed (Chittenden, cited by Cooke and Birchall, 1969).

The effect of blood or other intravenous (IV) fluids administered to an injured subject can be reasoned out. If nonalcoholic, they will dilute or reduce subsequent blood alcohol concentrations, but the effect will be insignificant once the fluids have circulated and equilibrated. For example, if a 150-lb man received 3 pt of blood or IV fluids, this would dilute his blood alcohol concentration by only about 3% (3 lb in 100, assuming that alcohol is distributed in the body water, which is about two thirds of a man's body weight).

In court, the witness should take enough time with his calculations to avoid errors. Some witnesses bring a pen and paper or calculator to the witness stand in case the questions asked or parameters given differ from those available when the witness made his initial calculations prior to trial. When presenting one's calculations to attorneys, judges, or the jury, it is helpful to explain the basis for the calculations so that the reasoning behind the conclusions can be followed. Showing one's calculations on a blackboard or easel is helpful. Juries may find this interesting, and it can do much to demystify the process by which a number or range of numbers is reached.

Finally, inexperienced or ill-prepared witnesses may fail to recognize that the number of drinks necessary to reach a given alcohol concentration is different for men and women of the same body weight, and less for obese people than for tall or muscular people of the same body weight.

COURTROOM LANGUAGE AND DECORUM

If it is necessary to speak to the judge, the witness should address him as "your Honor." Attorneys can be addressed as "counsel," "Sir" or "Ma'am." The witness should beware of answering questions that require legal definitions or conclusions (except when he or she has sufficient knowledge and information). If a question is asked to which an objection seems to be in order, the witness may pause and glance at the attorney who subpoenaed him. Hostile questions used to bait the witness, such as "Have you ever testified against an innocent man?," are likely to be objected to, and need not be answered if the judge rules them out of order. If there is an expert witness for the other side who contradicts one's testimony, the witness should avoid attacking him or her personally in rebuttal testimony. It is much better to argue the scientific facts than the credentials or reputation of the witness. A witness may help the attorney who called him by preparing appropriate questions about the other witness's experience and qualifications. The attorney may ask the witness to sit at the counsel table during the direct examination of the opposing witness in order to suggest questions for cross-examination. In this situation, the witness should write down comments and suggested questions, but should take care not to distract the attorney.

If asked whether he regards a particular text or scientist as "authoritative," the witness should answer in other terms, such as "Dr Smith is highly respected," or "that test is widely used." "Authoritative" implies that the text or person can be relied upon. It is likely that portions of texts will be obsolete or contain errors, and the same can happen with statements made or positions taken by individuals. A witness who has acknowledged a person or text as authoritative may find his opinion contradicted by the authoritative source!

In response to open-ended questions such as "Are those *all* the factors that can affect metabolism?" or "Are there *any other* sources of error in the test?," while it is necessary to tell the whole truth, an honest answer like "Those are the important ones" or "Those are all I can think of" may help to avoid a laborious search through the recesses of one's memory for a prolonged list of ever more fanciful and unlikely possibilities.

The proper role of the expert is to be an unbiased witness to the scientific truth and to help the jury understand that truth, not to take sides or help an attorney to win a case. The decision about the case belongs solely to the jury (or the judge, if there is no jury), who will have heard all the evidence. If the witness has taken sides or made a decision about the desirable outcome of the case, that bias is likely to show in his answers and demeanor, and may affect the jury's impression of his credibility. This certainly does not mean that the witness cannot have an opinion about the case based on the information given to him, but he should be cautious about how that opinion is presented. The witness should respond using alternative language when answering questions referring to "the side you are working for" or asking "how much you are being paid for your testimony." The witness should be compensated for his time and expenses, but no one should be able to buy his or her testimony or to allege or suggest that it has been purchased, without a respectful dissent from the witness.

It is evident that the expert witness has a key role to play in our legal system, and should conduct himself with honor and dignity.

REFERENCES

Bogusz, M., Pack, J., and Stasko, W. Comparative studies on the rate of ethanol elimination in acute poisoning and in controlled conditions. *J. Forensic Sci.* 22:446–451, 1977.

Chang, R.B., Smith, W.A., Walkin, E., and Reynolds, P.C. The stability of ethyl alcohol in forensic blood specimens. *J. Anal. Toxicol.* 8:66–67, 1984.

Chittenden, R.H., cited by Cooke, A.R., and Birchall, A. Absorption of ethanol from the stomach. *Gastroenterology* 57:269–273, 1969.

Coldwell, B.B., and Grant, G.L. A study of some factors affecting the accuracy of the Breathalyzer. *J. Forensic Sci.* 8:149–162, 1963.

Dubowski, K.M., and Essary, N.A. Response of breath-alcohol analyzers to acetone: Further studies. *J. Anal. Toxicol.* 8:205–208, 1984.

Goldfinger, T.M. A comparison of blood alcohol concentration using non-alcohol– and alcohol–containing skin antiseptics. *Ann. Emerg. Med.* 11: 665–667, 1982.

Kier, L. Private forensic toxicology. *In Introduction to Forensic Toxicology* (R.H. Cravey and R.C. Baselt, eds.), Biomedical Publications, Davis, Calif., 1981.

Winek, C.L., and Eastly, T. Factors affecting contamination of blood samples for ethanol determinations. *In Legal Medicine Annual* (C.H. Wecht, ed.), Appleton-Century-Crofts, New York, 1976, pp. 145–162.

Winek, C.L., and Paul, L.J. Effect of Short-term storage conditions on alcohol concentrations in blood from living subjects. *Clin. Chem.* 29:1959–1960, 1983.

The following references were not cited in the text but are informative on the role of the scientific expert witness:

Chamberlain, R.T. Medical legal aspects of breath alcohol analysis. American Association for Clinical Chemistry Therapeutic Drug Monitoring Continuing Education Program, 5:1–8, 1983.

Harris, P.C. Giving a deposition in a malpractice suit. *Med. Lab. Observer* September, 1986, pp. 39–44.

Kogan, J.D. Expert testimony. *In Introduction to Forensic Toxicology*. (R.H. Cravey and R.C. Baselt, eds.), Biomedical Publications, Davis, Calif., 1981, pp. 247–257.

Labowitz, D. Professional responsibilites and liabilities of the pathologist concerning the problem drinker. *Am. J. Clin. Pathol.* 74:751–754, 1980.

Van Duizend, R., and Saks, M.J. Scientific evidence in litigation: Problems, hopes, accommodations, and frustrations. *State Court J.* 7:1–9, 1983.

Wilber, C.H. Legal considerations for the clinical chemist. *Am. Clin. Prod. Rev.* November/December, 1983, pp. 20–28.

INDEX